FORMULATION AND ANALYTICAL DEVELOPMENT FOR LOW-DOSE ORAL DRUG PRODUCTS

FORMULATION AND ANALYTICAL DEVELOPMENT FOR LOW-DOSE ORAL DRUG PRODUCTS

Edited By

JACK ZHENG
Pharmaceutical Sciences R&D, Lilly Research Labs, Eli Lilly and Company

WILEY

A JOHN WILEY & SONS, INC., PUBLICATION

Published by John Wiley & Sons, Inc., Hoboken, New Jersey
Published simultaneously in Canada

Library of Congress Cataloging-in-Publication Data:

Formulation and analytical development for low-dose oral drug products /
[edited by] Jack Zheng.
p. ; cm.
Includes bibliographical references and index.
ISBN 978-0-470-05609-7 (cloth)
1. Drugs—Dose-response relationship. 2. Drugs—Dosage. 3. Oral medication. 4. Drug development. I. Zheng, Jack.
[DNLM: 1. Chemistry, Pharmaceutical—methods. 2. Administration, Oral. 3. Drug Evaluation, Preclinical—methods. 4. Drug Industry. QV 744 F726 2008]
RM301.8.F67 2008
615′.1—dc22

2009009573

Printed in the United States of America

10 9 8 7 6 5 4 3 2 1

Opportunities multiply as they are seized

—Sun Tsu

To my wonderful wife Lijuan and my talented children Karen and Allen for their love, encouragement, and support

CONTENTS

PREFACE

In November 2005, I co-chaired a symposium entitled "Analytical and Formulation Development Strategies, Challenges and Regulatory Considerations for Low-dose Drug Products" during the annual meeting of the American Association of Pharmaceutical Scientists. The goal of the symposium was to provide an overview on development of low-dose drug products from the perspective of pharmaceutical, analytical, and regulatory sciences, including formulation design, process development, analytical method development, and regulatory considerations. The presenters included Dr Norm Sesi from Eli Lilly and Company, Dr Ravi Harapanhalli from the U.S. Food and Drug Administration, Dr Mary am Ende from Pfizer Inc., and Dr Keith Hutchison from Capsugel, Division of Pfizer Inc. After the meeting, I was approached by John Wiley & Sons Inc. to discuss the publication of a book on analytical and formulation development of low-dose drug products. As a pharmaceutical scientist who has worked in product development for more than a decade, I know that product development scientists in the pharmaceutical industry and the graduate students in the pharmacy schools will benefit from a book that collects the existing knowledge, techniques, and strategies in development of low-dose drug products. After two years of diligent work, all contributors and the publisher, John Wiley& Sons Inc., have made the book available to our readers.

Formulation and Analytical Development for Low-Dose Oral Drug Products focuses on the key topics involved in the challenges and strategies in analytical, formulation, and regulatory perspectives for development of low-dose drug products. The book begins with eight chapters devoted to aspects of formulation and process development of low-dose drug products, including theoretical consideration of particle size of drug substance, micronization and physical characterization of drug substance, control of excipients, and different manufacturing platform technologies. Chapter 2 provides an overview of challenges and strategies in formulation development of low-dose drug products. Chapters 4–7 are concerned with formulation and process development of low-dose drug products. Commonly used manufacturing platform technologies for low-dose drug products are discussed, such as high-shear wet granulation, fluid bed granulation, direct compression, and roller compaction. Chapters 3, 8, and 9 deal with drug substance, ranging from theoretical consideration of particle size according dose strengths, the methods for micronization of drug substance, and quality and functionality of pharmaceutical excipients.

Chapters 10–13 focus on challenges in analytical method development for low-dose drug products, including physical characterization of the micronized powder and the solid state of API in dosage forms. Analytical issues related to low-dose assay and impurities are discussed together with some specific case studies. Chapter 11 provides guidance on how to run appropriate dissolution testing so that meaningful data can be obtained. Chapter 14 provides a particularly interesting perspective on how pharmaceutical excipients should be controlled in the development of low-dose drug products and how an excipients library can help formulation scientists select appropriate excipients for better control of product quality. There is also a chapter specifically addressing practical concerns in the pharmaceutical industry with respect to cleaning verification of manufacturing equipment, illuminated by many examples.

The last section of the book is devoted to a few very important topics in development of low-dose drug products, including regulatory perspectives and containment technologies used in analytical laboratories and manufacturing plants. I hope that this combination of topics will enable the readers to obtain a broad overview on development of low-dose drug products.

I sincerely acknowledge the contributing authors of this book and thank them for their cooperation in the timely preparation of their specialized chapters, which allowed me to produce a book that reflects state-of-the-art thinking in analytical and formulation development of low-dose drug products. I would especially like to thank Drs Joe Zhou, Ralph Lipp, and Paul Collins for stepping in at the final hour and writing chapters on the fluid bed granulation technology and micronization of drug substance. Without these chapters, the book would have been incomplete. Also, I give my appreciation to Drs Gus Hartauer, Dave Maclaren, Ralph Lipp, Eugene Inman, Bret Huff, and Tom Verhoeven for their tremendous support and encouragement for my preparing this book. My sincerest thanks to Ms Karen Boleyn, a senior technical writer, for reviewing and making editorial corrections for several chapters in this book. Special thanks are expressed to Drs David Long, Tim Woznik, David Moeckly, Paul Sirois, James Wood, and Thirumala Kommuru for peer review of book chapters. Further, I would like to thank the editors at John Wiley and Sons Inc., in particular Jonathan Rose, for his accessibility and helpfulness in all aspects of the book's production. Finally, I would like to thank my wife Lijuan (Susan) and my talented children, Karen (a Yalie) and Allen, for their love, understanding, and support in the time I have spent editing this book. Now I will have more time for them upon the completion of this project.

JACK ZHENG, PH.D.

Indianapolis, Indiana

FOREWORD

A few years ago, I sat in my office with Dr Jack Zheng as we discussed a technically challenging chemical stability issue we were having with a very-low-dose formulation of an early-phase clinical compound. There are unique challenges that a development team faces with low-dose compounds delivered orally; in effect, we agreed that it would be extremely useful to generate an internal guidance leveraging our collective in-house knowledge in this area. Jack not only acted on that idea, but has gone one better by recruiting a team of experienced scientists from multiple companies across the industry to author a book on this very topic.

At first glance, the thought of bringing forward a molecule with very low doses can have an appealing upside. One specific benefit is seen in reduced quantities of often very expensive active pharmaceutical ingredient (API) needed during the various stages of the development process, as well as impact on COPS. While this is definitely an advantage, this book clearly demonstrates that the hurdles present in developing a low-dose product can quickly offset that advantage. Time and expense can increase if the team does not robustly plan for and develop a formulation, manufacturing process, and analytical/API physical property control strategy to overcome those challenges. The most effective development plan in these cases arises from a multidisciplinary approach to bring to bear the best science and exploration of appropriate design space. This approach is reflected in the individual chapters of this book, where specific technical areas such as *in vitro* dissolution testing, physical transformation and containment techniques are discussed, but in the context of the ultimate goal of developing a commercial product.

The development of low-dose formulations is certainly not new to the pharmaceutical industry; one obvious example is the long-term clinical use of digoxin tablets. However, with the introduction of new technologies to identify molecular targets and the use of high-throughput screening techniques to select structures with increased selectivity and activity toward a given target, the trend has been toward an ever-increasing amount of candidates dosed in the submilligram range. The increase in candidates meeting this definition of low-dose, along with the combination of increasing regulatory (e.g., impurity specifications) and technical requirements for such products, makes this book a valuable and timely contribution to pharmaceutical sciences.

Recent estimates have approached $1.2 billion for the cost of development of a new chemical entity into a commercial drug product (i.e., medicine). This book is a systematic, technical collection on this relevant topic than can help lead to a more effective and efficient drug development process. I consider it to be a welcome addition to the library of all drug product developers involved in bringing new therapies to patients.

KERRY "GUS" HARTAUER, PH.D.

Director—Pharmaceutical Sciences R&D
Eli Lilly and Company

CONTRIBUTORS

AHMAD ALMAYA, PH.D., Pharmaceutical Sciences R&D, Lilly Research Labs, Eli Lilly and Company, Indianapolis, Indiana

H. GEORGE BERESFORD, Analytical Research & Development, Development Science & Technology, Global Research and Development, Pfizer, Inc., Groton, Connecticut

DANIEL O. BLACKWOOD, M.S., Pfizer Global Research & Development, Oral Products Center of Emphasis, Pfizer, Inc., Groton, Connecticut

JOYCE BRIDGES, Analytical Sciences R&D, Lilly Research Labs, Eli Lilly and Company, Indianapolis, Indiana

CHRISTOPHER L. BURCHAM, PH.D., Chemical Product R&D, Lilly Research Labs, Eli Lilly and Company, Indianapolis, Indiana

VICTORIA CATHCART, Scientific Safety, Global Operations Environmental Health & Safety, Pfizer, Inc., Groton, Connecticut

QING CHANG, PH.D., Analytical Sciences R&D, Lilly Research Labs, Eli Lilly and Company, Indianapolis, Indiana

PAUL C. COLLINS, PH.D., Chemical Product R&D, Lilly Research Labs, Eli Lilly and Company, Indianapolis, Indiana

MARY T. AM ENDE, PH.D., Pfizer Global Research & Development, Oral Products Center of Emphasis, Pfizer, Inc., Groton, Connecticut

DANIEL S. GIERER, PH.D., Pfizer Global Research & Development, Oral Products Center of Emphasis, Pfizer, Inc., Groton, Connecticut

VIVIAN A. GRAY, V. A. Gray Consulting, Inc., Hockessin, Delaware

Ravi S. Harapanhalli, Ph.D., Branch V, Division of Pre-marketing Assessment and Manufacturing Science, Office of New Drug Quality Assessment, Office of Pharmaceutical Science, Center for Drug Evaluation and Research. Food and Drug Administration, Silver Spring, Maryland

Ronald G. Iacocca, Ph.D., Analytical Sciences R&D, Lilly Research Labs, Eli Lilly and Company, Indianapolis, Indiana

Daniel J. Jarmer, Ph.D., Chemical Product R&D, Lilly Research Labs, Eli Lilly and Company, Indianapolis, Indiana

Kevin C. Johnson, Ph.D., Intellipharm, LLC, Niantic, Connecticut

Sarah Jones, Scientific Safety, Global Operations Environmental Health & Safety, Pfizer, Inc., Groton, Connecticut

Reena M. Joseph, Research Formulations, Research Science & Technology, Global Research & Development, Pfizer, Inc., Groton, Connecticut

Lisheng Kang, Ph.D., Pharmaceutical Sciences R&D, Lilly Research Labs, Eli Lilly and Company, Indianapolis, Indiana

Ralph Lipp, Ph.D., Pharmaceutical Sciences R&D, Lilly Research Labs, Eli Lilly and Company, Indianapolis, Indiana

Christopher P. Neu, M.S., Pfizer Global Research & Development, Oral Products Center of Emphasis, Pfizer, Inc., Groton, Connecticut

Beverly Nickerson, Ph.D., Analytical Research & Development, Development Science & Technology, Global Research & Development, Pfizer, Inc., Groton, Connecticut

Alex M. Opio, Analytical Research & Development, Development Science & Technology, Global Research & Development, Pfizer, Inc., Groton, Connecticut

Brian W. Pack, Ph.D., Analytical Sciences R&D, Lilly Research Labs, Eli Lilly and Company, Indianapolis, Indiana

Charles Palmer, Analytical Research & Development, Development Science & Technology, Global Research & Development, Pfizer, Inc., Groton, Connecticut

Margo Palmieri, Ph.D., Analytical Sciences R&D, Lilly Research Labs, Eli Lilly and Company, Indianapolis, Indiana

David S. Pattavina, Research Analytical, Research Science & Technology, Global Research & Development, Pfizer Inc., Groton, Connecticut

Nancy Sage, Chemical Research & Development, Development Science & Technology, Global Research & Development, Pfizer, Inc., Groton, Connecticut

Kevin D. Seibert, Ph.D., Chemical Product R&D, Lilly Research Labs, Eli Lilly and Company, Indianapolis, Indiana

Norman Sesi, Ph.D., Elanco Animal Health, Eli Lilly and Company, Indianapolis, Indiana

Gregory A. Stephenson, Ph.D., Pharmaceutical Sciences R&D, Lilly Research Labs, Eli Lilly and Company, Indianapolis, Indiana

Robert L. Ternik, Ph.D., Pharmaceutical Sciences R&D, Lilly Research Labs, Eli Lilly and Company, Indianapolis, Indiana

Keri Varner, Analytical Sciences R&D, Lilly Research Labs, Eli Lilly and Company, Indianapolis, Indiana

Jack Y. Zheng, Ph.D., Pharmaceutical Sciences R&D, Lilly Research Labs, Eli Lilly and Company, Indianapolis, Indiana

J. Joe Zhou, Ph.D., Engineering Technology Center, Eli Lilly and Company, Indianapolis, Indiana

CHAPTER 1

AN OVERVIEW

JACK Y. ZHENG
Pharmaceutical Sciences R&D, Lilly Research Laboratories, Eli Lilly and Company, Indianapolis, IN 40285

U.S. law defines a drug as any substance, other than a food or device, either (1) intended for use in the diagnosis, cure, relief, treatment, or prevention of disease or (2) intended to affect the structure or function of the body. The mission of pharmaceutical scientists is to continue developing safer and more effective new drugs to conquer various human diseases. However, successfully developing new medicines for patients requires significant collaboration of many interdisciplinary sciences, including:

- molecular biology;
- medicinal chemistry;
- pharmacology;
- toxicology;
- preformulation;
- formulation;
- clinical evaluation;
- synthetic chemistry;
- quality assurance/control;
- regulatory affairs;
- sales and marketing.

The objectives of formulation and analytical scientists are to develop new drug products for human use that are chemically and physically stable, bioavailable upon administration, manufacturable, cost-effective, elegant, and marketable.

Formulation and Analytical Development for Low-Dose Oral Drug Products. Edited by Jack Zheng

Pharmacologically, a drug should demonstrate its ability to:

- target the intended site or receptor (selectivity);
- remain attached to the receptor (affinity);
- show its effectiveness (efficacy);
- show its safety (adverse/side effects).

Ideally, a drug should be highly selective for its biological target, so that it has little or no effect on other physiological systems. The drug should also be very potent and effective, so that low doses of drug substance can be used, even for disorders that are difficult to treat. Finally, the drug should be administered orally, not only for patient compliance, but also for ease of production, distribution, and administration.

Drug product development is a process of transforming concept into reality. The process is not only science, but also art. After selecting a new drug candidate, drug development moves from preclinical studies to critical clinical investigation, and then to various stages of clinical and commercial product development. A drug candidate can become a drug product only when the compound is clinically efficacious and safe, and the developed product is bioavailable and stable, produces the desired pharmacological effects, and can be manufactured consistently with the identity, strength, quality, and purity it is represented to possess.

During development of an oral solid dosage form, dose strength is one of the critical product attributes that may have a significant impact on formulation and analytical development. Especially for a low-dose drug product, pharmaceutical scientists face great challenges in formulation, manufacture, analytical chemistry, and regulatory requirements.

This book addresses the challenges and strategies in developing low-dose oral solid drug products (i.e., less than 1 mg per dose unit), and aids development scientists in improving research and development productivity with a scientific and structured approach to product development. The information presented in the book is based on the extensive experience of the contributors, all of whom are actively working in the pharmaceutical industry and/or regulatory agency and have gained significant knowledge from their practical experience.

1.1 THE DRUG DISCOVERY AND DEVELOPMENT PROCESS

Drug discovery and development is a time-consuming and unpredictable process as well as an expensive venture. Today the average cost to research and develop each successful drug is estimated to be somewhere between \$1.2 billion and \$1.5 billion.[1] The whole adventure is highly innovative, highly risky, highly regulated, and highly technology- and information-intensive. Typically, it takes 10–15 years to develop a safe and effective new medicine from the early stage of discovery until the drug is available to treat patients.[2] This process, as illustrated in Fig. 1.1,

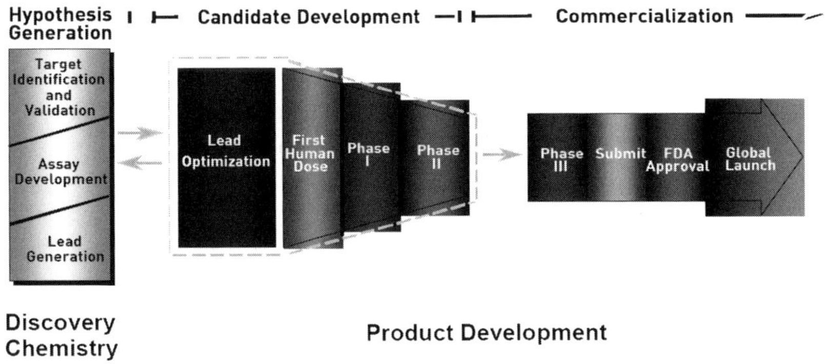

Figure 1.1 New drug discovery and development process. (See color insert.)

is normally divided into two key phases: discovery and development. During these phases, scientists have to:

- understand disease status, hypothesize "targets" that new drugs might be able to affect, and validate the targets;
- discover the molecule(s) to interact with the target hypothesized;
- assess the new compound (drug candidate) in the laboratory and clinic for safety and efficacy;
- develop the right drug product/dosage form for the intended use;
- gain regulatory approval and get the new drug into the hands of physicians and patients.

1.1.1 The Discovery Phase

Before discovering any new drug, scientists strive to understand the disease needing treatment and unravel the underlying cause of the condition. To do this, they investigate:

- how the genes are altered;
- how that alteration affects the proteins they encode;
- how those proteins interact with each other in living cells;
- how those affected cells change the specific tissue they are in;
- how the disease affects the patient.

This knowledge is the critical foundation for hunting a new medicine and treating the disease.

In 2001, scientists completed the sequencing of the human genome. They found that the genome of *Homo sapiens* consists of 24 distinct chromosomes (22 autosomal and the sex-determining X and Y chromosomes). There are approximately 3 billion

DNA base pairs containing an estimated 20,000–25,000 genes.[3,4] Each gene codes for a protein, and these proteins carry out all the functions of the human body, laying out how it grows and works. These genes and proteins can also be involved in disease. Hence, scientists are able to understand the inner workings of human disease at both the tissue level and the molecular level.

Once scientists understand the underlying cause of a disease, they can select a "target" for a potential new drug. A target is generally a single molecule, such as a gene or protein, which is involved in a particular disease state. Scientists call this earliest step in drug discovery "target identification."

After identifying a potential target, scientists must demonstrate that it actually is involved in the disease and that a drug can act on it. This process is called "target validation." Target validation is a crucial step in the drug discovery process that helps scientists minimize research paths that look promising, but that ultimately lead to dead ends. Target validation involves proving that DNA, RNA, or a protein molecule is directly involved in a disease process in vitro and in vivo, and that it can be a suitable target for a new therapeutic drug. Scientists use several methods to validate a target.

One type of target validation uses computer models. They are a fast, relatively cheap option for initial screening of both targets and potential drugs. The models usually focus on how the two types of candidate structures interact with each other.[5] Sense reversal is another route to target validation. It hinges on disrupting gene expression to reduce the amount of the corresponding protein, thereby identifying the physiological role of the target. Examples of this technique include gene knockouts, antisense technology, and RNA interference (RNAi).

One disadvantage of doing target validation at the genetic level, however, is that many genes produce several different protein isoforms that can have subtly different functions. Post-translational modifications can also give protein variations. To address these issues, a developing approach in target validation, proteomics, focuses on manipulating the activity of the potential target protein itself. Proteomics investigates and manipulates the protein make-up of a cell so it is easier to distinguish and target just one specific form of a protein.

In vivo target validation involves more complicated experiments in animal models of diseases.[5] However, animal models for certain diseases, such as psychiatric illnesses, are extremely difficult to develop. The alternative is to use gene knockouts, in which genes are deleted or disrupted to halt their expression in vivo. This can be a powerful method of predicting drug action. This method is based on the assumption that knocking out the gene for the potential target has the same effect as administering a highly specific inhibitor of the target protein in vivo. Once the target is validated, it can then be used for screening potential new drug candidates.

Scientists screen thousands of compounds (either by synthesizing or choosing from libraries) to find a molecule, or "lead compound," that may interact with the target to alter the disease course. De novo and high-throughput screening are methods commonly used to find a lead compound.[6,7] Promising lead candidates are called "hits." Hits go through a series of tests to provide an early assessment of the safety, efficacy, and pharmacokinetic properties.

Lead compounds that survive the initial screening are then "optimized" or altered to improve their drugability and developability (that is, they are developed to achieve better physicochemical and biopharmaceutical properties and more effective and safer profiles in animals). Scientists make and laboratory-test hundreds of different variations or "analogs" of the initial lead compounds to evaluate the structure–activity relationship (SAR) of the hits.

New techniques have revolutionized the ability of scientists to optimize potential drug molecules. These new techniques include magnetic resonance imaging, X-ray crystallography, and powerful computer modeling capabilities. These tools allow scientists actually to "see" the target in three dimensions. This allows them to design potential drugs to bind more powerfully to the active sites of the target where they can be most effective.

After optimization, scientists test the lead compounds in more sophisticated models including pharmacokinetics, pharmacodynamics, and toxicity. The optimal molecule selected from these assessments is then declared a new drug candidate and moves on to the next phase (development). If a program is successful, it may take a total of 3–6 years from target selection and validation through lead generation, lead optimization, and preclinical evaluation in animals to candidate selection for a potential new medicine.

In recent years, biologists have explored more therapeutic targets related to human diseases (for example, nuclear hormone receptor resources). This exploration led to the discovery of many drug candidates that are more highly specific and more active, and, consequently, can be delivered in lower doses than before. Examples include ligands for peroxisome proliferator-activated receptor, thyroid hormone receptor, mineralocorticoid receptor, and glucocorticoid receptor. The clinically efficacious dose for these compounds could be as low as a few milligrams or even micrograms. As expected, this leads to more challenges to pharmaceutical scientists during product development.

1.1.2 The Development Phase

A potential new drug candidate faces a well-defined clinical and product development process that has been refined over several decades. The development phase of a new drug product usually consists of two main activities: clinical evaluation (safety and efficacy), and product development (drug substance and dosage form). As shown in Table 1.1, the process can last as long as 7–9.5 years and the cost can be approximately 50% of the entire expense for development of a new medicine.[8] At this stage, some programs would be terminated for various reasons, such as lack of clinical efficacy, clinical toxicity, or drug developability.

Clinical investigations are clearly the most critical and demanding stage in the new drug development phase. When a drug company believes it has sufficient preclinical testing data to show that a new drug candidate is adequately safe for initial small-scale clinical studies, the company assembles and submits an investigational new drug (IND) application in the United States or a clinical trial application (CTA) in the European Union. The IND or CTA is the prerequisite for a company to obtain

TABLE 1.1 Clinical Evaluation and Drug Product Development Process for a New Drug Candidate

Attributes	Clinical Evaluation and Drug Product Development (IND)			NDA Submission and Approval	Process Validation and Launch
Length		6–7 years		0.5–2 years	0.5 year
No. of compounds	20	4	1–2	1	1
Percentage of total expense	5.8	11.7	25.5	6.9	
Clinical development	Phase I	Phase II	Phase III		
	• 20–100 healthy volunteers. • SDSS/MDSS • Safety and pharmacokinetic profiles	• 100–500 patients • Proof-of-concept • Efficacious dose range finding • Possible short-term side effects	• 1000–5000 patients. • Efficacy and safety evaluation • Randomized, double-blind placebo-controlled studies (two required) against a standard comparator	Submit clinical data package	Develop the plan for phase IV clinical study, i.e. postmarketing surveillance

Product development	• Design API synthesis route • Develop simple formulation for phase I clinical trials • Manufacture GMP materials	• Optimize API synthetic process • Develop commercial prototype dosage forms • Develop analytical method and control strategy • Supply clinical trial materials	• Scale-up and manufacture API on large scale • Optimize/scale-up commercial dosage form, manufacturing process and finalize control strategy • Prepare three registration batches • Supply clinical trial materials	Submit chemistry manufacturing control information	• ≥3 batches produced in manufacturing sites per proposed validation protocol • Develop/implement line extension strategy
Regulatory affairs	• Review preclinical/animal testing and plan for clinical testing • Approve to test the drug candidate in humans			• Review all clinical and preclinical findings, proposed labeling and manufacturing plans • Solicit opinion of an independent advisory committee • Determine if the drug can be approved for patients to use	

regulatory permission to begin testing a new drug in human subjects. Although there is no regulation that mandates a specific clinical trial structure and design, clinical evaluation of a new drug most often proceeds in at least three phases:

- *Phase I*—phase I trials consist of the cautious use of a new drug in 20–100 normal human volunteers to gain basic safety and pharmacokinetic information. The trials include a single-dose safety study (SDSS) and multiple dose safety study (MDSS). The main goal of a phase I trial is to discover if the new drug is safe in humans. These studies help scientists determine toxicity, absorption, metabolism, elimination, and other pertinent pharmacological actions, and to find the safety dosing range. Recently, the U.S. Food and Drug Administration (FDA) endorsed "microdosing," or the "phase 0 trial," which allows scientists to test a small drug dose in fewer human volunteers to quickly weed out drug candidates that are metabolically or biologically ineffective.[8]
- *Phase II*—during phase II, the drug candidate is given to a small number of patients—100–500—who have the disease or condition under study. Phase 2 trials give additional safety data, and provide the first indication of a drug's clinical effectiveness in its proposed use. Clinical researchers strive to understand some fundamental questions about the new drug: Is the drug working by the expected mechanism? Does it improve the disease condition? What are the effective dose range and dosing regime? If the new drug continues to show promise, the new drug moves into much larger phase III trials.
- *Phase III*—in phase III trials, the new drug is used in a significantly larger group of patients (about 1000–5000) who suffer from the condition that the drug is proposed to treat. This phase of clinical evaluation is key in determining whether the drug is safe and effective. It also provides the information for labeling instructions to ensure proper use of the drug. Phase III trials are both the costliest and longest trials. Hundreds of clinical sites (centers) around the United States and the world participate in the trials to get a large and diverse group of patients. Certain phase III trials, called "pivotal" trials, will serve as the primary basis for the drug approval. These studies must meet more rigorous standards, such as having a randomized, double-blind placebo-controlled study design, or having a comparator. Two pivotal clinical trials are required for a new drug application (NDA) with a regulatory agency.

The formulation, manufacturing process, analytical development, and long-term toxicology studies in animals are parallel to the clinical investigation (Table 1.1). Clinical trial materials should be developed, manufactured, tested, and released before conducting a phase I clinical trial. Process chemists may redesign the synthetic route for the drug candidate to meet the requirements of large-scale production in a pilot plant. Preformulation scientists complete the activities of salt selection, polymorphism studies, and physicochemical characterization. Formulation scientists develop less time-consuming formulations, such as drug-in-bottle or drug-in-capsule, for the first human dose (FHD) clinical trials.[9]

If a drug candidate survives phase I trials, the process chemists start to optimize the synthetic process for the drug substance and the formulation scientists develop near-market-image dosage forms for phase II clinical trials. Preliminary control strategies for both drug substance and drug product are developed.

Following successful phase II clinical trials, the manufacture of the drug substance is scaled up to meet commercialization needs. In addition, the prototype formulation and process is optimized and scaled up to greater than one-tenth of the commercial batch size.

The optimized formulation then is prepared for phase III pivotal clinical trials. Followed by manufacturing process optimization and scale-up, the three batches of the drug product are manufactured for primary stability evaluation at product launch sites. The information on the manufacture, scale-up, control, and stability is used for product registration with regulatory agencies.

During development, pharmaceutical scientists work to achieve an ideal drug product—one that is bioavailable after administration; physically/chemically stable through its shelf-life; and able to be manufactured reproducibly and reliably with high quality.

Upon completion of preclinical, clinical, and drug product development, the drug company submits to the FDA for approval an NDA containing a meticulous, well-indexed, comprehensive, and readable document. The document should satisfy the requirements of the Food, Drug, and Cosmetic Act and the code of Federal Regulations (CFR) used by the FDA in the review and approval of safe and effective drug products in the United States. The FDA's NDA review process may last approximately two years. Multiple review teams are involved in the review process including:

- clinical reviewer;
- pharmacology/toxicology reviewer;
- chemistry reviewer;
- statistical reviewer;
- microbiology reviewer;
- biopharmaceutics reviewer.

The NDA filing also triggers a division request for FDA field offices to conduct a preapproval inspection of the manufacturing facilities of the drug company (sponsor). During this check, FDA inspectors exam a sponsor's production facilities to audit sponsor statements and commitments made in the NDA against actual manufacturing practices employed by the sponsor.

During the drug review process, the FDA may seek advice and comment from the members of its drug advisory committees. The expert committees provide the agency with independent, nonbinding advice and recommendations.

At the end of the review process, the agency issues one of three letters: approval, approvable, or not-approvable. An approval letter means that the agency formally approves the new drug for marketing. An approvable letter most likely indicates that the sponsor must make certain revisions or submissions to the NDA, and probably submit final printed labeling before the agency grants marketing authorization. A not-approvable letter states that the agency cannot approve the NDA and identifies the relevant deficiencies.

The development phase for low-dose drug products is similar to any other drug product. At a minimum, the drug product developed should be clinically efficacious, safe, and chemically/physically stable no matter how low the dose strength. Needless to say, scientists who work in chemistry, manufacture, and control (CMC) encounter even more challenges. Therefore, this book focuses on strategies and solutions to the challenges from both theoretical and practical aspects.

1.2 CHALLENGES AND STRATEGIES IN DEVELOPMENT OF LOW-DOSE DRUG PRODUCTS

Over the last 15 years, the pharmaceutical industry has discovered and developed increasingly more low-dose drug products. Table 1.2 shows some low-dose drug products from the *Physician's Desk Reference*.[10] The dose strength of a low-dose product can be as low as 0.25 μg. Dosage forms include tablet, hard gelatin capsule, and soft elastic capsule; product types include both mono- and combo-drug substance(s). More than a few therapeutic areas use low-dose drug products.

Although development of new normal-dose and low-dose drug products follows a similar path (as discussed in the previous section), the increase in potency and decrease in dose with low-dose drug products creates increasing challenges. In particular, pharmaceutical scientists and production operators must meet the stringent regulatory standards required for formulation, manufacturing process, and analytical chemistry.

From a formulation perspective, a low-dose drug product means low drug concentration, or low drug load, which can be less than 0.01% (w/w). In other words, the low-dose formulation likely has a very high ratio of excipients to drug substance. These characteristics present many hurdles during formulation and process development, including:

- difficulty achieving content uniformity due to low drug concentration;
- low potency due to manufacturing loss;
- instability due to the huge ratio of excipients to drug substance (which increases the likelihood of incompatibility);
- chemical instability due to a micronized drug having greater surface exposure to excipients, moisture, and manufacturing equipment;
- instability due to physical transformation to a less stable solid form during manufacture or long-term storage.

TABLE 1.2 Marketed Oral Solid Low-Dose Drug Products

Brand Name	Chemical Name	Dose Strengths	Dosage Form	Indication	Pharmacological Action Mechanism	Ingredients	Manufacturer
Flomax®	Tamsulosin HCl	0.4 mg	Capsule	Benign prostatic hyperplasia	$Alpha_{1A}$ adrenoceptor antagonist	Methacrylic acid copolymer, polysorbate 80, SLS, MCC, triacetin, calcium stearate, talc	Boehriner Ingelheim
Avodart™	Dutasteride	0.5 mg	SEC	Benign prostatic hyperplasia	A selective inhibitor of both the type 1 and type 2 isoform of steroid 5α-reductase	Mono-di-glycerides of caprylic/capric acid, butylated hydroxytoluene	Glaxosmithkline (GSK)
Mavik®	Trandolapril	1, 2, 4 mg	Tablet	Hypertension	The ethyl ester prodrug of a nonsulfhydryl angiotensin converting enzyme (ACE) inhibitor	Corn starch, croscarmellose sodium, hypromellose, iron oxide, lactose, povidone, sodium stearyl fumarate	Abbott Laboratories
Tarka®	Trandolapril/verapamil HCl	1 mg/240 mg 2 mg/180 mg 2 mg/240 mg 4 mg/240 mg	Extended release tablet	Hypertension	ACE inhibitor	Corn starch, dioctyl sodium sulfosuccinate, ethanol, HPC, HPMC, lactose, magnesium stearate, MCC, polyethylene glycol, povidone, purified water, silicon dioxide, sodium alginate, sodium stearyl fumarate, talc, sytnetic iron oxides, titanium dioxide	Abbott Laboratories
Catapres®	Clonidine HCl USP	0.1, 0.2, 0.3 mg	Tablet	Hypertension	Alpha-adrenoreceptor agonist	Colloidal silicon dioxide, corn starch, dibasic calcium phosphate, gelatin, glycerin, lactose, magnesium stearate, methylparaben, propylparaben	Boehriner Ingelheim (Mylan)

(*Continued*)

TABLE 1.2 *Continued*

Brand Name	Chemical Name	Dose Strengths	Dosage Form	Indication	Pharmacological Action Mechanism	Ingredients	Manufacturer
Arimidex®	Anastrozole	1 mg	Tablet	Breast cancer	A selective nonsteroidal aromatase inhibitor	Lactose, magnesium stearate, HPMC, PEG, povidone, sodium starch glycolate, titanium dioxide	AstraZeneca
Avandamet™	Rosiglitazone maleate/ met-formin HCl	1 mg/500 mg 2 mg/500 mg 2 mg/1000 mg 4 mg/500 mg 4 mg/1000 mg	Tablet	Type II diabetes	Rosiglitazone: insulin sensitizing agent; metformin: decreasing endogenous hepatic glucose production	Hypromellose 2910, lactose monohydrate, magnesium stearate, MCC, PEG 400, povidone, sodium starch glycolate	GSK
Prandin®	Repaglinide	0.5, 1, 2 mg	Tablet	Type II diabetes	Stimulating the release of insulin from the pancreas. ATP-dependent K-channel blocker	Calcium hydrogen phosphate, MCC, maize starch, polacrilin, potassium, povidone, glycerol (85%), magnesium stearate, meglumine, poloxamer	Novo Nordisk
DDAVP®	Desmopressin acetate	0.1 mg, 0.2 mg	Tablet	Central diabetes insipidus	A synthetic analog of the natural pituitary hormone 8-arginine vasopressin	Lactose, potato starch, povidone, magnesium stearate	Aventis
ACTIQ®	Fentanyl citrate USP	200, 400, 600, 800, 1200, or 1600 μg	Oral Trans-mucosal	Analgesia	Opioid mu-receptor agonist	Hydrated dextrates, citric acid, dibasic sodium phosphate, berry flavor, magnesium stearate, modified food starch, confectioner's sugar	Cephalon
AMERGE®	Naratriptan HCl	1, 2.5 mg	Tablet	Migraine	5-HT1D/1B receptor agonist	Croscarmellose sodium, hypromellose, lactose, magnesium stearate, MCC	GSK

ORAP®	Pimozide	1, 2 mg	Tablet	Tourette's disorder	Blockade dopaminergic receptors in the CNS	Calcium stearate, MCC, lactose anhydrous, corn starch	Gate
Lanoxicap®	Digoxin	50, 100, 200 μg	SEC	Heart failure, atrial fibrillation	Na-K ATPase inhibitor	PEG 400, ethyl alcohol, propylene glycol, purified water	GSK
Tikosyn®	Dofetilide	125, 250, 500 μg	Capsule	Maintenance of normal sinus rhythm and conversion of atrial fibrillation/ flutter	Cardiac ion channel blocker/ antiarrhythmic drug	MCC, corn starch, silicon dioxide, magnesium stearate	Pfizer
LOTRONEX®	Alosetron HCl	0.5, 1 mg	Tablet	For women with severe diarrhea–predominant irritable bowl syndrome	A potent and selective 5-HT3 antagonist	Lactose anhydrous, magnesium stearate, MCC, pregelatinized starch	GSK
Mirapex®	Pramipexole 2HCl	0.125, 0.25, 0.5, 1 and 1.5 mg	Tablet	Parkinson's disease	Nonergot dopamine agonist	Mannitol, corn starch, colloidal silicon dioxide, povidone, magnesium stearate	Boehriner Ingelheim
Requip®	Ropinirole HCl	0.25, 0.5, 1, 2, 3, 4, 5 mg	Tablet	Parkinson's disease	A nonergoline dopamine agonist with high relative *in vitro* specificity and full intrinsic activity at the D2 and D3 dopamine receptor subtypes	Croscarmellose Na, lactose hydrous, magnesium stearate, MCC	GSK
Permax®	Pergolide mesylate	0.05, 0.25, 1 mg	Tablet	Parkinson's disease	D1 and D2 dopamine receptor agonist	Croscarmellose Na, lactose, magnesium stearate, povidone, L-methionine	Valeant Pharmaceuticals

(*Continued*)

TABLE 1.2 *Continued*

Brand Name	Chemical Name	Dose Strengths	Dosage Form	Indication	Pharmacological Action Mechanism	Ingredients	Manufacturer
Risperdal® M-TAB	Risperidone	0.5, 1, 2 mg	Orally disintegrating tablet	Schizophrenia	A selective monoaminergic antagonist (5HT2, dopamine type 2 (D2), α1, and α2 adrenergic, and H1 histaminergic receptors	Amberlite resin, gelatin, mannitol, glycine, simethicone, carbomer, sodium hydroxide, aspartame, red ferric oxide, peppermint oil	Janssen Pharmaceuticals
Risperdal®	Risperidone	0.25, 0.5, 1, 2, 3, 4 mg	Tablet	Schizophrenia	A selective monoaminergic antagonist (5HT2, dopamine type 2 (D2), α1 and α2 adrenergic, and H1 histaminergic receptors	Colloidal silicon dioxide, hypromellose, lactose, magnesium stearate, MCC, propylene glycol, sodium lauryl sulfate, corn starch	Janssen Pharmaceuticals
Decadron®	Dexamethasone USP	0.5, 0.75, 4 mg	Tablet	Replacement therapy in adrenocortical deficiency, anti-inflammatory	A synthetic adrenocortical steroid-potent anti-inflammatory effects	Calcium phosphate, lactose, magnesium stearate, starch	Merck & Co. (Roxane Laboratories and Par)
Propecia®	Finasteride	1 mg	Tablet	Male pattern hair loss	A specific inhibitor of steroid type II 5α-reductase	Lactose monohydrate, MCC, pregelatinized starch, sodium starch glycolate, docusate sodium, magnesium stearate, Hypromellose 2910	Merck & Co.

Dostinex®	Cabergolin	0.5 mg	Tablet	Hyperprolactin-emic disorders	A dopamine receptor (D2) agonist in CNS	Leucine USP, lactose	Pfizer
ProSom™	Estazolam	1, 2 mg	Tablet	Insomnia		Lactose, povidone, colloidal silicon dioxide, stearic acid, sodium starch glucolate	Abbott Laboratories
Xanax®	Alprazolam USP	0.25, 0.5, 1, 2 mg	Tablet	Anxiety disorder	Binding at stereo specific receptor/CNS active agent	Cellulose, corn starch, docusate sodium, lactose, magnesium stearate, silicon dioxide, sodium benzoate	Pfizer (Mylan)
Hivid®	Zalcitabine	0.375, 0.75 mg	Tablet	HIV	A synthetic nucleoside analog (DNA replacement)	Lactose, MCC $<$ croscarmellose Na, magnesium stearate, hypromellose, PEG, polysorbate 80	Roche
Klonopin®	Clonazepam	0.5, 1, 2 mg	Tablet	Panic disorder		Lactose, magnesium stearate, MCC, corn starch	Roche
Klonopin® Wafers	Clonazepam	0.125, 0.25, 0.5, 1 mg	Orally disinte-grating tablet	Panic disorder	Gamma aminobutyric acid (GABA) enhancement	Gelatin, mannitol, methylparaben sodium, propylparaben sodium, xanthan gum	Roche
Kytril®	Granisetron HCl	1 mg	Tablet	Nausea and vomiting	A selective 5-HT3 receptor antagonist	Hypromellose, lactose, magnesium stearate, MCC, polyethylene glycol, polysorbate 80, sodium starch glycolate, titanium oxide	Roche
Agrylin®	Anagrelide HCl	0.5, 1 mg	Capsule	Thrombo-cythe-mia and myelo-pro-liferative disorders	Inhibition of cAPM phosphodiesterase, ADP-collagen-induced platelet aggregation	Anhydrous lactose, crospovidone, lactose monohydrate, magnesium stearate, MCC, povidone	Shire

(Continued)

TABLE 1.2 *Continued*

Brand Name	Chemical Name	Dose Strengths	Dosage Form	Indication	Pharmacological Action Mechanism	Ingredients	Manufacturer
Synthroid®	Levothyroxine sodium	25, 50, 75, 88, 100, 112, 125, 137, 150, 175, 200, 300 μg	Tablet (USP)	Hypothyroidism, pituitary TSH suppression	Thyroid receptor agonist	Acacia, confectioner's sugar, lactose monohydrate, magnesium stearate, povidone, talc	Abbott Laboratories
Cytomel®	Liothyronine Na (T3)	5, 25, 50 μg	Tablet	Hupothyroidism, euthyroid goiters	Hormone, TSH suppressant	Calcium sulfate, gelatin, starch, stearic acid, sucrose, talc	King Pharmaceu-ticals
Hectorol®	Doxercal-ciferol	0.5, 2.5 μg	SEC	Secondary hyperpara-thyroidism	Vitamin D2 analog to regulate blood calcium	Fractionated triglyceride of coconut oil, ethanol, and butylated hydroxyanisole	Bone Care International
Rocaltrol®	Calcitriol	0.25, 0.5 μg	SEC	Secondary hyperpara-thyroidism and resultant metabolic bone disease, hypocalcemia	A synthetic vitamin D analog	A fractionated triglyceride of coconut oil	Roche
PLAN B®	Levonorgestrel	0.75 mg	Tablet	Emergency contraceptive	A synthetic progestogen	Colloidal silicon dioxide, potato starch, gelatin. Magnesium stearate, talc, corn starch, lactose monohydrate	Barr Laboratories
Seasonale®	Levonorgestrel/ ethinyl estradiol	0.15 mg/0.03 mg	Tablet	Oral contraceptive	Inhibition of ovulation	Anhydrous lactose, HPMC, MCC, PEG, magnesium stearate, polysorbate 80, titanium dioxide	Barr Laboratories

Yasmin®	Drospirenone/ ethinyl estradiol	3 mg/0.03 mg	Tablet	Oral contraceptives	Suppression of gonadotropins	Lactose monohydrate, corn starch, modified starch, povidone 25000, magnesium stearate, HPMC, Macrogol 6000, talc, titanium dioxide, ferric oxide pigment, yellow NF	Berlex
Cenestin®	Synthetic conjugated estrogens A (a blend of nine synthetic estrogenic substances)	0.3, 0.45, 0.625, 0.9, 1.25 mg	Tablet	Estrogen replacement therapy	Estogen receptors (two nuclear receptors identified)	Ethylcellulose, hypromellose, lactose monohydrate, magnesium stearate, PEG, polysorbate 80, pregelatinized starch, titanium dioxide, triethyl citrate	Duramed Pharmaceuticals
VAGIFEM®	Estradiol	25 μg	Vaginal tablet	Atrophic vaginitis	Estrogen receptor agonist	Hypromellose, lactose monohydrate, maize starch, magnesium stearate	Novo Nordisk
Ortho Micronor®	Norethindrone	0.35 mg	Tablet	Prevent conception	Suppressing ovulation/ progestin receptor	Lactose, magnesium stearate, povidone, starch	Ortho-McNeil
Estratest® H.S.	Esterified estrogens/ methyltesto-sterone	0.625 mg/1.25 mg	Capsule	Vasomotor symptoms from menopause	Estrogen/testosterone receptor	Acacia, calcium carbonate, citric acid, colloidal silicon dioxide, gelatin, lactose, magnesium stearate, MCC, glaze, povidone, sodium benzoate, sodium bicarbonate, carboxymethylcellulose sodium, sorbic acid, starch, talc, titanium dioxide, tribasic calcium phosphate, alcohol denatured 3A	Solvay Pharmaceuticals

(Continued)

TABLE 1.2 *Continued*

Brand Name	Chemical Name	Dose Strengths	Dosage Form	Indication	Pharmacological Action Mechanism	Ingredients	Manufacturer
Femtrace®	Estrodiol acetate	0.45, 0.9, 1.8 mg	Tablet	Vasomotor symptom from menopause	Estrogen receptor	Povidone, lactose monohydrate, MCC, croscarmellose Na, silicon dioxide, magnesium stearate	Warner Chilcott
Alesse®-28	Lenonorgestrel and ethinyl estradiol	0.10 mg/0.02 mg	Tablet	Oral contraceptives	Estrogen/progestin receptor	Cellulose, hypromellose, lactose, magnesium stearate, polacrilin potassium	Wyeth
Lo/Ovral®-28	Norgestrel and ethinyl estradiol	0.3 mg/0.03 mg	Tablet	Oral contraceptives	Estrogen/progestin receptor	Cellulose, lactose, magnesium stearate, polacrilin potassium	Wyeth
Ovrette®	Norgestrel	0.075 mg	Tablet	Oral contraceptive	progestin receptor	Cellulose, lactose, magnesium stearate, polacrilin potassium	Wyeth
Premarin®	Conjugated estrogens USP	0.3, 0.45, 0.625, 0.9, 1.25 mg	Tablet	Vasomotor symptom from the menopause	Estrogen receptor	Calcium phosphate tribasic, calcium sulfate, carnauba wax, cellulose, glyceryl monooleate, lactose, magnesium stearate, hypromellose, glaze, PEG, stearic acid, sucrose, tinanium dioxide	Wyeth

Low potency, the most common issue for a low-dose drug product, is most likely related to platform-dependent manufacturing loss. Physical properties of the drug substance (particle size, shape, and density) and poor mixing of trace amounts of drug substance with excipients can cause lack of content uniformity. Product instability can be associated with impurities in excipients, physical transformation of drug substance to a less stable form during manufacture, and nonoptimal container-closure systems. Thus, formulation design, optimization, and selection of manufacturing platform become a different set of challenges for a low-dose drug product in comparison with a conventional drug product.

There are also enormous challenges for analytical chemists in analytical method development, method validation, and control of product quality. It can be very difficult to develop robust methods for assaying trace amounts of drug substance and impurities in dosage forms, resolving testing interferences of impurities from excipients, and determining the residue of drug substance on manufacturing equipment after cleaning. Extraction of trace amounts of drug from the formulation matrix and maintaining drug stability in the testing medium can also be very challenging. Analytical chemists have to make extra efforts to improve the method sensitivity and selectivity of the equipment used. For example, higher sensitivity for impurity testing using high-pressure liquid chromatography (HPLC) can be obtained from the following approaches:

- sample preparation (derivatization and preconcentration techniques);
- enhanced detection systems (electrochemical/fluorescent detector, mass spectrometry);
- large volume injection loop.

For in vitro dissolution methods, a small volume vessel using 100 mL of medium can also offer a significant sensitivity gain. Nevertheless, equipment modification may be needed to develop analytical methods for low-dose drug products.

In addition to technical challenges in formulation and analytical development, developing a containment strategy is another issue as the exposure limits for highly potent compounds become increasingly low. Product development areas, manufacturing areas, and analytical laboratories can encounter containment control issues. Containment control in pharmaceutical manufacturing and R&D processes is very important in minimizing exposure potential for workers involved in the process, controlling migration of materials for potential cross-contamination, and preventing any leakage of materials from environmental contamination in water and air.

Therefore, the book will cover a wide range of issues associated with low-dose drug product development, including drug substance, formulation design, manufacturing process, analytical control, regulatory consideration, and containment. Together, this book will result in overall scientific understanding of "state-of-the-art" low-dose oral drug product development. Our approach is to teach graduate students, pharmaceutical scientists, process engineers, process chemists, analytical chemists, and regulatory scientists what to do and how to do appropriate CMC activities. However, this book covers only oral solid dosage forms for low-dose drug products. Solution and soft-elastic capsule formulation development of low-dose products will be, for sure, the focus and interest of other pharmaceutical scientists.

1.3 SUMMARY

Since the beginning of this decade, research and development of new medicines in today's pharmaceutical industry have faced increasing challenges. Developing low-dose drug products from candidate selection to market poses a different set of challenges to pharmaceutical scientists in comparison with developing "normal"-dose products. These challenges include continuing to improve existing processes and introducing new cutting-edge technologies, worthy of the best minds and most innovative scientists.

Regardless of the challenges, involvement in new drug product development aimed at bettering human health is one of the greatest careers. The goal of pharmaceutical scientists is to reduce product development time and control development costs effectively without compromising safety and quality. In doing this, pharmaceutical scientists help achieve the goal of providing innovative, tailored, and affordable therapies to patients as early as possible.

ACKNOWLEDGMENTS

The author wish to thank Dr Paul Sirois at Eli Lilly and Company for review of the manuscript. Special thanks are expressed to Ms Karen Boleyn for help with preparation of the manuscript.

REFERENCES

1. Knudson L. 2007. The pursuit of productivity. http://www.ngpharma.com/pastissue/article.asp?art=270804&issue=212. Accessed July 30, 2007.
2. Harman RJ. 1999. The drug development process: introduction and overview. Pharm. J. 262: 334–337.
3. International Human Genome Sequencing Consortium. 2001. Initial sequencing and analysis of the human genome. Nature 409(6822): 860–921.
4. International Human Genome Sequencing Consortium. 2004. Finishing the euchromatic sequence of the human genome. Nature 431(7001): 931–945.
5. Smith C. 2003. Hitting the target. Nature 422(6929): 341–347.
6. Burbaum JJ, Sigal NH. 1997. New technologies for high-throughput screening. Curr. Opin. Chem. Biol. 1(1): 72–78.
7. Hann MM, Oprea TI. 2004. Pursuing the leadlikeness concept in pharmaceutical research. Curr. Opin. Chem. Biol. 8: 255–263.

8. Pharmaceutical Research and Manufacturers of America. 2007. Pharmaceutical Industry Profile 2007. Washington, DC: PhRMA, March 2007.
9. Hariharan M, Ganorkar LD, Amidon GE, Cavallo A, Gatti, P, Hageman MJ, Choo I, Miller JL, Shah UJ. 2003. Reducing the time to develop and manufacture formulations for first oral dose in human. Pharm. Technol. 27(10): 68–84.
10. Physician's Desk Reference, 60th edn. New Jersey: Thomson, 2006.

PART I

CHALLENGES AND STRATEGIES IN FORMULATION DEVELOPMENT OF ORAL LOW-DOSE DRUG PRODUCTS

CHAPTER 2

CHALLENGES AND STRATEGIES IN FORMULATION DEVELOPMENT OF ORAL SOLID LOW-DOSE DRUG PRODUCTS

JACK Y. ZHENG
Pharmaceutical Sciences R&D, Lilly Research Laboratories, Eli Lilly and Company, Indianapolis, IN 40285

2.1 INTRODUCTION

Over several decades, pharmaceutical scientists in both academia and industry have developed alternative drug delivery systems that target drugs more effectively and efficiently to the therapeutic site. These efforts have led to many new pharmaceutical delivery technologies, including pulmonary systemic delivery, nasal delivery, injectable formulations, and transdermal delivery. However, oral administration is still the preferred route when developing a conventional dosage form for a new drug.

Oral dosage forms have several advantages. They are easy to administer; they allow the patient to feel in complete control; and they are more cost-effective to manufacture as compared with alternative dosage forms. Because the manufacturing requirements are less rigorous than for parenteral dosage forms, well over 80% of the marketed drug products in the United States are oral dosage forms. Table 2.1 shows that more than 49% of new chemical entity applications approved by the U.S. FDA between 2000 and 2006 were solid oral dosage forms.[1] Oral dosage forms can also have a variety of choices, but the most common solid oral dosage forms are tablets or capsules (Table 2.2).

In vivo absorption of a drug from an oral solid dosage form into the general circulation after administration is a four-step process:

1. delivery of dosage forms into the stomach and disintegration into smaller particles;
2. drug dissolution/solubilization of the drug in the gastric intestinal fluid;

Formulation and Analytical Development for Low-Dose Oral Drug Products. Edited by Jack Zheng

TABLE 2.1 Dosage Forms of the New Molecule Entity Approvals by U.S. FDA from 2000 to 2007

Year	No. of Tablets	No. of Capsules Approved	No. of Injectable Dosage Forms Approved	No. of Other Dosage Forms Approved	Percentage of Approved Tablets and Capsules (%)
2000	8	5	11	3	30
2001	9	3	6	6	50
2002	8	2	5	2	59
2003	8	5	6	2	61
2004	12	2	13	4	45
2005	4	2	11	1	33
2006	8	4	2	4	67
2007	8	2	4	2	63

3. permeation of dissolved drug through the biological membranes of the intestinal tract;
4. distribution or movement of the absorbed drug away from the membrane into the general circulation.

Figure 2.1 illustrates this absorption process. The slowest of the four steps determines the rate of availability of the drug from an oral dosage form. Many factors in each step influence the rate and extent of availability of a drug. Physical, chemical, and biopharmaceutical properties of the drug, as well as the design and production of the dosage form, play a very important role in its bioavailability after administration. The goal of pharmaceutical scientists is to screen drug candidates with good

TABLE 2.2 Types of Solid Oral Dosage Forms

Type of Oral Dosage Form	Characteristics
Immediate release tablets	Disintegrate in stomach after taken orally
Delayed release tablets	Enteric coated tablets to keep tablets intact in stomach and disintegrate in intestines for absorption
Sustained/controlled release tablets	Release drug slowly for a period of time to reduce administration times
Chewable tablets	Tablets are broken by chewing before swallowing with water
Orally disintegrating tablets	Disintegrate in oral cavity without drinking water to form a suspension for ease of swallowing
Hard gelatin capsule (HGC)	Two-piece capsule shells filled with granules, powders, pellets, minitablets, sprinkles, semisolids, oils
Soft elastic capsule (SEC)	One-piece capsules filled with oily liquid
Sachets	Single-dose unit bag containing granules

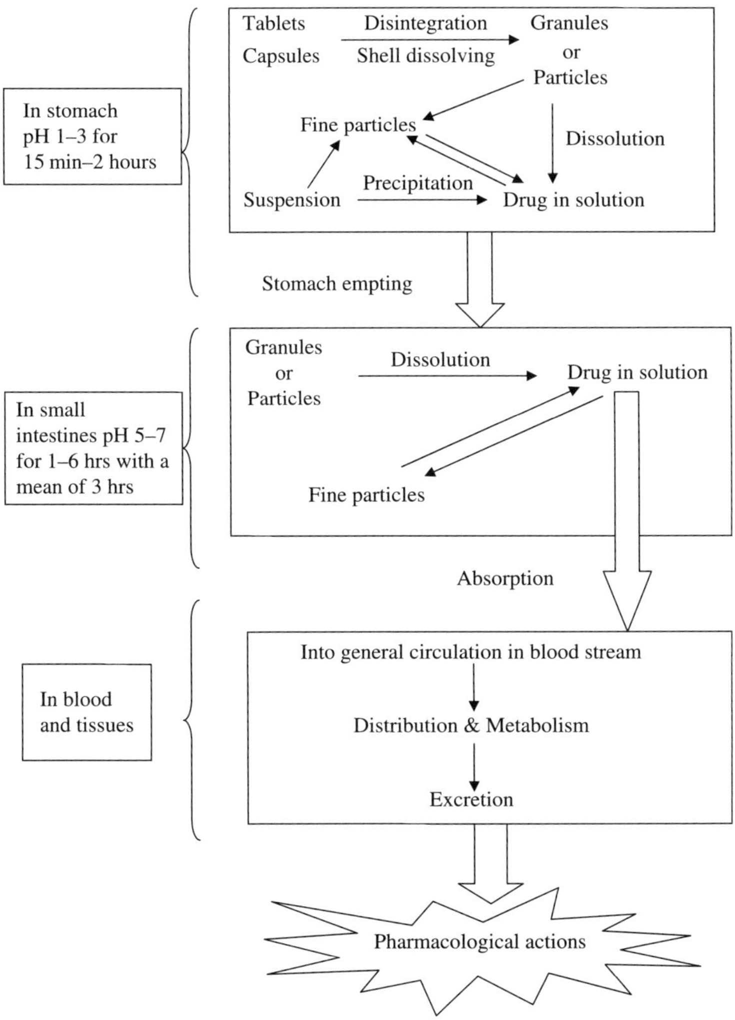

Figure 2.1 *In vivo* absorption of a drug from a solid oral dosage form.

pharmaceutical profiles (that is, excellent drugability), design a stable formulation with good bioavailability, and develop a robust manufacturing process for production.

In recent years, scientists in drug discovery have investigated many very potent small molecule drug candidates. The efficacious dose of such drugs for pharmacological action can be very low. Pharmaceutical development of such low-dose drug products poses significant challenges in product design and optimization, including technical difficulties involved in consistently producing drug products to meet patients' needs. The new regulatory environment that continues to raise the bar for assuring product quality and safety presents another challenge.

Common issues sometimes encountered during low-dose formulation and process development include:

- understanding patients' needs;
- selecting manufacturing platform technology;
- achieving blend uniformity;
- achieving dosage unit uniformity;
- understanding critical product quality attributes;
- controlling critical process parameters;
- understanding process analytical technology (PAT);
- controlling excipients for manufacturability and product stability;
- optimizing container/closure system for product stability;
- achieving quality by design (QbD) and risk assessment.

On the other hand, new product development is always an exciting field. It is innovative, creative, intellectually challenging, and organizationally demanding, but also highly rewarding. This chapter focuses on the following four areas:

1. overview of the impact of today's regulatory environment on drug product development;
2. insight into the strategies and challenges in low-dose formulation development;
3. selection of manufacturing platform technologies for a drug product;
4. current approaches to potent compound containment during drug product handling and manufacture.

2.2 CURRENT REGULATORY ENVIRONMENT AND ITS IMPACT ON NEW DRUG PRODUCT DEVELOPMENT

New drug discovery, development, and approval in the pharmaceutical world follow a reasonably well-defined process that has been refined over several decades. Each phase falls within one of three types of activities:

1. scientific studies designed to generate data on the safety, effectiveness, or toxicity of a new drug product;
2. preparation and submission of these data and other information in regulatory applications;
3. review and approval of the regulatory submission by the FDA.

The FDA regulates pharmaceutical manufacturing to ensure that the drug products in the United States are safe and of consistently high quality. Their major emphasis is on basic procedures and record keeping over decades. Usually, only limited development information is included in the regulatory submission in the United States, with slightly more included in the European Union (EU). However, the agency's recent initiatives and guidance documents provide more in-depth analyses along with their current thinking on new drug development (Table 2.3).[2–6] These initiatives and guidances have had a significant impact on the development and approval process for new drugs.

In August 2002, the FDA put together a significant new initiative, "Pharmaceutical Current Good Manufacturing Practices (cGMPs) for the 21st Century." This initiative enhances and modernizes the regulation of pharmaceutical manufacturing and product quality.[2] It creates a new framework for the regulatory oversight of manufacturing quality that is based on modern quality systems and risk management approaches. Implementing modern and comprehensive quality systems can help pharmaceutical manufacturers achieve compliance with 21 CFR parts 210 and 211.[3]

A robust quality system has the following characteristics:[3]

- science-based approaches;
- decisions based on an understanding of the intended use of a product;
- proper identification and control of areas of potential process weakness;
- responsive deviation and investigation systems that lead to timely remediation;
- sound methods for assessing and reducing risk;
- well-defined processes, control systems, and products, starting from development and extending throughout the product lifecycle;

TABLE 2.3 New Initiatives on Pharmaceutical Product Development by Regulatory Agencies

Time	Agency	Initiatives
August 2002	U.S. FDA	Pharmaceutical cGMPs for the 21st century
March 2004	U.S. FDA	PAT—a framework for innovative pharmaceutical development, manufacturing, and quality assurance
March 2004	U.S. FDA	Challenge and opportunity on the critical path to new medical products
September 2004	U.S. FDA	Pharmaceutical cGMPs for the 21st century, Final Report
May 2006	ICH	Q8: Pharmaceutical development
June 2006	ICH	Q9: Quality risk management
September 2006	U.S. FDA	Quality systems approach to pharmaceutical cGMP regulations
March 2007	U.S. FDA	Target product profile—a strategic development process tool (draft guidance)
May 2007	ICH	Q10: Pharmaceutical quality system (draft guideline)

- systems for careful analysis of product quality;
- supportive management (philosophically and financially).

It is important to maintain product quality throughout the product lifecycle. The attributes that are important to the quality of the drug product should remain consistent with those used in clinical studies. Without doubt, the manufacturing, distribution, inspection, and use of a drug product, including its components, necessarily entails some degree of risk. This risk is a combination of the probability of occurrence of harm and the severity of that harm. An effective quality risk management approach provides a proactive means to identify and control potential quality issues during development and manufacturing. This further ensures the high quality of the drug product to the patient.[4]

Pharmaceutical quality risk management must be a systematic process based on scientific knowledge. It must ultimately link the protection of the patient (by assessing, controlling, communicating, and reviewing risks) to the quality of the drug product. This must occur across all phases in the life of the product (from the initial development through marketing until the product's discontinuation). Quality risk management is a valuable component of an effective quality system.

To support innovation and efficiency in pharmaceutical development, manufacturing, and quality assurance, a PAT guidance document encourages manufacturers to use the latest scientific advances in pharmaceutical manufacturing and technology.[5] PAT is a system for designing, analyzing, and controlling manufacturing of raw and in-process materials and processes. It uses timely measurements (for example, during processing) of critical quality and performance attributes, with a goal of ensuring final product quality. Recognize, however, that quality cannot be tested into products; rather, quality should be built in by design.[6]

Quality by design means that a marketed product should consistently attain a predefined quality at the end of the manufacturing process. A new drug product developed in a QbD system uses the information and knowledge gained from pharmaceutical development studies and manufacturing experience. This information and knowledge provides scientific understanding and supports establishing the design space, specifications, and manufacturing control (Fig. 2.2).[7]

At a minimum, it is important to determine the aspects of drug substances, excipients, container closure systems, and manufacturing processes critical to product quality and to justify control strategies for them. Identification of critical formulation and process parameters generally occurs through assessing the extent to which their variation can affect the quality of the drug product. QbD, in conjunction with a robust quality system, provides a sound framework for transferring product knowledge and process understanding from drug development to the commercial manufacturing processes, and for postdevelopment changes and optimization.

Overall, these new initiatives and guidelines are critically shifting the FDA position towards innovation and continuous improvement during drug product development and its entire lifecycle. It is obvious that under the new regulatory environment the pharmaceutical industry must change the traditional way of developing and manufacturing drug products to meet more stringent regulatory requirements.

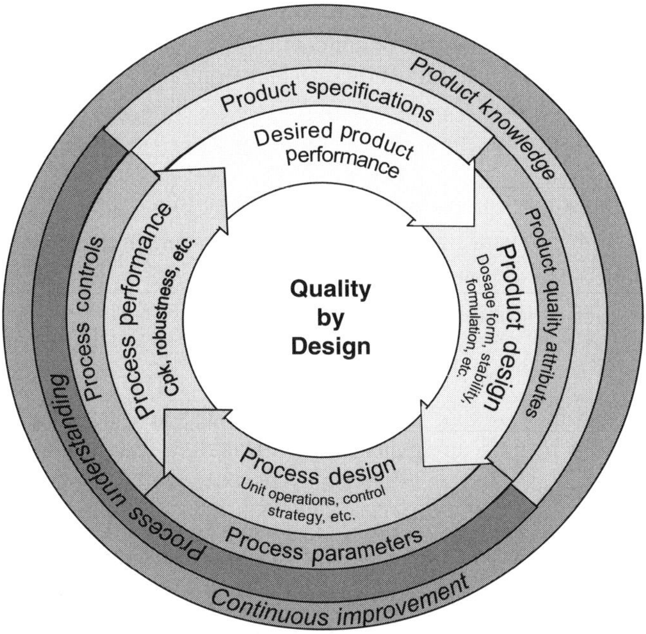

Figure 2.2 Product development in quality-by-design system.

2.3 CHALLENGES IN DEVELOPING LOW-DOSE FORMULATIONS

A formulation is the composition of a drug product that contains the drug substance (active pharmaceutical ingredient, API), and other inactive ingredients. Each inactive ingredient included in the formulation serves a specific purpose to ensure product performance and conformance. For example, inactive ingredients in a tablet formulation may include fillers/diluents, binders, disintegrants, wetting agents, glidants, lubricants, colorants, and other special ingredients to modify drug release rates or enhance in vivo absorption of a drug.

The goal of formulation development is to design a quality product and its manufacturing process to deliver consistently the intended performance of the product. A good formulation must be manufacturable, chemically and physically stable throughout the manufacturing process and product shelf-life, and bioavailable upon administration. It also must meet many other quality standards and special requirements to ensure the efficacy and safety of the product.

A target product profile (TPP) reflects the formulation goals. A TPP is a summary of a drug development program described in terms of labeling concepts.[8] Information on indications and usage, dosage and administration, dosage forms and strengths, use in specific populations, and clinical studies described in a TPP is very important to a formulation scientist. The TPP can help formulation scientists establish formulation strategies and keep formulation efforts efficient and focused.

For a low-dose drug product, drug substance in the dosage unit can be as low as a few micrograms. The ratio of inactive ingredients (excipients) to drug can be between 1000 and 10,000, which is significantly different from a common drug product. The characteristics of the formulation composition may have a significant impact on critical quality attributes of the product such as:

- content uniformity in powder blend and finished product;
- stability in manufacturing process and product shelf-life;
- low potency due to manufacturing loss;
- disintegration/dissolution;
- containment.

These issues are common to all low-dose drug products and independent of platform technologies used in manufacturing the products. Therefore, it is important to understand and evaluate the factors affecting these quality attributes during product development.

2.3.1 Content Uniformity in Powder Blend and Finished Product

According to 21CFR §211.110(a), pharmaceutical manufacturers are legally required to demonstrate the adequacy of mixing to ensure uniformity of in-process powder blends and finished dosage units. The uniformity of dose unit is usually a product specification for oral solid dosage forms and is tested to ensure it meets the compendial acceptance criteria.

To ensure the consistency of dosage units, a homogeneous powder blend is obtained prior to tablet compression or capsule filling. Most platform technologies for manufacturing oral solid dosage forms have a blending or mixing unit operation, including high-shear wet granulation, fluid bed granulation, dry granulation, and direct compression. From a formulation scientist's perspective, the uniformity requirements of the powder blend immediately lead to the following questions:

- How can acceptable uniformity of the final blend be achieved?
- How can blending uniformity be demonstrated or tested?
- How can validation and control of the blending operation be correlated to in-process testing of the dosage unit in production?
- What is the expectation of the regulatory agency?

In October 2003 the FDA published a Draft guidance[9] that addresses the use of stratified sampling of blend and dosage units to demonstrate adequacy of mixing for powder blends. Stratified sampling is the process of sampling dosage units at predefined intervals and collecting representative samples from specifically targeted locations in the compression/filling operation that have the greatest potential to yield extreme highs and lows in test results. The test results are used to develop a single control procedure to ensure adequate powder mix and uniform content in finished products.

Traditional powder blend sampling and testing is first used to demonstrate the adequacy of the powder mix. A series of studies are performed on the blending process and homogeneous testing procedure as follows:

- optimum blending time, speed, and load level of the blender;
- sampling locations and numbers in blenders and intermediate bulk containers (IBC) with an understanding of dead spots in the blenders and segregation areas in the IBCs;
- sampling thief selection and sample size (e.g., 1–10 times dosage unit range);
- analytical method for drug substance and appropriate statistical analyses (e.g., relative standard deviation, RSD).

In a low-dose formulation, typical problems associated with blending are high variability of potency (high RSD) and outliers (stray values) in assay for blending samples or finished products. Significant within-location variance in the blend data is an indication of one factor or a combination of factors such as insufficient blending, sampling error, segregation, aggregates or large particle size of drug substance, and analytical method error.[10–12] Significant between-location variance in the blend data can indicate that the blending operation is inadequate.

After developing a blending and sampling procedure, verify and correlate the results of powder mix uniformity to stratified in-process dosage unit data during capsule filling or tablet compression. Next, assess the normality and RSD from the results of stratified in-processing dosage unit samples. Collect a minimum total of 140 capsules or tablets for analysis (at least 20 sampling points with seven tablets or capsules each).[9] Collect an additional seven dosage units when significant process events occur (for example, hopper changeover, filling, or machine shutdown, and the beginning and end of the compression or filling operation). Compare the in-process dosage-unit data with the powder mix uniformity to see if there is any discrepancy. If there is a discrepancy, possible investigation and correction may range from improving powder characteristics in formulation to process optimization.

Finally, test the uniformity of dosage unit of the finished product according to an appropriate procedure. Usually, the USP <905> Uniformity of Dosage Units criteria are used as proof that the product is adequately uniform.[13] If the uniform content of the finished dosage units is comparable with the results of stratified in-process dosage unit analysis, assessment of powder mix adequacy and the stratified in-process sampling provide assurance of uniform content of the finished drug product. The developed mixing operation parameters and sampling plan are finalized through three process validation batches in the manufacturing area.[9,14] The adequacy of powder mixing is therefore demonstrated by the mix homogeneity and content uniformity of the in-process and finished dosage units through correlation and assessment of data from development, validation, and manufacturing batches. More specific discussion on this topic is located in the chapters of this book that deal with different manufacturing platform technologies.

While a better understanding of methodology to evaluate content uniformity is important for low-dose drug products, it is equally important to design a manufacturable formulation and develop robust manufacturing processes to ensure the content uniformity of the finished products. Although product quality attributes could depend on manufacturing platform technology, control of particle size of drug substance is critical for low-dose drug products unless the manufacturing process involves complete solubilization of drug substance spraying onto excipients. If one or more large particles or aggregates of fine particles exist in the bulk drug and are found in a single dosage unit, the observed potency can easily fall outside the required potency limits. Mixing cannot solve this problem, and the larger drug particles must be reduced in size before attempting to make a homogeneous blend.[15–17] Therefore, a control strategy for the particle size of the drug substance should be in place as early as possible when developing a low-dose drug product.

As mentioned earlier, a low-dose formulation has a very high ratio of excipient(s) to drug. Therefore, the quality of excipients in the formulation is vital to ensure quality of the finished dosage form. However, careful characterization and control of excipient quality is often neglected. Over the years, there has been limited progress in developing standard methods for characterizing pharmaceutical excipients and in creating reliable databases and predictive relationships of properties for commonly used excipients. The impact of specific material properties depends on the amount and function of a particular excipient used in the dosage form, as well as a particular manufacturing platform technology. In general, the impact of an excipient greatly decreases when it is present in a relatively low concentration, but there are some notable exceptions, such as lubricant and glidant. Table 2.4 shows a list of critical material properties, along with their potential impact on product attributes and processing behavior.[18]

TABLE 2.4 Impact of Material Properties on Critical Product Quality and Critical Process Parameters for Solid Oral Dosage Forms

Attributes	Mixing	Drying	Flowability	Mechanical	Uniformity	Dissolution	Wettability	Stability
Particle size and size distribution	•	•	•	•	•	•	•	•
Surface area	•		•					
Particle shape	•		•	•	•			
Bulk and tapped density	•		•	•	•			
Pore size				•			•	
Flow	•		•					
Cohesiveness	•		•		•			
Adhesiveness					•			
Compactibility				•				
Brittleness				•				
Static charge	•		•		•			
Amorphous content				•		•		•
Hygroscopicity		•	•	•			•	•

When manufacturing a tablet formulation by direct compression, the particle size and size distribution of excipients have a significant impact on blending homogeneity, powder segregation, and flowability. This can result in unacceptable content uniformity and high tablet weight variation. In such situations, control of excipients can be critical to product quality.

2.3.2 Stability of Drug Substance During Manufacturing Process and Product Shelf-Life

Stability is another significant issue for a low-dose drug product due to the huge ratio of excipients to drug substance. In general, multiple factors govern the product stability of a solid oral dosage form, including the following:

- physical and chemical properties of drug substance itself;
- manufacturing platform technology used;
- drug–excipient compatibility and impurities in excipients;
- container closure system;
- storage condition.

Manufacturing platform technology and trace amounts of impurities in excipients are particularly important for low-dose product stability. If a drug substance is highly soluble in aqueous media and has multiple polymorphic forms, wet granulation may lead to dissolution of the drug, which may cause polymorphic transformation during processing to form amorphous or another less stable crystal form.[19,20] The crystal form change can have a significant effect on long-term product stability.

Pharmaceutical excipients are increasingly considered important quality attributes of a drug product. They have an effect not only on product manufacturability, but also on product stability. The physical characterization of excipients has received the most attention, as discussed earlier. Excipient functionality testing and multisource excipient equivalence have been reviewed in the literature.[21] However, chemical impurity profiles of excipients have not, in general, received similar attention.

Excipients, like drug substances, contain process residues, degradation products, or other structural derivatives formed during manufacturing. Lactose is one of the most widely used excipients in solid oral dosage forms. In spray-dried lactose, there is a hexose degradant (5-hydroxymethyl furfuraldehyde), which can interact with primary amine for Schiff base formation and color development.[22,23] Fluoxetine, an antidepressant containing secondary amine, can be degraded by Maillard reaction with lactose.[24] Oxidative degradation is another important pathway for the loss of drug potency over time. Themanufacture of lactose may involve treatment with sulfur dioxide,[25] a powerful oxidizing agent. However, there are no reports of complications from the residues.

Higher levels of hydroperoxide (HPO) impurities have been found in several commonly used excipients (Table 2.5),[26] including povidone, polysorbate 80, polyethylene glycol 400, and hydroxypropyl cellulose. The level of HPO may vary

TABLE 2.5 Level of Hydroperoxides in Commonly Used Pharmaceutical Excipients

Excipient	No. Lots Tested	Average Hydroperoxides (nmol/g)	Range (nmol/g)
Povidone	5	7300	3600–11000
Polyethylene glycol 400	4	2200	1000–3300
Polysorbate 80	8	1500	180–4600
Hydroxypropyl cellulose	21	300	50–890
Poloxamer 188, 338, 407	7	30	10–50
Polyethylene glycol 3400, 4600, 6000	4	20	<10–40
Medium chain glyceride	3	<10	<10–<10
Microcrystalline cellulose	5	<10	<10–10
Mannitol	5	<10	<10–<10
Lactose	5	<10	<10–10
Sucrose	5	<10	<10–20

Data adapted from Ref. 26.

across different grades and between manufacturers of the same grade of excipients. Therefore, the role of HPOs in the oxidative degradation of a drug substance necessitates monitoring the HPO content in both excipients and drug product. Unfortunately, most pharmacopeial monographs do not list such organic contaminants. A good understanding of chemical impurity profiles of excipients may be included in the technical agenda to better control excipients used in low-dose drug products in the pharmaceutical industry.

On the other hand, drug–excipient interaction between functional groups of the molecules is commonly recognized as an issue for product stability. If a drug is incompatible with an excipient, the product stability could be problematic, with a decrease in dose strength. Drug substances containing primary, secondary, or tertiary amine have the propensity to react with aldehydic groups in reducing sugars or residual aldehydes present in excipients. The chemical reactions can cause degradation of the drug substance with rapid loss of efficacy because of the trace amounts of active drug present in a low-dose formulation.

Some excipients contain a certain amount of amorphous form such as spray-dried lactose,[27] and others are hygroscopic, such as microcrystalline cellulose.[28] These excipients will adsorb water, which causes a change in the micro-environment of the formulation. If the drug substance is moisture-sensitive, degradation may occur quickly. Therefore, consider both drug–excipient compatibility and excipient impurity profile in selecting excipients for low-dose drug products.

2.3.3 Low Potency Value

Low potency value due to manufacturing loss is another common issue in developing low-dose drug products. Loss of drug during manufacture of the product is highly related to the physical properties of the drug and specific unit operations associated with its manufacturing process. Because the quantity of drug substance is small in a low-dose formulation, loss of a small amount of the drug could cause a big potency drop. For a low-dose formulation, drug substance is usually micronized to achieve acceptable blending homogeneity and content uniformity. Micronized drug with a small particle size could be static, cohesive, adhesive, and fluffy with low density. Thus, the chance for loss of drug may have several different origins:

- loss during transfer of drug from a container to processing equipment;
- loss on equipment surface due to the static and adhesive behavior of the drug;
- loss during drying process due to higher inlet air volume or inappropriate filter bag;
- loss resulting from chemical degradation during manufacturing process.

When a low potency value is observed, conduct a thorough investigation to understand the root cause. If low potency is the result of an unavoidable processing-related operation that produces a quantitatively consistent loss of drug, then an overage can be justified. Perform a well-designed study to ascertain the reason for drug loss and to ensure that minimum overage of the drug substance is used. However, if the loss is due to instability of the drug during processing or an inappropriate analytical method, do not pursue such overage in the formulation.

2.3.4 Disintegration and *In Vitro* Dissolution

The rate of tablet disintegration and the size of the resulting aggregates can be the rate-limiting step in the dissolution process. Disintegration becomes even more important when the tablets are coated by polymer materials. If a coated tablet fails to disintegrate, the drug substance will not be able to dissolve for absorption, thereby affecting the efficacy of the drug product. For a low-dose formulation, deaggregating large disintegrated particles into fine particles may also affect the drug dissolution rate. Thus, formulate a tablet dosage form to have an appropriate range of disintegrations that will produce similar dissolution profiles between batches.

Over decades, in vitro dissolution testing has gradually been recognized as a tool for formulation screening, batch quality control, and prediction of *in vivo* product performance. The dissolution method and test conditions should therefore be selected to best serve their purpose. In most cases, dissolution testing assesses the release rate of drug substance from the formulated dosage form to ensure complete release. During development of a low-dose formulation, challenges in drug dissolution come from two different aspects: formulation design and testing method. Physical interactions between drug and excipient in a formulation can have an impact on drug release. Adsorption of drug by microcrystalline cellulose results in drug dissolution being less than complete and thus may decrease *in vivo* drug absorption.[29]

The difficulty in dissolution testing lies with analyzing very low concentrations of the drug, even when the most well-established apparatus described in the pharmacopeias for solid oral dosage forms is used. A number of noncompendial methods, such as a minivessel, have been discussed in the literature.[30] Use of a minivessel dissolution apparatus in combination with large-volume HPLC injection can significantly improve analytical method sensitivity suitable for low-dose drug products.[31] A separate chapter in this book, "In Vitro Dissolution Testing and Method Development," provides more detail on dissolution for low-dose drug products.

2.4 MANUFACTURING PLATFORMS FOR LOW-DOSE DRUG PRODUCTS

The nature and properties of a drug substance dictate the design of formulation composition and the choice of manufacturing platform technology. The most commonly used manufacturing platforms for solid oral dosage form include:

- high-shear wet granulation;
- direct compression;
- roller compaction;
- fluid bed granulation;
- melt granulation;
- semisolid/solid melt for capsule filling;
- soft gelatin capsules.

Each manufacturing platform has unique characteristics and complexity in terms of unit operations. Table 2.6 presents a fairly comprehensive (but by no means exhaustive) list of unit operation, process parameters, and quality attributes. Since more than one platform technology can be used to manufacture a drug product, selection of the most appropriate manufacturing platform is affected by many factors, such as:

- physical, chemical, and biopharmaceutical properties of the drug substance;
- capabilities at launch sites (experience, facility, equipment and volume);
- dose;
- cost and development duration;
- critical product quality attributes;
- process and in-process control strategy;
- technology transfer to launch sites.

As discussed earlier, one of the most important quality attributes for low-dose drug products is uniformity of dose unit. Usually, dose strength of a drug product is important in selecting a manufacturing platform technology. A simple decision tree on platform selection according to dose strength is described in Fig. 2.3 and is discussed below.

TABLE 2.6 Typical Unit Operations, Process Parameters, and Quality Attributes for Tablet Manufacture

Unit Operation	Process Parameter	Quality Attributes
Mixing	Types of mixer	Blend uniformity
	Mixer load level	Bulk/tapped density
	Number of rotations (time and speed)	Flow properties
	Agitating bar (on/off pattern)	Compression profile in lubrication step
Milling	Mill type	Particle size
	Milling speed	Particle size distribution
	Blade configuration	Particle shape
	Screen size	Bulk/tapped density
	Feeding rate	Flow properties
High-shear wet granulation	Impeller speed, configuration	Power consumption
	Chopper speed, configuration	Blend uniformity
	Spray nozzle type and location	Flowability
	Method of binder addition	Moisture content
	Binder fluid temperature	Particle size and distribution
	Binder addition rate and time	Granule size and distribution
	Postgranulation mix time	Uniformity of dosage unit
		Compression profile
		Dissolution profile
Fluid bed drying	Inlet air volume, temperature, dew point	Granule size and distribution
	Exhaust air temperature	Granule strength, and uniformity
	Filter properties	Particle size
	Shaking intervals	Flowability
	Product temperature	Bulk/tapped density
		Moisture content
Roller compaction	Roll speed	Appearance
	Roll gap	Ribbon density, strength, and thickness
	Roll pressure	Compression profile
	Auger screw rate	
	Roller surface type	
Tableting	Compression speed	Weight uniformity
	Compression main force	Content uniformity
	Precompression force	Breaking strength/solid fraction
	Ejection force	Thickness
	Feed frame type and speed	Friability
	Hopper design, height, and vibration	Disintegration
	Depth of fill	Dissolution
Film coating	Product temperature	Visual appearance
	Spray nozzle type and number	Percentage weight gain
	Gun to bed distance	Film thickness
	Spray rate	Color uniformity
	Solid content in coating suspension	Dissolution
	Pan rotation speed	Disintegration
	Atomization air pressure	
	Exhaust air temperature	
	Inlet air temperature	

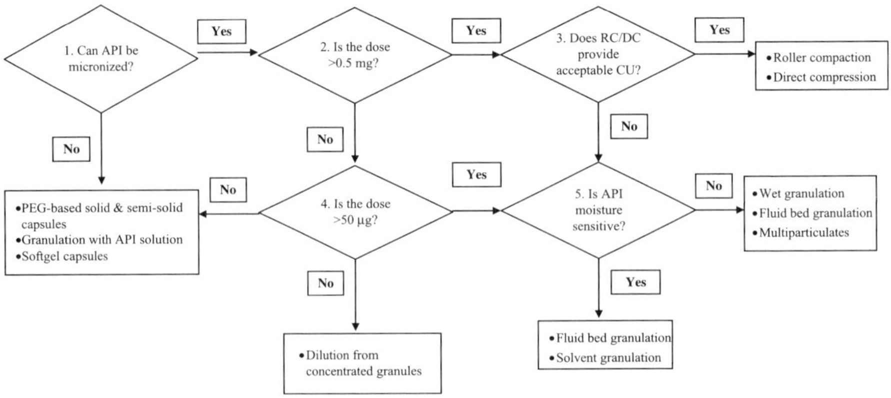

Figure 2.3 Solid oral formulation decision tree for low-dose drug product (<1 mg).

Can API be Micronized? The particle size of drug substance at the micron level is critical to achieving blending uniformity and uniformity of dosage unit.[16,17] If the drug substance cannot be micronized due to physicochemical stability or material properties, consider dissolving the drug in solution for forwarding processes.

First, evaluate the feasibility of solid dispersion such as a polyethylene glycol (PEG)-based semisolid or solid hard gelatin capsule formulation.[32,33] When the molecular weight of PEG used in the formulation is greater than 3350 Da, PEG exists as a solid. Prerequisites for this formulation approach include (1) adequate solubility and (2) thermal-stability of the drug in molten PEG during processing.

For general processing, dissolve the drug into molten PEG, and fill the melt into a hard gelatin capsule at a higher temperature. The melt solidifies in the capsule when the temperature of the melt decreases. If the solubility of a drug is not high enough in molten PEG, add co-solvents and surfactants to the formulation to improve the wettability and solubility. This resultant formulation could be a semisolid form (paste-like). In this case, use the minimum amount of solvent or surfactant necessary for drug solubility to avoid incompatibility with the hard gelatin capsule shell. Also, banding capsules may be needed for a semisolid formulation. In general, higher molecular weight PEG (>3350 Da) is recommended. Other appropriate polymers may replace the PEG.

A second approach for unmilled drug substance is soft gelatin capsules if the drug substance is lipophilic. Dissolve the drug in oily vehicles such as vegetable oils, mineral oils, medium chain triglycerides, and acetylated glycerides. Fill the resultant liquid into individual capsules by a positive-displacement pump in one operation.[34] Because the capsules are filled with liquids, excellent drug content uniformity can be achieved even at a very low dose level. Also, dissolving the drugs in a liquid vehicle reduces the risk of operator exposure to dusts, a common issue in tablet and capsule manufacturing operations.

Another option is to dissolve large particles of drugs in aqueous or organic solution followed by wet granulation or fluid bed granulation. Compress the granules into tablets or fill into hard gelatin capsules. Nevertheless, solubilization of unmilled drug substances is a necessary processing step to assure dose accuracy for low-dose products.

Are Doses Greater than 0.5 mg? If a drug substance can be micronized and the dose strength is greater than 0.5 mg, direct compression (DC) or roller compaction (RC) could be the appropriate choice of manufacturing platform. Direct compression and roller compaction offer economic advantages through eliminating intermediate granulating and drying steps. Direct compression and roller compaction platforms do not involve water during manufacture, and thus provide advantages for a drug substance that has physical and chemical stability problems when exposed to moisture and high temperature.

Because blending or mixing is the key unit operation, a homogeneous blend with less tendency to segregation must be obtained by careful selection of excipients and optimization of formulation and manufacturing process.[35] In an ideal situation, the ordered mixing by design may offer good blending homogeneity required in direct compression or roller compaction.[36,37]

If dose strength is less than 0.5 mg, direct compression or roller compaction may present significant challenges in achieving acceptable product content uniformity. In this case, explore other platform technologies.

Does Roller Compaction or Direct Compression Provide Acceptable Content Uniformity? If the dose is greater than 0.5 mg and direct compression/roller compaction cannot provide acceptable content uniformity, choose other manufacturing platform technologies such as wet granulation, solvent granulation, or multiparticulates. In general, fluid bed granulation and/or solvent granulation can be used for a moisture-sensitive compound as further discussed below.

Are Doses Greater Than 50 μg? If the dose strength is less than 50 μg, an obvious problem in development is product content uniformity. Dissolving the drug substance for the manufacturing process can provide a good solution to the content uniformity issue and the drug product can be PEG-based solid or semisolid capsules, soft gelatin capsules, or tablets made by wet granulation. Another approach may also be very effective: dilution of concentrated granules to low-dose drug products. Concentrated granules can be manufactured by high-shear wet granulation or fluid bed granulation, and a filler such as microcrystalline cellulose, spray-dried mannitol, and spray-dried lactose can be used for further dilution. Determine an optimum dilution factor by experiment; however, three to five times dilution should be a good starting point.

If the dose ranges between 50 μg and 0.5 mg, evaluate the granulation process or multiparticulates, including high-shear wet granulation, fluid bed granulation, and multiparticulates by beads coating.

Is the Drug Substance Moisture-Sensitive? A moisture-sensitive compound can be degraded when exposed to moisture during the manufacturing process. In this case, do not select high-shear or low-shear wet granulation since the process involves water and high temperatures for drying. However, solvent granulation is still a viable option since the granulation solution uses organic solvent, rather than water. In addition, explore fluid bed granulation because the duration of exposure of the drug substance to moisture in fluid bed granulation is relatively short and minimal. Aqueous binding solution is sprayed onto the powder bed and dried simultaneously.[38]

If a drug substance is not moisture-sensitive and the dose strength ranges between 50 μg and 0.5 mg, consider wet granulation, fluid bed granulation, or multiparticulates by beads coating. The literature contains many successful examples.[39–44]

Selecting the manufacturing platform technology is the first stage of process development for product commercialization. It is very important to involve the production site in selecting the platform during the commercial product design phase. The eventual technology transfer and process validation are likely to be smoother if there is communication between R&D scientists and production staff. If considering a platform new to manufacturing sites, production can plan ahead to cope with the requirements to the facility and new processes needed for the product.

2.5 USE OF EXPERIMENTAL DESIGN IN FORMULATION AND PROCESS DEVELOPMENT

Pharmaceutical formulation and process development should provide sufficient information and knowledge to understand and support establishment of the design space, specifications, and manufacturing control. The design space of QbD is defined as the multidimensional combination and interaction of input variables (e.g., material attributes) and process parameters that have been demonstrated to provide assurance of quality.[6] Because multiple variables in formulation and process can be encountered, it is important to use an effective methodology to define the design space.

Design of experiments (DOE) and statistical analysis have been applied widely to formulation and process optimization. The main advantage of using DOE in formulation and process development is that interaction effects between variables, as well as the main effects of the individual variables, can be identified and quantified simultaneously, systemically, and quickly. When the formulation and manufacturing process of a drug product are optimized by a systematic approach using DOE, scale-up and process validation can be very efficient due to the robustness of the formulation and manufacturing process. Table 2.7 gives an example of some important factors of a low-dose tablet formulation evaluated by DOE studies. A detailed discussion of the statistical principles underlying DOE is beyond the scope of this book. However, a few DOE design examples are highlighted below which serve to illustrate the utility of DOE in defining design space,[45] including:

- full factorial design;
- fractional factorial design;
- response surface design;
- mixture design.

TABLE 2.7 Factors and Response of a Tablet Formulation Using Design of Experiment Studies

Factor	Responses	Design of Experiment
Percentage drug load	Impurity	Full factorial
Percentage filler or ratio of fillers	Uniformity (content and weight)	Fractional factorial
Percentage binder	Compactibility	Central composite
Percentage wetting agent	Ejection force	Mixture
Percentage disintegrant	Flowability	D-optimal
Percentage glidant	Disintegration	Response surface
Percentage lubricant	Dissolution profile	Box–Behnken
	Stability	

A full factorial design consists of studying several factors, with each factor having a low level and a high level. All combinations of the low and the high level of each of the factors are studied with each of the other factors. Thus, if there are four factors, there are a total of 2^4, or 16, trials. This design allows one to estimate all main effects, two-factor interactions, and any higher order interactions among the factors. If a middle level is relevant for each of the factors, repeat independent trials are often performed with each of the factors set at their mid level in an attempt to assess whether there is evidence that at least one of the factors may have curvature associated with it. This is assessed by comparing the average of the center point trials to the average of the factorial trials. If there is strong evidence of a difference between these two quantities, there is evidence of curvature due to at least one of the factors. If a factor only has two levels and does not have a middle level (e.g., type of disintegrant), it is common to perform two or more center point replicates at each of the different levels of the factor. However, the use of three-level factorial design adds considerably to the number of experimental runs required.

In many situations, it is not feasible to perform a full factorial, as the number of combinations becomes too large. In addition, it is often assumed that the system can be adequately modeled by the main effects and the two-factor interactions and that the higher-order interactions are not the primary drivers in the system. Fractional factorial designs are often an economical approach to evaluate several factors in this situation. A fractional factorial design consists of performing a specific subset of the full factorial trials so that each of the main effects and (typically) two-factor interactions can be evaluated. In these designs, the main effects and two-factor interactions are confounded with higher-order interactions, which means they are being estimated, assuming that the higher-order interactions are negligible.

One limitation of two-level factorial designs is the assumption of linearity of the effects. If it is possible that the effect of one or more of the factors is nonlinear, a response surface design may be selected. A central composite response surface design is a full factorial or fractional factorial design that is supplemented with additional trials to allow for estimation of curvature from the factors of interest. For each factor of interest to be studied for curvature, two additional trials are performed: (1) one trial with all of the factors at their middle level except for the factor of interest, which is set at its low level; and (2) a second trial with all of the factors at their middle level with the factor of interest at its high level. Thus, for each factor studied for curvature, there are two additional trials to be performed.

Mixture designs are applied in cases where the levels of individual components in a formulation require optimization, but where the system is constrained by a maximum value for the overall formulation. In other words, a mixture design is often considered at this stage when the quantities of the factors must add to a fixed total. In a mixture experiment, the factors are proportions of different components of a blend. Mixture designs allow for the specification of constraints on each of the factors, such as a maximum and/or minimum value for each component, as well as for the sum and/or ratio of two or more of the factors. These designs are very specific in nature and are tied to the specific constraints that are unique to the particular formulation. However, as with the discussion of the fractional factorial designs, in order to be most efficient, it is important to provide realistic prior expectations on anticipated effects so the smallest design can be set up to fit the simplest realistic model to the data.

The use of appropriate DOE can be an invaluable tool to optimize use of resources at all stages of product development, and to shorten the development time from formulation/process screening to optimization. When the formulation and manufacturing processes of a pharmaceutical product are designed and optimized by a scientific and systematic approach, the scale-up, technology transfer between manufacturing sites, and process validation can be more efficient because of the robustness of the formulation and manufacturing process.

2.6 CONTAINMENTS

New drug substances in low-dose products, in many cases, are highly potent. An increase in potency indicates higher requirements on containment during handling and processing the drug substance. The importance of containing highly potent compounds is appreciated much more today in the pharmaceutical industry. Good containment of potent drugs can reduce employees' exposure to avoid health and safety consequences, minimize cross-contaminations to other products for GMP compliance, and decrease the risks of environmental pollution.[46] The three main approaches used for containing highly potent compounds are engineering controls, administrative controls, and personal protective equipment (PPE).

The most conservative and safest potent-compound containment strategy depends on the use of engineering controls in both the processing equipment and the manufacturing facility. Specific design features of a high-containment facility should include the following:[46]

- utilize airlocks to segregate processes that pose different levels of exposure risk;
- provide airlock-isolated gowning/degowning areas with a shower/mist installation;

TABLE 2.8 Containment Technologies and Exposure Level Control

Level of control	Technology	Design
<0.01 μg/m^3	Automation	Remote operation; fully automated; no human contact
<5 μg/m^3	Barrier technology	Negative pressure; hard shell, soft shell and glove bag; transfer using double posting ports
5.0–20 μg/m^3	Laminal flow technology	Transfers using high-containment valves (e.g., split butterfly valves; containment for every disconnect
50–100 μg/m^3	Local or point exhaust	Fan, filter and dust system to remove airborne particles

- provide capability for facility decontamination and surface cleaning [i.e., installation of floor drains, high-efficiency particulate air (HEPA) vacuums, and cleanable room surfaces];
- incorporate design features for safety maintenance activities (e.g., "through the wall" control module mounting, bag in/bag out HEPA filters);
- use "one-pass air" for general ventilation of potent drug areas;
- design local exhaust ventilation exhaust stacks to eliminate reintrainment of contaminated exhaust air back into the facility.

Many containment technologies are available. The criteria for selection of the technology should be based on an exposure limit (Table 2.8).[47] When designing manufacturing unit operations for a low-dose compound, the first and most important principle is to minimize the number of material transfers. Using multiple-function process equipment such as intermediate bulk container (IBC) blenders and granulator-dryers, including the double-plinth IBC blender, accomplishes this best. Many tablet machines now have wet-in-place or clean-in-place capability, which is coupled with isolators for dedustor, metal detector, and tablet hardness tester. These integrated designs have made containment manufacturing more process-friendly.[48]

Overall, the trend toward high-potency and low-dose drug products is leading to an increased use of containment technology. Use of multiple-function process equipment as well as containers that are compatible with all unit operations is preferred. Any plan for a new or renovated facility that will include contained manufacturing must account for these features.

2.7 SUMMARY

This chapter summarized some of the key challenges and strategies during the development of low-dose drug products. To successfully develop a low-dose drug product for today's market, extra effort should be made in the control of drug substance and excipients, design of formulation and process, selection of manufacturing platform, and considerations for containment. Different chapters of this book provide detailed discussion on the development of low-dose drug products using different platform technologies, and readers interested in learning more about this subject are encouraged to consult the related contents.

ACKNOWLEDGMENTS

The author wishes to thank Dr Paul Sirois at Eli Lilly and Company for review of the manuscript. Special thanks are expressed to Ms Karen Boleyn for help with preparation of the manuscript.

REFERENCES

1. U.S. Food and Drug Administration. Drug Approval Report. http://www.fda.gov. Accessed June 8, 2007.
2. U.S. Food and Drug Administration. 2004. Pharmaceutical cGMPs for the 21st century—a risk-based approach, final report. http://www.fda.gov/cder/guidance/index.htm. Accessed June 8, 2007.
3. U.S. Food and Drug Administration. 2006. Guidance for industry: Quality systems approach to pharmaceutical cGMP regulations. http://www.fda.gov/cder/guidance/index.htm. Accessed June 8, 2007.
4. International Conference on Harmonization. 2006. Q9: Quality risk management. http://www.fda.gov/cder/guidance/index.htm. Accessed June 8, 2007.
5. U.S. Food and Drug Administration. 2004. Guidance for industry: PAT—a framework for innovative pharmaceutical development, manufacturing, and quality assurance. http://www.fda.gov/cder/guidance/index.htm. Accessed June 8, 2007.
6. International Conference on Harmonization. 2006. Q8: Pharmaceutical Development. http://www.fda.gov/cder/guidance/index.htm. Accessed June 8, 2007.
7. Nasr MM. 2006. Pharmaceutical quality assessment system (PQAS) in the 21st century. Presentation at PhRMA API Workshop. Denver, Colorado.
8. U.S. Food and Drug Administration. 2007. Guidance for industry and review staff: Target product profile—a strategic development process tool. http://www.fda.gov/cder/guidance/index.htm. Accessed June 8, 2007.
9. U.S. Food and Drug Administration. 2003. Guidance for industry: Powder blends and finished dosage units—stratified in-processing dosage unit sampling and assessment. http://www.fda.gov/cder/guidance/index.htm. Accessed June 8, 2007.
10. Prescott JK, Garcia TP. 2001. A solid dosage and blend content uniformity trouble shooting diagram. Pharm. Technol. 25(3): 68–88.
11. Berman J. 2001. The compliance and science of blend uniformity analysis. PDA J. Pharm. Sci. Technol. 55(4): 209–221.
12. Muzzio FJ, Robinson P, Wightman C, Brone D. 1997. Sampling practices in powder blending. Int. J. Pharm. 155: 153–178.

13. United States Pharmacopeia. 2007. <905> Uniformity of Dosage Unit. 30-NF 25.
14. Geoffroy JM, LeBlond D, Poska R, Brinker D, Hsu A. 2001. Unit dose sampling and final product performance: an alternative approach. Drug Dev. Ind. Pharm 27(7): 731–743.
15. Yalkowsky SH, Bolton S. 1990. Particle size and content uniformity. Pharm. Res. 7(9): 962–966.
16. Zhang Y, Johnson KC. 1997. Effect of drug particle size on content uniformity of low-dose solid dosage forms. Int. J. Pharm. 154: 179–183.
17. Rohrs BR, Amidon GE, Meury RH, Secreast PJ, King HM, Skoug CJ. 2006. Particle size limits to meet USP content uniformity criteria for tablets and capsules. J. Pharm. Sci. 95(5): 1049–1059.
18. Hlinak AJ, Kuriyan K, Morris KR, Reklaitis GV, Basu PK. 2006. Understanding critical material properties for solid dosage form design. J. Pharm. Innov. 1(1): 12–17.
19. Curatolo W, Singhal D. 2004. Drug polymorphism and dosage form design, a practical perspective. Adv. Drug Deliv. Rev. 56: 335–347.
20. Zhang GZ, Law D, Schmitt EA, Qiu Y. 2004. Phase transformation considerations during process development and manufacture of solid oral dosage forms. Adv. Drug Deliv. Rev. 56: 371–390.
21. Bolhuis GK, Chowhan ZT. 1996. Materials for direct compaction. In: Alderborn G, Nystrom C, editors. Pharmaceutical powder compaction technology. New York: Marcel Dekker; 473–476.
22. Brownley CA Jr, Lachman L. 1964. Browning of spray processed lactose. J. Pharm. Sci. 53: 452–454.
23. Janicki CA, Almond HR Jr. 1974. Reaction of haloperidol with 5-(hydroxymethyl)-2-furfuraldehyde: an impurity in anhydrous lactose. J. Pharm. Sci. 63: 4143.
24. Wirth DD, Baertschi SW, Johnson RA, Maple SR, Miller MS, Hallenbeck DK, Gregg SM. 1998. Maillard reaction of lactose and fluoxetine hydrochloride, a secondary amine. J. Pharm. Sci. 87: 31–39.
25. Campina BV. Stabilization of crystalline lactose. Netherlands Patent Application: NL8301220A841101 and NL83-1220 830407. DMV.
26. Wasylaschuk WR, Harmon PA, Wagner G, Harman AB, Templeton AC, Xu H, Reed RA. 2007. Evaluation of hydroperoxides in common pharmaceutical excipients. J. Pharm. Sci. 96(1): 106–116.
27. Winfield AJ. 2006. Lactose, spray-dried. In: Rowe RC, Sheskey PJ, Owen SC, editors. Handbook of pharmaceutical excipients, 5th ed. London and Washington, DC: Pharmaceutical Press and American Pharmaceutical Association; 396–401.
28. Armstrong NA. 2006. Mannitol. In: Rowe RC, Sheskey PJ, Owen SC, editors. Handbook of pharmaceutical excipients, 5th ed. London and Washington, DC: Pharmaceutical Press and American Pharmaceutical Association; 449–453.
29. Senderoff RI, Mahjour M, Radebaugh, GW. 1992. Characterization of adsorption behaviour by solid dosage form excipients in formulation development. Int. J. Pharm. 83: 65–72.
30. Crail DJ, Tunis A, Dansereau R. 2004. Is the use of a 200 mL vessel suitable for dissolution of low dose drug products? Int. J. Pharm. 269: 203–209.

31. Sesi NN. 2005. Low-dose drug products: analytical challenges and strategies. Annual Meeting of American Association of Pharmaceutical Scientists, Nashville, TN.
32. Law D, Wang W, Schmitt EA, Long MA. 2002. Prediction of poly(ethylene) glycol–drug eutectic compositions using an index based on the van't Hoff equation. Pharm. Res. 19(3): 315–321.
33. Lloyd GR, Craig DQM, Smith A. 1997. An investigation into the melting behavior of binary mixes and solid dispersions of paracetamol and PEG 4000. J. Pharm. Sci. 86(9): 991–996.
34. Berry IR. 1985. One-piece, soft gelatin capsules for pharmaceutical products. Pharm. Engng 5(5): 15–25.
35. Venables HJ, Wells JI. 2001. Powder mixing. Drug Dev. Ind. Pharm. 27(7): 599–612.
36. Hersey JA. 1975. Ordered mixing: a new concept in powder mixing practice. Powder Technol. 11: 41–44.
37. Mort PR, Riman RE. 1995. Determination of homogeneity scale in ordered and partially ordered mixtures. Powder Technol. 82: 93–104.
38. Thiel WJ, Nguyen LT, Sberna FJ. 1986. Content uniformity of microdose tablets (dosage 1 μg–10 μg) produced by fluid bed granulation of interactive mixtures. J. Pharm. Pharmac. 38: 335–343.
39. Vromans H, Poels-Jassen HGM, Egermann H. 1999. Effect of high-shear granulation on granulate homogeneity. Pharm. Dev. Technol. 4(3): 297–303.
40. Kornchankul W, Parikh NH, Sakr A. 2000. Effect of process variables on the content uniformity of a low dose drug in a high-shear mixer. Pharm. Ind. 62: 305–311.
41. Hausman DS. 2004. Comparison of low shear, high-shear, and fluid bed granulation duign low dose tablet process development. Drug Dev. Ind. Pharm. 30(3): 259–266.
42. Crooks MJ, Schade HW. 1978. Fluidized bed granulation of a microdose pharmaceutical powder. Powder Technol. 19: 103–108.
43. Matinez L, Tchoreloff P, Leclerc B, Besnard M, Couarraze G. 2001. Active layering and direct compression of sugar spheres: content homogeneity in low-dosage tablets. Pharm. Technol. Eur. October issue: 38–46.
44. Greaves FC, Beasley MW, Suddith AW, Swarbrick J. 1995. Novel approaches to the preparation of low-dose solid dosage form. Pharm. Technol. 19: 60–64.
45. Box GEP, Hunter WG, Hunter JS. 1978. Statistics for experiments, an introduction to design, data analysis, and model building. New York: John Wiley & Sons; 291–302.
46. Newton C. 2006. Controlling worker exposure to potent compounds in pharmaceutical development pilot plant. Am. Pharm. Rev. 9(1): 70–80.
47. Rahe H. 2001. Selecting the correct technology. In: Wood JP, editor. Containment in the pharmaceutical industry. New York: Marcel Dekker; 115–127.
48. Herreman G. 2003. Current technology for contained manufacturing. Pharm. Technol. 27(10): 132–146.

CHAPTER 3

PARTICLE SIZE OF DRUG SUBSTANCE AND PRODUCT CONTENT UNIFORMITY—THEORETICAL CONSIDERATIONS

KEVIN C. JOHNSON
Intellipharm, LLC, PO Box 644, Niantic, CT 06357

3.1 INTRODUCTION

Judging from the questions asked after having presented numerous times on the topic to be covered in this chapter, it would seem that sufficient confusion exists to warrant a chapter dedicated to this one aspect of content uniformity: the effect of drug particle size on content uniformity. Now drug particle size can have many effects on content uniformity but only one particular effect will be discussed. This is not to say that the other effects are not important, but if the drug particle size is not conducive to good content uniformity, nothing can be done through mixing, processing, switching excipients, changing the size of the dosage form, or changing the relative ratio of drug to excipients to achieve good content uniformity unless the necessary drug particle attrition occurs during mixing and processing. The author suspects that actual content uniformity problems have been resolved through unintended drug particle size reduction during processing without the formulator realizing the cause of the problem or the real reason it was solved. Other formulation scientists may have not yet encountered the problem if they have never worked on a low-dose formulation, because it would be unlikely that the typical drug particle size would be so large as to cause a problem with a high-dose drug. However, the author has encountered the problem at a 10 mg dose, even though he understood the topic at the time that the content uniformity problem was observed. But understanding the issue allowed him to quickly rectify the problem.

The goal of this chapter is to describe the effect of drug particle size on content uniformity using the concept of ideal mixing.[1] The intention is to provide a

Formulation and Analytical Development for Low-Dose Oral Drug Products. Edited by Jack Zheng

model to predict when poor content uniformity will likely occur, and thereby, provide a strategy to set drug particle size specifications to avoid the problem. The concept of ideal mixing will also be compared to the approach of Yalkowsky and Bolton.[2]

3.2 CONCEPT OF IDEAL MIXING

The concept of ideal mixing[1] attempts to make the drug particle size distribution in each dosage form the same as the lot of drug used to make the dosage forms. This is a reasonable goal, for if the particle size make-up of the drug in the dosage form did not match the drug itself, some segregation of drug particles would have to have occurred, leading to a lack of homogeneity. The previous statement ignores the possibility that some drug particle size attrition could occur during processing that would make the drug within the final dosage form smaller than the original drug. However, as will become apparent later, any drug particle size reduction after the original milling due to processing, such as blending, roller compaction, and further milling of the drug and excipient blend, in general will be favorable to content uniformity. But the intention of having a model for ideal mixing is to understand the effect of drug particle size on content uniformity, to be able to predict and set a drug particle size specification that will be conducive to good content uniformity before formulation begins, and not rely on the dosage form manufacturing process to achieve the necessary drug particle size.

Figure 3.1 presents a schematic representation of the concept of ideal mixing. The numbered ovals are intended to represent unit dosage forms, in this case, 40. Enclosed in the ovals are circles of three different sizes that are intended to represent drug particles. Taken together, the different sizes and number of particles in each size group represent the drug particle size distribution used to make the 40 unit doses. In the example shown in Fig. 3.1, assume that the pharmaceutical scientist made one weighing of the drug equal to the nominal amount needed for 40 unit doses. It contained 760 particles of the smallest particle group, 10 particles of the intermediate particle size group, and four of the largest particle size group.

As shown in Fig. 3.1, it is possible to evenly distribute the smallest particles among the 40 doses. Each unit gets exactly 19 particles. However, for the intermediate group, there are only 10 particles. This works out to one particle for every four doses so that in Fig. 3.1 one intermediate particle is added to every fourth unit dose. For the largest particles, one particle is added to every tenth unit dose.

In Fig. 3.1, it can be seen that every unit dose does not have the same number of particles for every particle size group, and therefore, the particle size distribution in each unit dose will not represent the particle size distribution of the drug used to make the dosage forms. When the drug particle size distribution within the dosage form cannot be made to match the distribution of the drug lot, the concept of ideal mixing will make drug particle size distribution within the drug–excipient blend match the particle size distribution of the drug lot at the smallest possible subdivision of the drug–excipient blend, which may be many times larger than the amount in a single dose. In the case shown in Fig. 3.1, the smallest subdivision of the

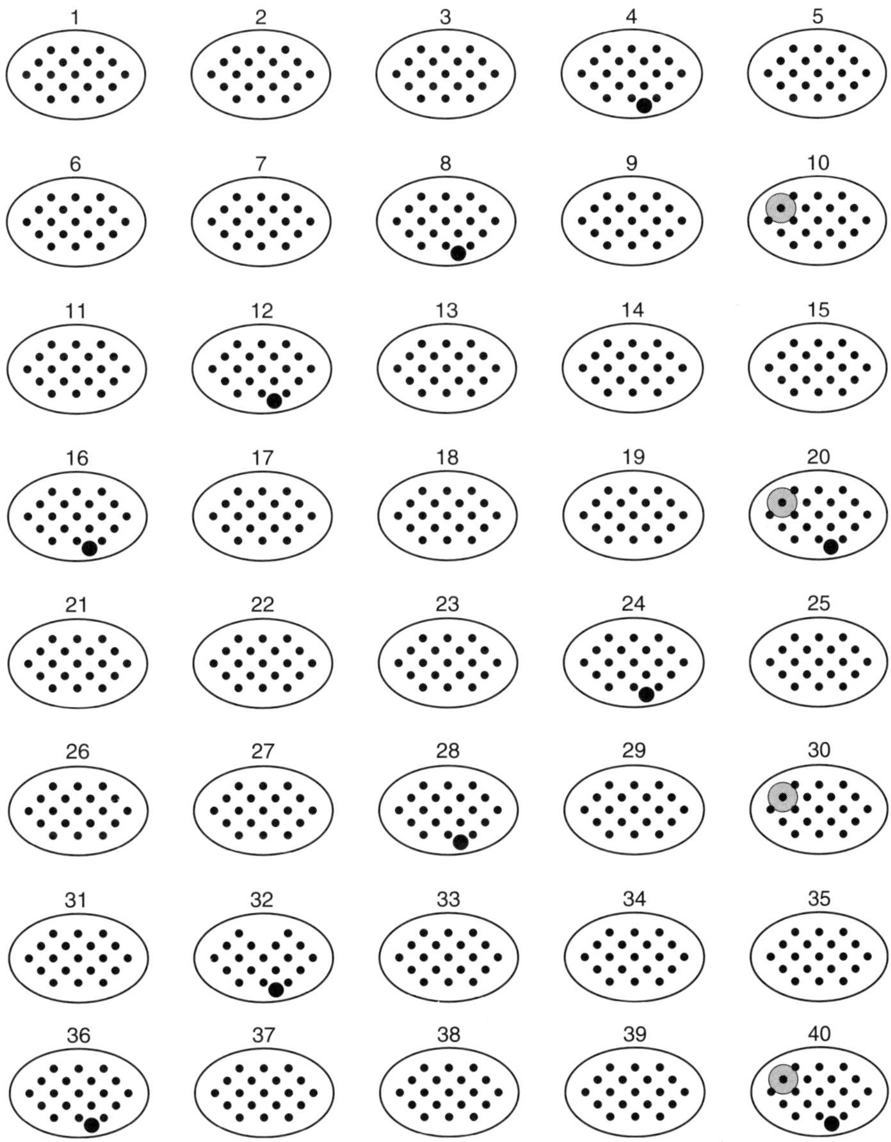

Figure 3.1 Schematic representation of the concept of ideal mixing.

drug–excipient blend that would match the drug itself would be 20 units. This treatment results in the best homogeneity for the blend overall.

Obviously, not all the unit doses in Fig. 3.1 will have the same potency. Most of the units, 28 out of 40, will be below in the intended potency because they only contain 19 of the smallest particles. Two of the units, units 20 and 40, contain 19 of the smallest drug particles plus one intermediate and one large particle. These two units will be above the intended potency.

Several points should be made that are important in understanding and solving real content uniformity issues. First, no amount of mixing would make the content uniformity represented by Fig. 3.1 get any better. If unit dose samples of the blend were analyzed for potency and the poor content uniformity revealed, one might be tempted to mix the blend longer, assuming the blend was poorly mixed, which is not the case. One might be tempted to think that moving some of the smallest particles out of a dosage form with a large particle would improve content uniformity. However, it should be realized that it would take numerous small particles to equal the mass of a large particle and that finding a dosage form with an unusually low number of small particles after mixing would be unlikely. The only way to improve the content uniformity in the given example is to break up the larger particles so that their mass can be evenly distributed throughout the blend. To achieve this, the best approach would be to apply a theoretical approach like the concept of ideal mixing before any drug formulation work begins, to set a particle size specification that is conducive to good content uniformity and then mill the drug to meet that specification. Poor content uniformity due to the presence of large drug particles is easy to avoid if one understands the concepts presented in this chapter and applies one of the approaches that will be discussed.

A second point is that a blend that is ideally mixed as defined above but still suffering the problem of poor content uniformity due to large drug particles will display characteristics that may help identify the problem. As mentioned above, if one observes that most of the potency samples are slightly below the intended potency with only a few samples displaying unusually high potency or "hot spots," then this suggests that the high end of the drug particle size distribution is too large and that mixing is not the problem. In this case, it would be wise to check the particle size analysis of the drug to make sure it is conducive to good content uniformity.

A third point is that an ideally mixed blend with poor content uniformity due to large drug particles will not display unusually low potency values or "cold spots" unless drug particles in the lower range of the particle size distribution are also too large. Again, one should check the drug particle size analysis to make sure the drug particle size is conducive to good content uniformity. If the drug particle size is conducive and "cold spots" are observed, this suggests that mixing is not ideal and that the mixing process should be improved instead of altering the drug particle size.

Lastly, it should be recognized that real mixing will not be as efficient as the concept of ideal mixing. Setting a particle size specification assuming ideal mixing provides an edge of failure. It guarantees that exceeding the particle size specification will lead to failure. It does not guarantee that being below the particle size specification will lead to success because real-life mixing may be far from ideal. For this reason, it would be prudent to set a particle size specification somewhere below the edge of failure.

Taking the concept of ideal mixing to the next level of detail, assume that a pharmaceutical scientist is attempting to make a 0.1 mg strength tablet of a certain

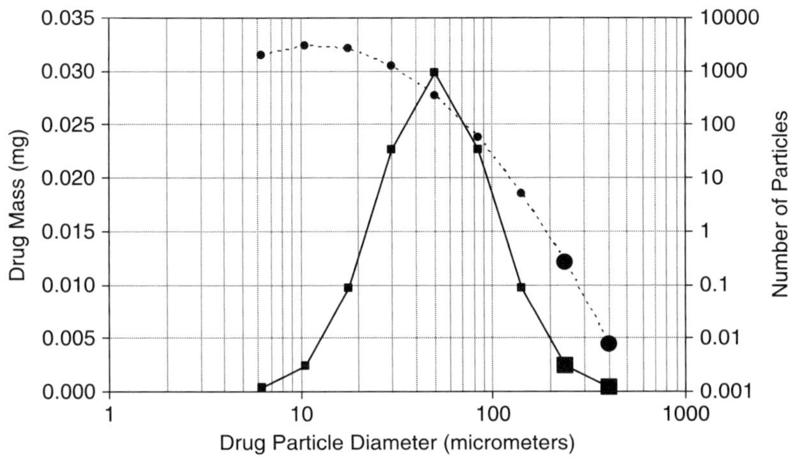

Figure 3.2 Drug particle size mass and number distribution normalized to a unit dose of 0.1 mg. Square symbols represent the mass distribution (left axis) and circular symbols represent the number distribution (right axis). The same data are also shown in Table 3.1.

drug, and that the drug has a particle size distribution as shown in Fig. 3.2. The particle size analysis was done using more drug than the unit dose of 0.1 mg but the particle size distribution shown in Fig. 3.2 has been normalized to the unit dose of 0.1 mg. The log–normal mass distribution represented by the bell-shaped profile (square symbols) utilizes the left vertical axis while the right vertical axis should be used to refer to the number of particles profile (round symbols). The same two profiles are also shown in tabular form in Table 3.1.

Commercially available particle size analyzers will typically report particle size data as mass distributions and assume that particle geometry is spherical. Particles that are similar in size will be grouped and represented by an average particle size for the range or the range may be specified. For the sake of space efficiency,

TABLE 3.1 Drug Particle Size Mass and Number Distribution for a 0.1 mg Dose

Particle Diameter (μm)	Mass Distribution (mg)	Number Distribution	Percentage of Dose for One Particle	Cumulative Percentage of Dose
6.25	0.000333	2000	0.000166	0.333
10.51	0.00238	3010	0.000790	2.71
17.68	0.00972	2580	0.00376	12.4
29.73	0.0226	1260	0.0179	35.0
50.00	0.0299	352	0.0851	65.0
84.09	0.0266	55.8	0.405	87.6
141.42	0.00972	5.05	1.93	97.3
237.84	0.00238	0.260	9.16	
400.00	0.000333	0.00763	43.6	

the particle size data given by Fig. 3.2 and Table 3.1 uses only nine particle size groups. In practice, more groups would be more realistic, but the use of fewer groups does not affect the explanation of the concept of ideal mixing.

The number distribution is derived naturally from the mass distribution. Knowing the drug particle diameter, the total mass of drug of that diameter, particle geometry, and the density of the drug, one can calculate the number of particles represented by each particle size group.[1,3] Because the mass distribution was normalized to the unit dose of 0.1 mg, the number distribution shown represents the number of particles in a unit dose.

Table 3.1 provides a guide for distributing particles of the same size evenly among the dosage forms in a given batch. For example, 2000 particles with a diameter of 6.25 μm should be added to each dosage form, 3010 particles with a diameter of 10.51 μm, and so forth. However, a dilemma is encountered when deciding how many 237.84 μm particles should be added. How can one add 0.260 particles to a unit dose? The answer is that one cannot. But by taking the reciprocal of the number of particles per unit dose for particle groups that have a number less than 1, the frequency of adding those particles to unit doses can be determined to evenly spread out the particles. For the 237.84 μm particles, the reciprocal of 0.260 is approximately 4, so that a 237.84 μm particle should be added every fourth unit dose. For the 400 μm particles, the reciprocal is approximately 131, so that a 400 μm particle should be added at intervals of 131 dosage forms. Following this pattern, at some point both a 237.84 and a 400 μm particle will be added to the same dosage form resulting in a super-potent dosage form.

What is the end result predicted by using the concept of ideal mixing? Automating the calculations by writing a computer algorithm,[1] Table 3.2 summarizes the simulation for 100,000 unit doses of the example given in Table 3.1.

Referring to Table 3.1, it should be noted that particles with a diameter of 141.42 μm and smaller can be added in whole numbers to all the dosage forms so that the minimum potency is 97.3% as reflected in both Tables 3.1 and 3.2. Adding a 237.84 μm particle to every fourth dosage form adds 9.16% for a total potency of 106.46%. Adding a 400 μm particle adds 43.6% of the intended dose to every 131 dosage forms for a total potency of 140.9%. However, 190 times out of 100,000, that 400 μm particle gets added to a dosage form that also has a 237.84 μm particle to yield a potency of 150.06%.

TABLE 3.2 Potency Distribution for a 0.1 mg Dose Simulated for 100,000 Unit Doses Using the Ideal Mixing Model and the Drug Particle Size Distribution in Fig. 3.2 and Table 3.1

Simulated Potency (Percentage of Intention)	Number of Dosage Forms with the Given Potency
97.3	74,427
106.46	24,810
140.9	573
150.06	190

As mentioned above, it should be noted that, in Table 3.2, the simulated potency values are not symmetrically distributed about the mean. There are "hot spots" of unusually high potency but no corresponding "cold spots." This skew toward high potency has been observed experimentally.[1,4]

The ability of the concept of ideal mixing to explain the observed skew reflects the strength of the approach. In converse, if one observes dosage forms of unusually low potency that cannot be explained by the concept of ideal mixing, or if poor content uniformity is observed that is not predicted by ideal mixing, then one can be fairly certain that the problem is incomplete mixing and not an unfavorable drug particle size. On the other hand, if one observes a higher frequency of potencies slightly below 100% of that intended, it might be an indication that the particle size distribution is not conducive to yielding good content uniformity and that hot spots might exist.

Perhaps the biggest danger in not routinely setting an appropriate drug particle size specification is that a problem may not be recognized and that some patient may eventually receive an overdose. Table 3.3 is a repeat of the simulation represented in Fig. 3.2 and Table 3.1. However, this time the number of particle size groups was increased from nine to 100 to be more realistic, and the total number of simulated dosage forms was increased from 100,000 to 200,000. Because of the increase in the number of particle size groups, the number of discrete potency values is too large to report. Instead, the number of doses in a particular range is reported in Table 3.3.

Only a small percentage of the doses fall outside the range that would trigger retesting or rejection of the lot. If only 10 dosage forms need to be tested initially,

TABLE 3.3 Potency Distribution of a 0.1 mg Dose Simulated for 200,000 Unit Doses Using the Ideal Mixing Model and a Similar Drug Particle Size Distribution to that in Fig. 3.2 and Table 3.1, Only with an Increase in the Number of Particle Size Groups to 100 from the Nine Shown

Potency Range (Percentage of Intention)	Number of Doses in Range	Percentage of Doses in Range
85–90	48,208	24.104
90–95	58,567	29.2835
95–98	13,335	6.6675
98–102	35,777	17.8885
102–105	5,725	2.8625
105–110	16,479	8.2395
110–115	9,245	4.6225
115–125	6,919	3.4595
125–150	5,240	2.62
150–175	429	0.2145
175–200	74	0.037
>200	2	0.001

and only a small percentage are problematic, then there is a good chance that the content uniformity problem will not be identified. From a safety point of view, this is a concern because some patient will eventually receive a dose that could be twice the nominal amount for the given example. If the drug has a narrow therapeutic window, the overdose could result in a serious adverse response from the patient. On the less dire side of possible events, the analyst could test a dosage form that would result in the rejection of the entire lot, or less severe side effects might reduce patient compliance.

On the positive side, setting a drug particle size specification somewhere below the edge of failure based on the concept of ideal mixing is straightforward, and controlling the drug particle size will eliminate the certain content uniformity problem that would result from using a drug particle size distribution that would never yield good content uniformity. Again, poor content uniformity can result from other causes, for example poor mixing, so that producing a drug with a particle size distribution conducive to good content uniformity does not guarantee that good content uniformity will result. However, once the particle size specification is met, the formulator can focus on determining a process that will yield good mixing and not be fooled by poor content uniformity unrelated to mixing.

3.3 IDEAL MIXING MODEL COMPARISON WITH THE YALKOWSKY AND BOLTON APPROACH

Another method for estimating the effect of particle size on content uniformity has been described by Yalkowsky and Bolton[2] and more recently updated by Rohrs et al.[4] The Yalkowsky and Bolton approach attempts to establish a particle size specification that would lead to a 99% chance of passing the USP Content Uniformity test. In this section, a comparison of their approach vs the ideal mixing model[1] will be made.

In the original presentation of the Yalkowsky and Bolton model,[2] no experimental results were given to validate the model. In the updated paper,[4] experiment data were provided, and particle size descriptors were changed to median diameter on a weight basis and geometric standard deviation, and content uniformity criteria were updated to current USP28/NF23 specifications. A graph is also included to provide an easy estimation of the upper limit for the particle size median diameter and geometric standard deviation over a range of doses that would lead to a high probability of passing content uniformity criteria.[4]

There are several significant differences between the Yalkowsky and Bolton[2] approach and the ideal mixing approach.[1] First, the Yalkowsky and Bolton approach assumes that the assayed values for the drug mass in a unit dose or potency will be normally distributed about the intended mean. In other words, the Yalkowsky and Bolton approach assumes that there is an equal likelihood of finding high or low potency values on either side of the mean. The ideal mixing model makes no assumptions about how the potency values are distributed, but allows them to follow naturally from the particle size distribution. Secondly, the Yalkowsky and Bolton approach assumes that the drug particle size distribution is described by a log–normal distribution. Although the log–normal distribution will be used in some simulations using the ideal mixing model, the ideal mixing model does not depend on the drug particle size distribution being of any particular form. The ideal mixing model could utilize experimental particle size data of any shape. The log–normal distribution will be used for convenience and for direct comparison to the Yalkowsky and Bolton approach, and not because the ideal mixing algorithm depends on it. Thirdly, the Yalkowsky and Bolton approach assumes that the number of drug particles in a unit dose sample obeys the Poisson distribution. Again, the ideal mixing model makes no such assumptions but lets the number of drug particles in a unit dose follow naturally from the drug particle size distribution, whatever that might be.

For comparison with the Yalkowsky and Bolton approach,[2] it is necessary to provide the ideal mixing model[1] with a particle size distribution representative of a unit dose. Because the Yalkowsky and Bolton approach assumes that the particle size is described by a log–normal distribution, simulated particle size data based on the log–normal function will be used by the ideal mixing model, although as stated above, this need not be the case. The log–normal function extends to infinity on either end of the mean, but this is not practical for milled drug powders that would have passed through some kind of opening of finite size. Calculations for setting the endpoints for the log–normal distribution have been reported[1,5] and will be used here. The author has extensive experience in measuring the particle size of milled drug from a variety of mills, including jet and hammer mills.[3,5] This experience has shown that a geometric standard deviation of 2 with endpoints calculated using an exponent of 3 for the geometric standard deviation in the following equations provides a reasonable representation of milled drug powders in general:

$$d_{\mathrm{max}} = d_{\mathrm{g}}\sigma_{\mathrm{g}}^{3} \tag{3.1}$$

$$d_{\mathrm{min}} = \frac{d_{\mathrm{g}}}{\sigma_{\mathrm{g}}^{3}} \tag{3.2}$$

where d_{max} is the maximum drug particle size diameter, d_{min} is the minimum drug particle size diameter, d_{g} is the geometric mean drug particle size, and σ_{g} is the geometric standard deviation.

As mentioned above, Rohrs et al.[4] provided a graph that gives the maximum volume median particle diameter predicted to pass the USP Stage I content uniformity criteria with 99% confidence as a function of dose and geometric standard deviation. This graph includes predictions for a geometric standard deviation of 2, and the corresponding dose and particle diameters taken from that graph are shown in Table 3.4. Also shown in Table 3.4 are the corresponding minimum and maximum diameters that were calculated from the median and Eqs. (3.1) and (3.2) above. Using the median particle diameter from Rohrs et al. and assuming the particle size distribution was log–normal with the minimum and maximum values as shown in Table 3.4, simulations were repeated using the ideal mixing model. This allows a comparison to be made of the Yalkowsky and Bolton approach[2] to the ideal mixing

TABLE 3.4 Maximum Volume Median Particle Diameter Predicted to Pass USP Stage I Content Uniformity Criteria with 99% Confidence for the Doses Listed and a Geometric Standard Deviation of 2 Taken from Figure 3.3 of Rohrs et al.[4] Also Shown are the Minimum and Maximum Particle Diameters Calculated for the Listed Maximum Median Diameters Using Eqs. (3.1) and (3.2)

Dose	Maximum Median Diameter	Minimum Particle Diameter	Maximum Particle Diameter
0.001	6.9	0.8625	55.2
0.01	14.8	1.85	118.4
0.1	31.9	3.9875	255.2
1	68.7	8.5875	549.6
10	148	18.5	1184

model[1] at a geometric standard deviation of 2. The results of the ideal mixing approach are summarized in Table 3.5.

Table 3.5 shows the predicted distribution of potencies based the ideal mixing model[1] using the maximum volume median particle diameter predicted to pass USP Stage I content uniformity criteria with 99% confidence for a geometric standard deviation of 2, as reported in figure 3 from Rohrs et al.[4] The ideal mixing model predicts that only about 1% of the dosage forms would be above 115% of intended value. However, it also predicts a significant number of dosage forms would be above 125%; significant from the point of view that those dosage forms would be released and eventually taken by a patient. It is important to remember that both the Yalkowsky and Bolton approach[2] and the ideal mixing model do not include the real-life error resulting from nonideal mixing, that both predictions represent the best case scenario, and that the real frequency of higher potencies could be greater than predicted.

TABLE 3.5 Predicted Potency Distributions Using the Ideal Mixing Model and the Maximum Volume Median Particle Diameters and Particle Distribution Minimum and Maximum Diameters from Table 3.4 and a Geometric Standard Deviation of 2

	Number of Units Out of 100,000 in the Given Potency Range for the Indicated Dose				
Potency Range (%)	0.001 mg	0.01 mg	0.1 mg	1 mg	10 mg
95–98	48,764	44,581	44,540	44,644	44,581
98–102	33,689	36,448	36,492	36,583	36,448
102–105	8,470	9,896	9,734	9,783	9,896
105–110	5,137	6,283	6,326	6,090	6,283
110–115	2,410	2,090	2,296	2,132	2,090
115–125	1,244	624	597	674	624
125–150	286	78	15	94	78

TABLE 3.6 Predicted Potency Distributions Using the Ideal Mixing Model for Progressively Smaller Mean Drug Particle Diameters and a Geometric Standard Deviation of 2

	Number of Units Out of 100,000 in the Given Potency Range for the Indicated Mean Particle Size in Micrometers				
Potency Range (%)	31.9	25	20	15	10
95–98	44,540	38,750	26,320	0	0
98–102	36,492	42,628	59,899	93,321	100,000
102–105	9,734	13,560	10,388	6,470	0
105–110	6,326	4,480	3,292	209	0
110–115	2,296	560	101	0	0
115–125	597	22	0	0	0
125–150	15	0	0	0	0

Table 3.6 singles out the 0.1 mg dose from Table 3.5 and repeats the ideal mixing model[1] simulations starting with the maximum diameter of Rohrs et al.[4] of 31.9 μm and including progressively smaller median diameters while keeping the geometric standard deviation constant at 2 and using Eqs. (3.1) and (3.2) to calculate the particle size distribution end points. Table 3.6 is intended to show how the ideal mixing model could be used to decide on a particle size specification as a tradeoff between reducing particle size vs the added benefit of decreasing the occurrence of high-potency dosage forms.

3.4 EXPERIMENTAL SUPPORT OF MODEL ASSUMPTIONS

The original report of the Yalkowsky and Bolton approach[2] did not provide any experimental support of their assumption that the content uniformity data would be normally distributed. The ideal mixing model[1] predicts that the distribution should be skewed toward higher potencies and this prediction was confirmed experimentally.[1] When Rohrs et al.[4] updated the Yalkowsky and Bolton approach, they generated experimental data and compared the predictions with their experimental data. Their data also showed an increasing skewness toward high potencies with decreasing dose while holding drug particle size constant.[4] This behavior is predicted by the ideal mixing model but not the Yalkowsky and Bolton approach. For the lowest strength made by Rohrs et al., one tablet had a potency of 160% of intent and another of 292% of intended value out of a total of 30 tablets assayed. For the next to lowest strength of tablets made, one tablet had a potency of 139% of intended value. Neither of the highest observed potency values for the two batches was predicted by the Yalkowsky and Bolton approach. However, simulations using the ideal mixing model with the experimentally reported median particle diameters and a geometric standard deviation of 2 did, as shown in Table 3.7.

TABLE 3.7 Predicted Potency Distributions Using the Ideal Mixing Model, a Geometric Standard Deviation of 2, and Experimental Doses and Corresponding Particle Diameters Reported by Rohrs et al.[4]

Potency Range (%)	1.3 μg Dose 29 μm Mean Particle Size	3.6 μg Dose 22 μm Mean Particle Size
0–75	27,472	0
75–85	21,359	19,484
85–90	8,863	16,367
90–95	4,313	25,853
95–98	7,763	3,744
98–102	2,552	7,033
102–105	3,804	5,957
105–110	2,988	4,554
110–115	3,132	5,369
115–125	5,224	5,613
125–150	6,510	4,689
150–175	2,324	867
175–200	1,131	346
>200	2,565	124

The particle size analysis of Rohrs et al. also showed that a geometric standard deviation of 2 gives a reasonable characterization of the distribution in the larger particle size region.

The frequency of the high-potency dosage forms observed by Rohrs et al.[4] is roughly the same magnitude as predicted by the ideal mixing model shown in Table 3.7, although the actual data have gaps. However, the experimental data of Zhang and Johnson[1] showed a higher frequency of high-potency units compared to the ideal mixing prediction. There could be several reasons why the data of Rohrs et al. agree better with the prediction of the ideal mixing model than that of Zhang and Johnson. It could be that the mixing achieved by Rohrs et al. was more ideal than that of Zhang and Johnson. Because of the personal observation by the author that real mixing was likely far less than ideal, and because of the limited amount of data available for analysis to provide more confidence in how closely real mixing approaches ideal mixing, the author would again recommend caution in setting particle size specifications close to the edge of failure.

Another piece of evidence to suggest that content uniformity data is not normally distributed can also be seen in the content uniformity data of Rohrs et al.[4] They report the content uniformity assay results for 11 batches of tablets. In every case except one, the actual mean potency is below the target value. If the content uniformity data were normally distributed, as assumed by the Yalkowsky and Bolton approach,[2] one might expect to see a more even distribution of mean values above and below the target. The one exception was for the lowest potency batch for which one tablet was assayed to be 292% of intented value, as mentioned above. This characteristic is more consistent with the ideal mixing model,[1] which would predict an average potency below the mean when the sample size is relatively low compared to the batch size due to the more numerous occurrences of dosage forms below 100% of intented value (see Tables 3.2, 3.3, 3.5–3.7).

Given that a commercial batch size of dosage forms could be in the range of 100,000–1,000,000 and that only 10 dosage forms need to be tested to release the batch, it is unlikely that the required testing will identify problems with content uniformity. Because it would be prohibitively costly and time-consuming to test enough dosage forms to adequately characterize a commercial batch, it would be better to apply either the Yalkowsky and Bolton approach[2] or the ideal mixing model[1] to design quality into the dosage form. Setting a rational particle size drug specification reduces development time by reducing one of the causes of poor content uniformity, increases the chances of passing the USP content uniformity test, and most importantly, increases the quality and safety of the finished dosage form.

From a safety and quality point of view, the ideal mixing model[1] is better than the Yalkowsky and Bolton approach[2] at describing the potential danger of unusually high potency dosage forms and can simulate the experimentally observed skew in content uniformity data toward higher potencies. And although the graph of Rohrs et al.[4] provides a quick and easy way of identifying a particle size specification, the author believes that being able to simulate content uniformity data through the use of a computer program based on the ideal mixing model provides a better method to understand and appreciate the effect of drug particle size on content uniformity. The ideal mixing model also has fewer assumptions that allow it to be applied to real drug particle size distributions that might not be described by a log–normal function.

3.5 ANALYTICAL AND PRACTICAL CONSIDERATIONS

Although an in-depth discussion of particle size analysis is beyond the scope of this chapter, some general comments are worthwhile. From the discussion of the ideal mixing model, it should be obvious that large drug particles, ones that represent a significant percentage of the dose, will cause poor content uniformity. It should also be noted that, because they could occur less frequently than once per unit dose, the analytical particle characterization technique might have to characterize more particles than would be found in a single dose to identify the problem. For example, if the offending particle only occurred once in every 100 dosage forms and the dose was 0.1 mg, then 10 mg of drug would have to be looked at on average to identify the problem. This could be a daunting task, and not all particle characterization instruments provide the necessary information. At the risk of being redundant, it would be much better to use one of the methods described in this chapter to determine a particle size distribution conducive to good content uniformity, choose a mill that experience has taught will likely provide the desired distribution, and only then use the particle size instrument to confirm that the particle size distribution is conducive. Keeping a database on mills, milling conditions, and the resulting particle size would be a good approach in selecting the best mill for the job.

Both the Yalkowsky and Bolton approach[2] and the ideal mixing model[1] teach that reducing the geometric standard deviation or "spread" of the distribution will lead to better content uniformity. Reducing the spread can even allow a larger mean drug particle size that will yield good content uniformity. This is because the mean and the spread together determine the upper range of the particle size distribution where the offending particles will be found. Removing just the offending particles by passing the drug through a wire mesh screen will be effective, although screening may not be a popular technique. Personal experience has shown that some drugs can be screened very easily while others cannot. Fortunately, the problem addressed in this chapter is most pertinent to low-dose drugs, and therefore, the amount of drug that needs to be milled or screened is relatively small. Any method that would remove just the large offending drug particles might also be advantageous because any method that reduces the size of all particles might generate extremely fine drug particles that can cause formulation problems of their own.

REFERENCES

1. Zhang Y, Johnson KC. 1997. Effect of drug particle size on content uniformity of low-dose solid dosage forms. Int. J. Pharm. 154: 179–183.
2. Yalkowsky SH, Bolton S. 1990. Particle size and content uniformity. Pharm. Res. 7(9): 962–966.
3. Hintz RJ, Johnson KC. 1989. The effect of particle size distribution on dissolution rate and oral absorption. Int. J. Pharm. 51: 9–17.
4. Rohrs BR, Amidon GE, Meury RH, Secreast PJ, King HM, Skoug CJ. 2006. Particle size limits to meet USP content uniformity criteria for tablets and capsules. J. Pharm. Sci. 95(5): 1049–1059.
5. Lu ATK, Frisella ME, Johnson KC. 1993. Dissolution modeling: factors affecting the dissolution rates of polydisperse powders. Pharm. Res. 10(9): 1308–1314.

CHAPTER 4

DEVELOPMENT OF LOW-DOSE FORMULATIONS USING FLUIDIZED BED GRANULATION

J. JOE ZHOU
Engineering Technology Center, Eli Lilly and Company, Indianapolis, IN 40285

RALPH LIPP
Pharmaceutical Sciences R&D, Lilly Research Laboratories, Eli Lilly and Company, Indianapolis, IN 40285

4.1 INTRODUCTION

Granulation is a physical process where small particles are combined to form larger particle agglomerates. These agglomerates must be strong enough to withstand substantial processing. The original particle identity is retained in the agglomerates. The reasons for granulation in pharmaceutical industry can be summarized as follows:

- improved material flowability—both flow rate and flow consistency may be favorably impacted, enabling more accurate control of dose weights;
- improved dose uniformity—when the desired dose is low, necessitating high dilution of the API, very fine particle sizes of API must be used and the creation of ordered mixes reduces the likelihood for segregation to occur; granulation produces uniform blends that do not easily segregate;
- improved compressibility—uniform incorporation of compressible components on the surface of less compressible API and excipients can improve inherent compressibility;
- increased density for shipping and storage;

Formulation and Analytical Development for Low-Dose Oral Drug Products. Edited by Jack Zheng

- improved wetting and *in vivo* dispersion—poorly water-soluble, hydrophobic materials may be granulated with hydrophilic materials to significantly improve wetting and *in vivo* dispersion;
- improved control of physical properties (dissolution rate, compression, porosity, surface:volume ratio);
- reduced dust loss and dust handling hazards;
- improved appearance;
- prevention of caking and lump formation.

Two types of granulators are widely used in pharmaceutical industry: high-shear granulators and fluidized bed granulators. High-shear granulation usually increases the bulk density of the material while fluidized bed granulation usually results in more porous, less dense material. Bulk density may impact material flow and segregation properties.

This chapter focuses on the use of fluidized bed granulation process in the development and preparation of low-dose granule formulations for further conversion to immediate release tablets for personal administration. As a reference document, the chapter does not cover some very common subjects such as process safety, material characterization techniques and basic process and instrumentation technologies. Because the authors' intention is to relate their experience in this specialized area, these areas are not discussed in any depth; however their omission does not reduce their importance.

The main advantage of a fluidized bed granulator is that it does preblending, granulation, and drying in a single piece of equipment. Samples can be easily obtained for analysis at any stage. It is also a mild process that produces granules with high porosity and narrow granule size distribution.

A fluidized bed is formed when a quantity of solid particulates is forced to behave as a fluid and is usually induced by the introduction of pressurized gas such as N_2 or air through a gas distributor. This results in particles with many of the properties and characteristics of normal fluids, including the ability to free-flow under gravity, or to be pumped using fluid-type technologies. The resulting phenomenon is called *fluidization*. In addition to granulation, fluidized beds are also widely used for drying and coating processes. Typically, pressurized gas enters the fluidized bed vessel through a distributor plate at the bottom of the fluidized bed. The gas flows upward through the bed, causing the solid particles to be suspended. When a stream of gas passes upward through the particles at a rate great enough to set them in motion, an expanded bed is formed. At this point, the frictional force between a particle and fluidization gas equals the weight of the particles. A few particles will visibly vibrate and move about in restricted regions. This process can also take place at elevated temperatures. Since granulation in pharmaceutical industry processes organic powders, there is a potential risk of dust explosion. Precautions must be taken against producing explosive vapors when using with this process.

In a general sense, single dosage forms with drug content of no more than 1 mg are considered to be low dose. Dosages below 100 μg per single dose are considered ultralow-dose and represent a real challenge to fluidized bed manufacturing operations. However, a real challenge of low-dose formulations lies in the ultralow-dose range at or below 100 μg, for example, ranging from 20 to 100 μg per single dose. The following considerations and comments focus on this demanding subset of low-dose formulations. Nevertheless, the formulations and processes being developed for this ultralow-dose range will, in practice, work for the remaining range of the low-dose formulation as well. The following considerations and comments focus on this demanding subset of low-dose formulations.

From a practical perspective, the nominal dose of the drug substance needs to be set into relation to the mass of a resulting final dosage form in order to better understand the particular boundary conditions of low-dose formulations in general. The dose is to be converted into a drug load factor, which is more meaningful to the formulator. The conversion itself is straightforward since one simply has to set the dose of the drug in relation to the desired tablet core weight. Large tablets usually require higher tablet weights and thus increase the dilution of the active pharmaceutical ingredient, which in turn increases the formulation challenge. Hence, the focus on small tablets.

However, the minimum size is also set by the patient's compliance. Tablets below a certain size are considered undesirable because of increased handling issues for

TABLE 4.1 Potential Formulation and FBG Process Risks and Challenges Triggered by Various Drug Loads

Drug Load Challenge/Risk	Ultra Low <0.2%	Low 0.3–1%	Mid 2–30%	High >30%
Homogeneity of blend	Severe challenge	Challenge	Moderate challenge	No challenge
Content uniformity of single unit dosage form	Severe challenge	Challenge	Moderate challenge	No challenge
Loss of activity during granulation	Very high risk	High risk	Moderate risk	Low risk
Chemical stability of API in formulated tablet[a]	High risk	Moderate risk	Low risk	Low risk
Tableting behavior	Mainly dependent on excipient selection	Mainly dependent on excipient selection	Potential problems depending on API	Potentially severe problems depending on API

[a]Stability of API in formulation depends on intrinsic stability of API and formulation as well as packaging characteristics. However, drug substances prone to degradation typically show higher relative loss on content in diluted (low drug load) formulations than in high drug load formulations.

patients. For any round biplanar or biconvex tablet this translates into a core of typically 5 or 6 mm in diameter as the lower limit. Considering standard height vs diameter ratios and typical densities of standard tablets, those diameters convert into minimal core weights of approximately 50–80 mg per tablet.[1] Simple division of the aforementioned low-dose example of a 20 μg drug substance by a theoretical tablet core weight of 50 mg leads to a drug load of 0.04%. Our discussion therefore focuses on formulations less than 100 μg drug substance or a 0.2% drug load, which are the more challenging in nature. Once drug loads significantly exceed 0.2%, the challenges of low-dose formulations decrease for a variety of reasons (see Table 4.1).

Pharmaceutical products such as tablets usually consist of active pharmaceutical ingredients. In the pharmaceutical industry, the API particle size has tended to become smaller in recent years and the needle shape has become very common. These small API particles usually belong to Group C according Geldart classification.[2,3] It is well known that the needle-shaped Group C particles are very cohesive. They do not flow easily and mix poorly with other particles.

4.2 GRANULATION FUNDAMENTALS

To help readers better understand our approach, some basic principles of granulation and fluidization are briefly introduced.

Granulation is an operation designed to create small grains or pellets from small particles, which are gathered into larger, permanent masses in which the original particles can still be identified. The granulation operation is a process intended to produce controlled growth of particles to form a uniform shape. The process utilizes dry powder materials and a liquid, the granulation solution. Binders may be dissolved in the granulation solution or incorporated into the dry powder blend. Agglomerates are formed by combining dry ingredients (powders and perhaps crystals) and granulation fluid, mixing to achieve uniform distribution of the granulation solution over the surface of the dry ingredients and allowing particle–particle interactions. This is a physical phenomenon.

4.2.1 Inter-Particle Forces

The inter-particle forces are responsible for the formation of stable granules. Below is the list of inter-particle forces:

- *Van der Waals forces.* This is the collection of all solids' molecularly based attractive forces. The range of van der Waals forces is usually wide compared to that of chemical bonds.
- *Surface tension.* Surface tension represents the attractive property of a liquid for itself, which results from the cohesive forces generated between neighboring molecules of the liquid. These forces are generally stronger than the attractive

force between the liquid molecules and the atmosphere. Due to differences in the magnitude of these forces, liquids do not spontaneously disintegrate into the vapor state unless energy is imparted to the material (as in the form of heat). Surface tension is the force that is responsible for the droplet formation.

- *Interfacial tension*. Interfacial tension is the forces generated at the interface changes as the composition of the materials at that interface changes. If the granulating solution and the powder mixture have compatible chemistries, it is possible for the liquid and the solid particles to generate sufficient attractive forces to allow the solution to wet the solid surface. The liquid–solid interface is not restricted to the exterior of the particle. If the attractive forces between the solid particle and the solution are great enough, the solution may be drawn into the pores of the solid and further strengthen the liquid bridge.
- *Electrostatic forces*. Particles may acquire electrostatic charge during particle–particle collision and frequent rubbing of particles against equipment surfaces. Charging characteristics of particles are affected by many physiochemical factors such as particle size, size distribution, density, morphology, hygroscopicity and energy level, and operational environmental conditions such as relative humidity and temperature.
- *Liquid bridge forces*. When the granulation solution wets the surface of the dry ingredients it forms liquid bridges, which contact, and adhere to, the surface of particles of the API–excipient mixture to produce agglomerates of particles. As a result of surface and interfacial tensions, these agglomerates have the strength to withstand the effects of the particle–particle collisions. The primary force responsible for the initiation of the agglomerative process is liquid bridge formation between particles. The net result of these various forces acting in concert is the formation of particle–particle liquid bridges that are able to withstand attrition on further mixing and ultimately provide a nucleolus from which permanent agglomeration may be affected. The mechanics of wet granulation is very much dependent upon the surface area and surface properties available for the interaction.
- *Solid bridge forces*. When a wet particle collides with another particle in the fluid bed a liquid bridge appears between the two particles. When subsequent drying occurs, the solvent evaporates and a solid bridge arises due to the solidification of the binder material. Solid bridge is the most important force holding dried solids together to form stable granules.

4.2.2 Granulation Mechanism

Newitt and Conway-Jones[4] found that there are four types of liquid state of granules depending on the liquid content in the granules. These states are known as pendular, funicular, capillary and droplet.

In the *pendular state*, the particles have been exposed to sufficient granulating solution for liquid bridges to begin to form. Since the pendular state is characterized by a small value of the liquid saturation factor, the total volume of liquid bridges is limited and the resulting granules are fairly friable. This granulation would likely be described as "too dry" by an experienced granulator.

As moisture content increases, surface coverage by the granulation liquid also increases in the *funicular state*. The liquid bridges joining adjacent particles are interspersed less frequently by air. Since larger percentages of the total particle surface area are participating in the agglomerative process, these agglomerates are characterized by greater strength than agglomerates formed in the pendular state.

Further addition of granulation liquid leads to essentially complete liquid coverage of the solid-phase surface. This is the *capillary state*. Resulting from even greater percentages of the total particle surface area in the liquid bridge formation, agglomerates in this phase are characterized by good strength and demonstrate minimal attrition on further processing.

Continued addition of granulation liquid leads to complete wetting of the entire solid surface. Any liquid added beyond this point has no possibility of adhering to the solid surface and becomes associated with the part of the liquid film that is covering the surface of the particles in the granulator. For wet granulation, it is generally understood that the formation of granules goes through three process steps, that is wetting/nucleation, growth/consolidation, and breakage.

Before preblended solids are wetted, the solids surface is in contact with air. The wetting process involves replacing the contacting air with the granulation suspension. This is an important step since it is critical for the formation of the liquid bridge(s). Wetting is necessary for nucleation, a step to form small granules or a nucleus by combining primary solids particles. Wetting of solids surface is impacted by the surface tension of liquid and the contact angle it forms on the surface of particle material. Generally speaking, good wetability makes granulation process easier to control and operate.

The coalescence of the nucleus provides the initial growth of granules. The granules will then consolidate to form bigger granules. Granule density increases during consolidation. Liquid saturation is an important factor affecting granule growth. The extent of consolidation depends on formulation and process variables.

Granule breakage also takes place during granulation process. Granule breakup and attrition during granule–granule collision and granule–equipment wall impact are responsible for granule breakage. Granule attrition is usually undesirable since it generates dusts. For granulation process, granule size and its distribution are controlled by managing granule growth and breakage.

4.3 THEORY OF FLUIDIZATION

4.3.1 Fluidization Fundamentals

As discussed earlier, fluidized bed granulators normally operate in a bubbling bed regime. The operating superficial gas velocity is above the minimum fluidization velocity and below the onset velocity for a turbulent bed. The preferred method for determining minimum fluidization velocity, u_{mf}, is to make a plot of pressure drop across the bed of particles vs superficial gas velocity. The minimum fluidization velocity can be obtained as superficial gas velocity corresponds to the join point between two nearly linear lines. Based on the work by Wen and Yu,[5] the minimum fluidization velocity can be calculated by the following set of equations:

$$Re_{mf} = \sqrt{C_1^2 + C_2 Ar} - C_1 \tag{4.1}$$

where

$$Re_{mf} = \frac{\bar{d}_p u_{mf} \rho_g}{\mu_g} \tag{4.2}$$

and

$$Ar = \frac{\rho_g(\rho_p - \rho_g) g \bar{d}_p^3}{\mu_g^2} \tag{4.3}$$

with ρ_p and ρ_g being the particle and gas density, μ_g the gas shear viscosity, g the acceleration due to gravity, and $\bar{d}_p$ the mean particle diameter. Values for constants C_1 and C_2 for minimum fluidization correlation are recommended to be 27.1 and 0.0408 by Grace.[6]

Based on the study on pressure fluctuation and the change in bubble size, Yerushalmi and Cankurt[7] proposed that the onset velocity to start the transition from bubbling bed to turbulent regime can be calculated as

$$u_c = 3\sqrt{\rho_p \bar{d}_p} - 0.17 \tag{4.4}$$

The minimum bubbling velocity is usually greater than the minimum fluidization velocity. Therefore, the fluidized bed dryer should be operated at superficial gas velocity that is greater than the minimum fluidization velocity, u_{mf}, but less than the onset velocity to turbulent regime, u_c.

It is worth noting that not every particle can be easily fluidized. Geldart[2] introduced a classification scheme to show that different fluidization behaviors of particles belong in groups A, B, C, or D depending primarily on particle size and particle density. Most feed particles to a fluidized bed granulator are usually group A, but sometimes there are also group C powders. Group A particles usually have a mean particle diameter between 30 and 120 μm for pharmaceutical powders, and are "aeratable." They are fluidized easily. Group C materials, on the other hand, are "cohesive." They are very fine powders, usually below 30 μm. It is very difficult to fluidize group C particles in a fluidized bed without other assistance. Obviously, it is very important to make sure the granulation materials are group A particles to ensure a good fluidization for fluidized bed granulation.

4.3.2 Fluidized Bed Granulation System

Figure 4.1 shows a top-spray fluidized bed granulator. It is usually made from stainless steel. For fluidized bed granulation, before granulation suspension spray starts, API and excipient particles are dry-blended through fluidization. Top-spray fluidized bed granulators are usually operated in a bubbling bed regime, which requires the superficial gas velocity to be higher than the minimum fluidization velocity and below the velocity to reach the turbulent regime. In a bubbling bed regime, gas velocity is usually high enough to provide good gas–solid heat and mass transfer as well as good mixing between API and excipient particles. Meanwhile, since the gas velocity is below the transition velocity to turbulent flow, the solid entrainment rate is greatly reduced. This improves solids mixing as well.

Fluidized bed granulators (FBG) are usually run as batch operations in the pharmaceutical industry. As shown in Fig. 4.2, the FBG system includes an air handling system, fluidized bed granulator HEPA filters and an induced fan. The air handling system controls the moisture and temperature of fluidization air into the FBG. It is usually equipped with humidity control, filtering, and heating components. In addition to filters inside the FBG, a HEPA filter is used to further remove particulates from the exhaust gas before it is goes to a blower, which provides the fluidization gas to the FBG.

The fluidized bed granulator consists of a gas plenum, which is the receiver for inlet fluidization air, a gas distributor, a product container, an expanded chamber, a set of

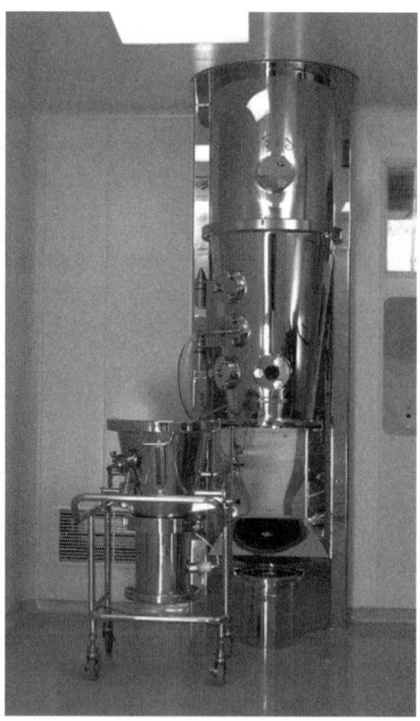

Figure 4.1 Top spray fluidized bed granulator.

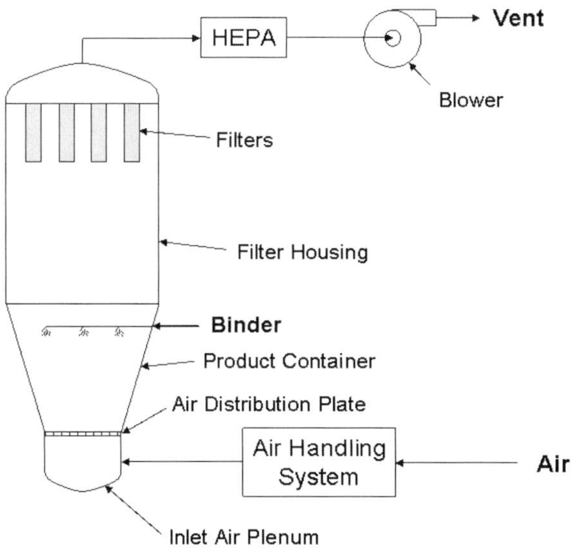

Figure 4.2 Schematic of fluidized bed granulaton system.

filter bags in the expansion chamber, and a binder spray system. There are many types of air distribution plates used by different equipment manufacturers. The main purpose of the plate is to distribute gas uniformly across the product bed. The factors considered for the plate design for pharmaceutical industry fluidized bed granulators include pressure drop across the plate, jet velocity to avoid excessive attrition, elimination of dead area, and mechanical integrity. To achieve a good fluidization, as a rule of thumb, the ratio of the pressure drop across the plate, Δp_{plenum}, to differential pressure across the product bed, Δp_{bed}, should be around 0.2–0.3. For fluidized bed granulators, there are usually several plates with different amounts of opening available. The selection of the plates should depend on the particle properties and the loading of products.

A cone-shaped container is usually employed to hold product materials. Compared to a cylinder-shaped product bed, for a conical-shaped product bed, the change in bed height is not as significant when the material loading changes. The advantage of the cone shape is that it provides better turn-down ratio compared to a straight-wall cylindrical container. During granulation, particles grow bigger and heavier. The expansion of a conical-shaped bed experiences fewer changes for the same reason. Observation windows are usually provided to monitor the movement of product bed solids. The bed surface during granulation is usually below the expansion chamber.

Granulation binder spray guns are placed above the product bed. They usually consist of several spray nozzles. Dual flow nozzles are widely used to atomize granulation binder before it reaches the solids bed. A good atomization is very important for granulation operation. The nozzles should also provide uniform spray across the bed surface.

In the expansion chamber, the superficial gas velocity is lower compared to that in the product bed. Particles entrained by the fluidization air slow down and return to the product bed. This reduces the solids entrainment rate significantly. Filter bags in the expansion chamber separate entrained solids from the exhaust air, which is further cleaned by a HEPA filter. The induced fan is generally used to perform the granulation under minor negative pressure to the atmosphere to prevent solids leaking out of granulators.

4.4 FORMULATION DEVELOPMENT

This chapter will familiarize the reader with the basic principles of how to develop low drug load formulations using fluidized bed granulation. While the practical development of those drugs aims at an integration of formulation development and pharmaceutical process development in order to achieve optimal results, the two areas have been separated within this chapter to provide the reader with information in a highly focused manner. However, in order not to oversimplify the depiction of what typically is a highly integrated development process, cross-references have been made between the formulation development and process development section in order to highlight the interdependencies between both areas.

One of the most intriguing tasks in drug development is the design of formulations. The scientist active in this area has to develop the drug with the end in mind which encompasses several aspects from the areas of quality, safety and efficiency as well as cost of goods. The development should be planned in a reverse-engineering fashion providing answers to the following questions:

- With the patient in mind, what are the desired *performance characteristics of the drug*? This question aims at topics like required dose as well as onset and duration of action of the medication, thus leading to the desired release profile of the active pharmaceutical ingredient. The conceptual development process needs to bridge chemical and physical product characteristics, pharmacokinetic performance and pharmacodynamic results. Combining information from all of the aforementioned areas, the formulator might consider various dosage forms. However, for the sake of clarity, this chapter focuses on immediate release low-dose formulations only.
- Which *quality attributes* need to be built into the dosage form? Dose accuracy, content uniformity, purity and stability are aspects to be evaluated, all of which are of particular interest to the scientist developing low-dose formulations.
- How can the *manufacturing process be designed for the dosage form* in order to achieve the desired attributes mentioned above in a reliable, robust, efficient, safe—from an integrated environment health and safety perspective—and cost-effective manner? When developing low-dose formulations this requires an insightful comparison of various manufacturing processes and unit operations.
- How can you *select excipients* which enable the design of robust and performing formulations and processes? The fundamental principles which apply to all

formulation aspects apply in the case of low-dose FBG formulations as well, thus specifically compatibility with the active and manufacturability has to be taken into consideration.

- How do you *design the physical properties of the API*? For the development of low-dose formulations, the design of the solid-state form of the drug substance is of utmost importance. Careful selection of a suitable salt form, co-crystal or clathrate (if applicable), crystal modification, habit, particle size and particle size distribution is of utmost importance.

Whilst planning the various steps of developing an FBG-based low-dose formulation largely benefits from applying the reverse-engineering conceptual development process, it also is in line with the currently emerging quality-by-design paradigm,[8] as outlined in the ICHQ8 guideline.[9] The actual drug development will be carried out in the sequence API definition, excipient selection and design of the manufacturing process, with the appropriate feedback loops included.

4.4.1 Physical Property Design of the Active Pharmaceutical Ingredient

In general, the selection of a suitable salt[10] or co-crystal[11] is mainly driven by biopharmaceutical and stability considerations. Where several modifications exist, the selection of the most suitable for formulation purposes is a general formulation issue as well.[12]

For low drug load formulations, however, content uniformity of the resulting single unit dosage forms is of particular relevance and comes with stringent requirements in the area of particle size and particle size distribution.[13,14] One of the major factors controlling the degree of homogeneity is the particle size distribution of the API. A high-level guide of how to achieve a coefficient of variation of not greater than 1% for drug content per tablet made from random, homogeneous mixtures was given by Johnson.[15] The particle size distribution of the API should contain no more than 20% of particles above the "limiting particle size" for this drug load and the maximum particle size within the distribution should not be greater than three times the "limiting particle size." The "limiting particle size" in dependence of the drug load level was calculated based on theoretical considerations. However, it should be noted that experimental potency data might not be as good as simulated potency data.[16]

Emphasis has also been placed on the particle size distribution and the uniform size distribution of the API rather than on the mean particle size alone by other authors.[14,16] Rohrs et al.[16] give a nomograph for identifying the maximum median particle diameter to pass USP 28 stage I content uniformity criteria with 99% confidence as a function of dose as well as width of particle size distribution (geometrical standard deviation).

In addition to the particle size of the API, the genesis of the material is of importance. Typically, the final step of the API preparation is a milling or micronization process, which determines physical properties like cohesiveness and the tendency to form agglomerates. These play an important role in the achievable content uniformity.[14,17,18] For formulations with a drug load below 0.1% or below 100 μg per dose, it has been reported that these phenomena become even more important than particle size distribution.[18]

Therefore, it has been concluded that the rate-limiting step in achieving the required homogeneity is the API particle randomization when using particles smaller than a critical size and hence the breakdown of the API agglomerates for particles below the critical particle size.[18] This means that the quality of blend and content uniformity for small amounts of micronized, cohesive API particles strongly depends on the success in de-agglomeration rather than on the mixing efforts.

Ultralow-dose formulations thus typically require micronized drug substances[19] with particle sizes (d_{50}) of approximately 3–5 μm. Those small particle sizes typically translate into very high specific surface areas of the related drug substance, for example approximately 10–20 m^2/g (Brunauer–Emmett–Teller method, BET). Whilst the use of micronized drug particles is highly beneficial from a content uniformity point of view, the significantly enlarged specific surface area of those drug substances often exacerbates potential chemical degradation issues of the molecule. This issue is further amplified by the fact that, even if degradation products are formed at a low absolute level, they might amount to a rather high relative level compared to the target dose, which is problematic from a purity and stability perspective.[20]

One other drawback of the utilization of micronized API in the context of fluidized bed granulation is the potential to lose a material fraction into the filters of the equipment due to the fact that smaller particles demand lower suspension velocities than large ones. More specifically, the potential loss of drug substance via the air current according to Eq. (4.1) is determined by the fact that the air current which is applied to suspend a particle is proportional to the square root of its diameter:[21]

$$u_{g,\max} \approx \sqrt{\frac{4d_p \cdot \rho_p \cdot g}{3\rho_g}} \tag{4.5}$$

where $u_{g,\max}$ is the suspension velocity, d_p is the particle size, ρ_p is particle density, ρ_g is gas density, and g is the gravitation constant.

Additionally, the enlarged surface area leads to a high electrostatic charge of the small particles. Whereas this charge might be advantageous in stabilizing blends by adhesion of the active particles to granule excipients, the charged material tends to stick to metal surfaces. This induces an unwanted loss of material in the granulator wall, where the adhesive forces form a material film on the surface. Especially in campaign production, this might lead to unwanted changes in the assay values from batch to batch.

Finally, given the fact that pharmaceutical excipients employed in low-dose formulations normally exhibit larger particle sizes[22] than the API, segregation of the finer API from the excipients after a successful initial blending might be an unwanted result. If the particle size chosen is very small, this process is pronounced and might jeopardize all efforts in the prior granulation processes.

These production issues, introduced by an extremely reduced drug substance particle size (typical d_{50} values ranging from 2 to 10 μm), can be tackled by a sophisticated granulation process strategy. One measure is to start the FBG process with a rather wet initial granulation phase (see below). Following these important guiding principles will lead to a robust process resulting in a drug product with 100% of the targeted assay value without the need for the application of any overages for potential process losses.

One rarely used but powerful means of maximizing both content uniformity (as mentioned above) and stability aspects of low-dose pharmaceuticals is the formation of inclusion complexes to increase both the drug load in the formulation as well as the stability of the API. One specific example is the complexation of ethinyl estradiol in the form of its β-cyclodextrin clathrate for use in pharmaceutical formulations.[23] This inclusion complex has been successfully applied in the development of an ultralow-dose formulation of this steroid.[24]

The aforementioned explanations of the design of physical characteristics of the API are obviously only of relevance as long as the FBG process is utilizing solid API without any dissolution step. While this holds true for most of the processes used today to manufacture low-dose drugs via FBG, some processes include a dissolution step for the drug [e.g., in (hydro-)alcoholic systems]. This method yields excellent blend uniformity results, but requires special precautions as all the equipment has to be installed in an explosion-proof manner. Additionally, due to environmental protection restrictions, exhaust air handling might be mandatory associated with supportive technical equipment and hence enhanced costs. Furthermore, the dissolving and subsequent precipitation during the manufacturing process increases the risk of yielding an unwanted polymorphic form with undesired properties such as limited stability or reduced dissolution characteristics.

4.4.2 Excipient Selection

Once the target dose of the active pharmaceutical ingredient is established and its physical properties as outlined above have been designed, the selection of the excipients from a qualitative and quantitative perspective becomes front and centre within the formulation development process. Given the specifics of process of interest (fluid bed granulation) and the desired intermediate product (granules for further processing toward tablets) excipients of choice stem from the typical excipient classes: filler, binder, and lubricant. Thus, the low-dose formulation development for the FBG process has a lot in common with traditional tablet development at the first glance. However, there are two important differences.

Given the fact that only a very low amount of drug is incorporated, its physical and mechanical properties typically do not alter the formulation characteristics and do not influence the downstream manufacturability to a large extent. While it is known for high drug load formulations that compressibility and tablet attributes such as hardness, friability, and disintegration are in some cases strongly dependant on the characteristics of the API, this is not true for low-dose formulations. The latter formulations thus can in principle be developed like placebos, as long as the compatibility with the drug substance is given.

In practical terms, this benefit leads to a high versatility of platform formulations in the low-dose formulation range. Those platforms typically stem from experience and previous knowledge of the formulation space with a variety of different drugs and thus can be further applied to a multitude of different drugs from various structural classes and with different physical properties.

While this is a very positive boundary condition for the development of low-dose formulations, the major drawback of the low-dose formulation range is, as mentioned earlier, the potential exacerbation of chemical instability of active pharmaceutical ingredients. Thus, stabilization techniques are of high interest to the formulator dealing with this formulation space. Specifically, stabilizers from various classes of antioxidants have been applied.[23,24] It is obvious that the specific knowledge of potential and actual degradation pathways of the drug will be crucial for the development of stable formulations.

Meaningful preformulation studies are needed to include elucidation of degradation pathways. These are enabled by structure elucidation of related substances, often via means of sophisticated analytical tools, for example HPLC-MS-systems. Furthermore, as in most areas of formulation development, preformulation experiments comprising stress stability studies based on binary and ternary mixtures of the API with excipients are highly recommended for the development of low-dose formulations. In planning those experiments, the low drug load factor of the target formulation has to be mimicked in order to produce meaningful results during the course of the short-term stress stability testing. One clear benefit in the development of low-dose formulations is that the miniformulation approach, which is considered to be an augmenting route in preformulation, is easily applicable. This is due to the aforementioned suitability of platform formulations for low-dose drug products.

As described before, the homogenous distribution of the API is a major challenge of low-dose formulation. Here, the excipient functions as diluents for the API, stabilized by an adsorption of the microfine particles on the surface of coarser excipient carrier particles. This has been described as ordered mixing, which is contrary to noncohesive, noninteracting particulate systems produced by a randomization concept.[25] The ordered mixing concept has been suggested for the production of low-dose pharmaceutical products in order to guarantee optimal homogeneity and to reduce

TABLE 4.2 Particle Size Comparison (d_{50}) of Typical Formulation Components for an FBG Granulation

$\leq$10 μm	>10–50 μm	>50–200 μm	>200 μm
Micronized drugs; e.g., ethinyl estradiol	d_{50}: 20–50 μm lactose monohydrate; milled; e.g., Pharmatose 150M–450M™	d_{50}: 55–180 μm Lactose monohydrate, sieved; spray dried lactose; e.g., Pharmatose DCL21™	d_{50}: 290 μm Lactose monohydrate, sieved; e.g., Pharmatose 50M™

TABLE 4.3 Component Classes and Formulation Example for Low-Dose FBG Formulations

Phase	Component Class	Typical Ranges	Example[29]
Inner phase	Drug	Up to 1%	Ethinyl estradiol: 0.0375% Drospirenone: 3.75%
	Filler	30–80%	Lactose: 60.2%
	Dry binder	10–50%	Corn starch: 18.0%
	Wet binder	2–10%	PVP 25: 5.0%
	Disintegrant	0–20%	Mod. starch: 12.0%
	Stabilizers	0–5%	—
Process aid		q.s.	q.s. to form a 16% solution of the wet binder
Outer phase	Filler	0–50%	—
	Binder	0–50%	—
	Disintegrant	0–10%	—
	Lubricant	0.5–3%	Mg stearate: 1.0%

the potential for segregation.[26,27] A synonym for ordered mixing used in literature is interactive mixing.

Therefore, the excipient selection will not only be performed based on the preformulation results, but also based on a careful consideration of physical parameters such as particle size and surface characteristics.

Table 4.2 provides an overview of standard FBG excipients together with their typical particle size in comparison to the particle size of micronized drugs. Table 4.3 shows that the design of low-dose formulations for FBG processes can be performed in a rather flexible manner. On the one hand, formulations might be designed in a very straightforward fashion, consisting of an inner phase—which resembles essentially the material to be granulated—and lubricant only. On the other hand, more complex formulations containing additional excipients in the outer phase might be designed as well. The standard process aid for FBG processes is water, but organic solvents are utilized in order to dissolve lipophilic components such as drugs and stabilizers as well. A further process aid is air or, where an inert atmosphere is required, nitrogen. The gas is used in order to create the fluidized bed as well as to spray the binder solution into the bed. If nitrogen is applied, this necessitates the employment of closed loop processes, whereas the air is often utilized as process gas in an at least partly open fashion.

4.5 PROCESS DEVELOPMENT

4.5.1 Preblending Process

Immediate release tablets, and thus the granules they are based on, typically consist of several different materials, including APIs and various excipients. Uniform representation of the materials in the granules is very important. A uniform mixture of powders is needed before granulation starts. This can be achieved either through a separate preblending process or a prebend in the fluidized bed granulator. For preblend in the fluidized bed granulator, the starting material needs to belong to group A according to Geldart's classification to ensure good fluidization. For very small or light starting materials that are difficult to achieve very good fluidization with, an external preblend might be needed. Proper selection of preblend process is critical for low-dose products since it is usually challenging to uniformly mix small quantity of API with excipient particles. Product uniformity and the loss of fine API particles are two main potential problems to avoid during fluidized bed granulation for the manufacture of low-dose products. The problem of losing fine API powder through entrainment during dry blending can be overcome by shortening the time for dry blending before spraying the granulation solution onto the dry powders. This also reduces the risk of dust explosion.

The second option is to perform the preblend in a fluidized bed granulator. The advantage of performing preblend in a fluidized bed granulator is the elimination of preblending equipment and the transfer from the preblend equipment to the fluidized bed granulator. It also eliminates the requirement to address containment around the transfer process and reduces overall processing time. To use this method, powders must have the proper properties for achieving good fluidization during preblending. This is especially important for low-dose drug products. The fluidization velocity during preblending is also very important to avoid the excessive loss of API through entrainment. This approach is highly recommended for low-dose products.

The third option is to incorporate API in a granulation liquid. This is also a preferred method for the manufacture of low-dose product. However, many APIs have a solubility problem in water. The application of a solvent for a granulation liquid involves the capability of the granulation system and causes some safety concerns. The selection of granulation method should consider the properties of the starting materials, formulation, product specification, the availability of equipment, and personal and equipment safety.

Wan et al.[28] suggested that dissolving the API in a granulation liquid was preferable for low-dose drug production in a fluidized bed granulation. For API with reasonable solubility in a granulation liquid, API can also be dissolved first and sprayed onto the mixture of excipient particles. In a fluidized bed granulator, when granules are formed out of starting materials with a granulation liquid, they are bigger and heavier. These big and heavy granules tend to move towards the bottom, which leaves small and lighter granules or starting material on the top to be sprayed with the granulation liquid and form bigger and heavier granules. This mechanism helps create uniform granules in terms of particle size and composition.

However, API solubility in water may be an issue. For API with poor solubility in water, slurry preparation and spray uniformity can create serious problems for operation. It is even more challenging for low-dose products, which require good uniform spray throughout the granulation process. In some cases, the use of surfactants or other stabilizers is needed to keep the API-containing liquid uniform. The use of solvent can improve the solubility problem, but it may cause some safety concerns since it increases the risk of dust explosion. Not every fluidized bed granulation system is designed and built to handle the use of solvent as granulation liquid. Another potential drawback of incorporating API in a granulation liquid is the loss of the solid-state form of the API. Physical and chemical instabilities are another concern to be addressed when the API is dissolved in a granulation liquid.

In summary, the second option, which is to perform a dry blend in a fluidized bed granulator in a very short time followed by spraying the granulation liquid onto the mixed dry powders, is recommended as the first choice for the manufacture of low-dose products.

4.5.2 Atomization and Spray Guns

Atomization of granulation liquid is mostly achieved by using a set of dual fluid nozzles. The main advantages of dual fluid nozzles include:

- good atomization at wide range of spray rate;
- the ability to adjust spray properties at a given spray rate;
- capability to atomize highly viscous liquids;
- greater resistance to blockage.

For dual fluid nozzles, there are usually two channels for fluids, one for granulation liquid and the other for atomization air, which provide the energy for atomizing the liquid. The atomized liquid droplet size is a function of liquid spray rate, atomizing air pressure and liquid viscosity. For fluidized bed granulation, it is most convenient to use atomizing air pressure to adjust droplet size, which increases with reducing atomizing air pressure, increasing liquid viscosity, and increasing spray rate.

However, when an organic solvent is used as granulation liquid, the solvent may evaporate too rapidly before it contacts granulation particles. In this case, pressure/hydraulic nozzles can be used. Granulation liquids in pressure nozzles are delivered to the nozzle under high pressure. The atomization of the liquids is achieved by applying its own kinetic energy. The droplet size increases with reducing liquid delivering pressure, increasing liquid viscosity and increasing spray rate.

The spray properties that affect granulation are mainly spray angle, droplet size, and its distribution. During granulation, it is desirable to spray evenly on the bed surface without touching the equipment walls. Overlap of spray can lead to overwetting, which may lead to unwanted oversized granules. It may also result in wide granule size distribution.

Since a large droplet is able to bind more particles, bigger granules are usually formed. Schaefer and Wotis[29] also reported wider granule size distribution for large droplets. Waldie[30] found the following relationship between droplet size and granule size.

$$d_{\mathrm{g}} \propto d_{\mathrm{drop}}^{n} \tag{4.6}$$

where n is 0.80 for lactose.

Obviously, granule size increases with increased spray rate of the granulation liquid, a reduction in atomizing air pressure, and an increase in liquid viscosity for FDG with dual fluid nozzles. Crooks and Schade[31] reported that the distribution of granulation liquid is more uniform among larger granules, implying that, for low-dose products when the API is dissolved in granulation, the production of big granules improves dose uniformity. They also found that, with more granulation liquid, the distribution of API in granules was more uniform among granules of different sizes. At a low spray, the API was more concentrated in both coarse and fine fractions with less in the intermediate fraction. Schaefer and Wotis[29] also found that increasing granulation liquid quantity resulted in a narrower granule size distribution.

A term called "spray drying" is often used to describe the process when the droplets of granulation liquid are dried before they contact the particle bed. Spray drying generates a lot of fines. When the API is incorporated into the granulation liquid, spray drying will generate a lot of API fines, which will be lost through the entrainment carried by the fluidization air. For low-dose product, attention needs to be paid to droplet size and nozzle location to avoid excessive spray drying to maintain the effectiveness of the product.

For top-spray fluidized bed granulators, spray guns are usually placed above the product bed surface and spray the granulation liquid downwards. When the location of the spray nozzles is too far from the bed surface, the problem of excessive spray drying may be experienced. On the other hand, when the spray nozzles are too close to the bed surface, it may cause localized overwetting, which may generate undesirable large agglomerates. Decreasing the nozzle height can also lead to larger granules. Therefore, the selection of nozzle height should be based on expanded granule bed height, spray droplet size, and spray angle. After the spray gun location is selected, it is recommended to keep the bed expansion relatively constant for the whole granulation process.

4.5.3 Fluidized Bed Granulation Process and Controls

During the granulation process, granules grow bigger and heavier. To keep the same bed expansion, an increase in fluidization superficial velocity is needed. The expansion of the bubbling fluidized bed is mainly caused by bubbles in the bed. The increase in voidage in the dense phase is usually not a big factor. When the entrained fines and solids in freeboard and bubbles are neglected, the balance of solids material gives the following expression for expanded bed height.

$$\frac{H}{H_{\mathrm{mf}}} = \frac{1 - \varepsilon_{\mathrm{mf}}}{(1 - \varepsilon_{\mathrm{d}})(1 - \bar{\varepsilon}_{\mathrm{b}})} \tag{4.7}$$

where H is the expanded bed height, H_{mf} is the bed height at minimum fluidization, $\varepsilon_{\mathrm{mf}}$ is the bed voidage at minimum fluidization, ε_{d} is the voidage in dense phase and $\bar{\varepsilon}_{\mathrm{b}}$ is the average bubble hold-up in the expanded bed, which can be calculated by integration of the local value of ε_b along the bed height:

$$\bar{\varepsilon}_b = \int_0^H \varepsilon_b \mathrm{d}h \tag{4.8}$$

The balance of the gas going through the bed in the form of bubble gives the following equation:

$$\varepsilon_b = \frac{\dot{V}_b}{u_b} \tag{4.9}$$

where $\dot{V}_b$ is volumetric flux of gas going through the bed in bubbles, and u_b is bubble velocity. To complete the bed expansion calculation, further calculation on bubble properties is needed. There is much literature available on performing calculations on bubble behaviors such as size, velocity, flux, and fraction.[32–38]

During process development, samples at various stage of granulation should be obtained and analyzed. To maintain similar bed expansion throughout the whole granulation process, the superficial gas velocity should be increased based on granule properties. The amount of fluidization gas required for the bed expansion can be estimated from Eqs. (4.6)–(4.8). The inlet airflow was found to have little impact on granule size.[37]

For fluidized bed granulation that preblends API solids with excipient particles in the granulator, careful consideration must be paid to the selection of fluidization airflow to ensure good and uniform blending while avoid entrainment of API particles. A low airflow is used for this stage. The preblending usually takes only a few minutes to complete. Attention should also be paid to the loading process. Mostly, API powders have electrostatic charge and tend to stick to the equipment surface This can lead to low assay values of API in final products. To avoid this problem, fine excipient solids can be first loaded into the granulator before loading the API material. The fine excipient material will stick to the equipment surface first and work as a "cushion" to reduce the amount of API powders that stick to the equipment surface. The reduction in electrostatic charge by adjusting upstream operation such as minimizing agitating dry powder during processing is also effective in minimizing the problem.

Several researchers[38] found that an increase in inlet temperature of fluidization air led to smaller granule size. However, the experimental data from Gao et al.[37] showed that inlet temperature had little effect on granule size. At elevated inlet air temperature, the viscosity of granulation liquid is lower, which leads to weaker liquid bridges. Granule size could be smaller due to weaker bonding forces at higher inlet air temperature. For the same reason, a high inlet temperature leads to weaker agglomerates.[29] More and faster evaporation of granulation liquid may also be responsible for it.

Granulation in the fluidized bed starts after dry starting materials are preblended for a very long time interval or up to several minutes, depending on the formulation. The last stage after granulation is drying. Figure 4.3 shows inlet air humidity, product humidity, fluidization airflow rate, and granulation liquid spray rate vs time during the whole process.

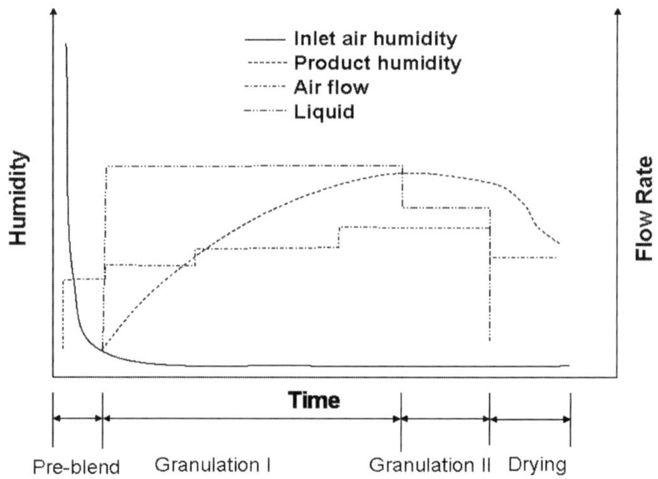

Figure 4.3 Inlet air humidity, product humidity, fluidization airflow rate and granulation liquid spray rate vs time.

As discussed earlier, the purpose of preblending is to achieve uniform mixture of all the starting materials including excipient particles and possibly API particles. The starting materials need to have the appropriate physical properties such as particle size and particle density to achieve good fluidization. At this stage, superficial gas velocity should be just high enough to achieve good fluidization, which is required for good mixing of the starting materials. However, the superficial gas velocity is low to avoid excessive particle entrainment. This is especially important to avoid the loss of API material for low-dose products. When operated properly, good mixing can be readily achieved.

Fluidization airflow is usually increased when granulation starts to maintain the bed expansion for wetter, heavier, and bigger granules. The superficial gas velocity is often increased a few times during the whole granulation. The amount of increase in fluidization air depends on the change in granule properties. The granulation stage is often operated in two phases. For the first phase, the liquid spray rate is high and product bed moisture increases significantly. Figure 4.4 shows the typical trends of inlet air temperature, product temperature, and granules over time in the granulator. As shown in Fig. 4.4, granule size increases significantly as well in phase I.

In phase I, the product moisture increases. In this phase, the amount of moisture that is removed by drying gas is smaller compared to the liquid that is sprayed on product bed. After preblending, when the product is heated up to a preset granulation temperature, the granulation liquid spray starts. The product bed temperature decreases slightly after liquid spray starts and then reaches a relatively stable temperature throughout the whole stage.

After the granules grow to a certain size, the liquid spray rate is often reduced. Starting from this point, the granulation goes to phase II. In this phase, the fluidization gas removes slightly more liquid compared with the spray liquid that granules receive.

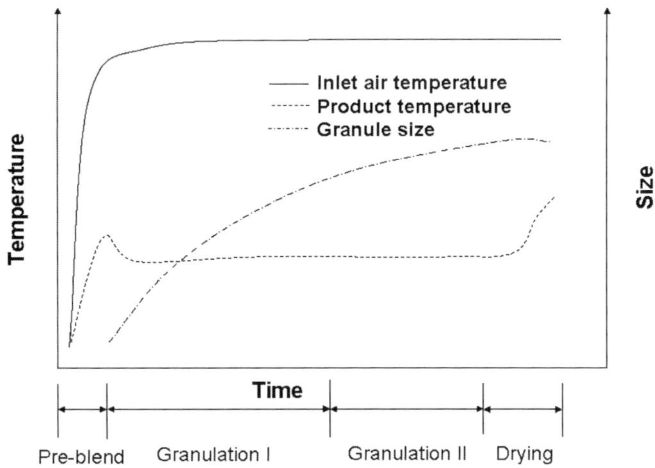

Figure 4.4 Inlet air temperature, and granule size vs time.

The moisture in the granules decreases slightly and granules are usually dried. The growth rate of granule size slows down significantly. The granule attrition rate remains stable. The product bed temperature is usually stable.

After granulation phase II, the spray of granulation liquid stops and drying starts. This is especially important for low-dose formulation processes. During this stage, because of attrition and breakage, fines are generated and particle size is reduced slightly. Compared to the airflow for phase I granulation, drying is usually operated at lower air flow to minimize granule attrition and breakage. The drying stage is usually short to avoid excessive loss of products. As shown in Fig. 4.2, shortly after drying takes place, the product bed temperature rises. Since *in-situ* granule moisture measurement technology is not commercially reliable yet, similar to fluidized bed drying operation, the product bed temperature can be used to determine the end point of the drying stage. The drying stage is usually very short. It normally takes just a few minutes to reach the end point.

4.5.4 Process Variables

Table 4.4 summarizes the main important parameters for the fluidized bed granulation process and their impact. Granule properties can be affected by several parameters. Granule size, for example, can be affected by starting material properties, atomization, spray liquid properties, and attrition. It is very important to take a comprehensive review of all the process parameters for process development.

In addition to have a good fluidization, it is essential to monitor the bed temperature, granule size, and density during operation of fluidized bed granulation process. The bed temperature is mainly controlled by adjusting spray rate. Samples can be obtained during operation for the measurements of granule size and density. Online analyzers to monitor granule size and density can also be very helpful. However, it is difficult to have a precise control on final granule size distribution.

TABLE 4.4 Key Process Variables

Operating or Material Variable	Comment
Particle size and density	Proper superficial gas velocity for good fluidization and minimum entrainment and attrition
Product loading	Granule density and strength, Proper differential pressure drop across the gas distribution plate is needed for good fluidization
Relative humidity	Fluidization, granule growth when a critical value is exceeded
Granulation liquid atomization	Granule size and its distribution, spray drying
Spray rate	Granule size, size distribution, granule strength, de-fluidization
Superficial gas velocity	Product bed expansion, solids attrition, solids entrainment
Temperature	Granule strength and granule size, it is often used for determining the end point of drying stage

4.5.5 Troubleshooting

Common problems associated with fluidized bed granulation process for low-dose drug products are:

- excessive entrainment;
- defluidization;
- excessive oversized agglomerates;
- spray nozzle blockage and material build-up around spray nozzle tips.

For low-dose drug product, the loss of API particles caused by excessive particle entrainment can lead to the problem of low potency. As discussed early, high operating air velocity is usually the main reason for the problem. In many cases, the air distribution plate is not properly designed so that low differential pressure is experienced under proper superficial velocity. To overcome the poor fluidization problem, many process development scientists and enginners choose to increase the superficial air velocity to improve the fluidization, which leads to excessive solids entrainment. The first step to solving the problem is to review the unit specifications. One can put in a proper distribution plate for the process or chose batch size and granule properties based on existing equipment properties if modifying existing equipment is not an option.

The formation of large dry and/or wet agglomerates can lead to defluidization. Large wet agglomerates are often caused by localized overwetting. From spray nozzle operation point of view, it is often associated with high spray rate or low atomization airflow. The problem can be fixed by increasing atomization airflow, reducing spray rate and/or adjusting the nozzle position.

The formation of cake around nozzle tip can significantly change the spray droplet size and spray pattern, which can lead to the formation of large agglomerates. In addition to considering proper nozzle location, spray properties, and reducing solids entrainment, the selection of nozzle can minimize the problem. Dripping of granulation solution is another cause of large, wet agglomerates. Poor fluidization such as channeling can also be the result of improper superficial air velocity and a poor air distribution plate.

Large dry agglomerates are usually the result of uncontrolled granule growth. Solving the problem usually involves adjusting superficial air velocity, spray conditions, and spray nozzle arrangement.

The blockage of spray nozzles causes many problems, especially for slurry feed. Usually, the earlier the problem is identified, the easier it is to unplug the nozzle. It is always a good idea to use simple nozzles to eliminate assembly problems. Nozzles that can be cleaned *in-situ* or easily removed are preferable.

After granulation, bed materials are discharged either by gravity or by pneumatic transfer. Usually low fluidization air is needed to ensure a full discharge. No manual scrubbing is required if the process is well operated. Selection of a good discharge valve eliminates the problems of blockage and excessive granule attrition.

4.5.6 Process Scale-Up

Once a fluidized bed granulation process is well developed, its scale-up is relatively easy compared to a high-shear granulation process. If the process is properly scaled up, the granule size, size distribution, and granule density do not change significantly during scale-up.

To be able to scale-up a fluidized bed granulation process, the process has to be developed in a unit that is big enough to minimize issues like wall effect and slugging. The typical size should be at least 0.3 m in diameter. Two units should geometrically be similar. The state of fluidization should be kept the same. In fluidized bed operation, bubble behavior plays a very important role. Although bubbles tend to be bigger in larger units, fluidization air should be distributed in the unit in a similar way.

For pharmaceutical processes, similar static bed height and bed expansion should be maintained during scale-up. To be able to produce granules of similar properties, significant changes in bed level should be avoided during scale-up. Then, the spray coverage should be scaled up according the increase in bed surface area. If the bed height has to be increased during scale-up, more attention should be paid to the change in fluidization, which is dependent on pressure drop across the distribution plate and superficial air velocity. Granules made in deeper beds tend to be denser.

It is very important to use the same type of nozzle and operate the nozzles under the same operating conditions during scale-up. When dual fluid nozzles are used, the spray rate and atomization airflow should be kept the same so that spray properties such as spray angle, droplet size, and its distribution stay the same. If superficial air velocity remains the same during scale-up, the relative position of nozzle to bed and nozzle-to-nozzle positions should be kept the same. The number of spray nozzles used should correlate with the bed surface area.

Obviously, bed temperature should be kept the same during scale-up as well. Bed moisture content needs to be similar. Because of the difference in gas–solids flow pattern, including bubble behavior, the time for each granulation phase may vary.

It is important to develop the range for operating conditions during initial process development.

For low-dose drug product, when a dry blend is required, the biggest challenge during scale-up is the initial dry blend. At a larger scale, it is more difficult to achieve uniform blending before the spray of the granulation liquid is started. During process development, more attention is needed in this early stage of granulation. Process analytical technologies such as near infrared (NIR) will be very helpful in scale-up this stage.

4.6 SUMMARY

In this chapter, the author's practical experience in developing formulations and manufacturing processes for low-dose pharmaceutical products is shared. To be able to successfully develop a process, it is necessary to pay attention to the details of every step of the whole process including formulation selection, preblending, granulation, and drying.

Fluidized bed granulation technology is very different from high-shear granulation. It is an important process for the making products with low-dose formulations for the pharmaceutical industry. Good content uniformity and stability can be achieved. Granules produced by fluidized bed usually have low particle density with good particle size distribution. The compressibility is usually excellent. With more products requiring low-dose formulation and high containment, fluidized bed granulation processes will play a more and more important role in pharmaceutical industry.

REFERENCES

1. Hilmann J, Heil W, Lipp R, Heithecker R. 2004. Pharmaceutical composition for use as a contraceptive. U.S. patent 6,787,531.
2. Geldart D. 1972. The effect of particle size and size distribution on the behaviour of gas-fluidized beds. Powder Technol. 6(4): 201–215.
3. Geldart D. 1973. Types of gas fluidization. Powder Technol. 7(5): 285–292.
4. Newitt DM, Conway-Jones JM. 1958. A contribution to the theory and practice of granulation. Trans. IChemE 36: 422–441.
5. Wen CJ, Yu YH. 1966. A generalized method for predicting the minimum fluidization velocity. AIChE 12(3): 610–612.
6. Grace JR. 1982. Fluidized-bed hydrodynamics. In: Hetsroni G, editor. Handbook of multiphase systems. New York: Hemisphere.
7. Yerushalmi J, Cankurt NT. 1990. Further studies on the regimes of fluidization. Powder Technol. 24: 187–201.
8. Nasr MM. 2006. Pharmaceutical quality assessment in the 21st century. http://www.fda.gov/ohrms/dockets/ac/06/briefing/2006-4241B1-02-12-FDA-QbD%20PQAS1%20103_Nasr.pdf.

9. ICH Q8. Guideline note for guidance on pharmaceutical development. EMEA/CHMP/167068/2004.
10. Gould PL. 1986. Salt selection for basic drug. Int. J. Pharm. 33: 201–217.
11. Morisette SL, Almarsson O, Peterson ML, Remenar JF, Read MJ, Lemmo AV, Ellis S, Cima MJ, Garner CR. 2004. High-throughput crystallization: polymorphs, salts, co-crystals and solvates of pharmaceutical solids. Adv. Drug Deliv. Rev. 56: 275–300.
12. Thiel WJ, Nguyen LT, Sberna FJ. 1986. Content uniformity of micro dose tablets (dosage 1 μg–10 mg) produced by fluid bed granulation of interactive mixtures. J. Pharm. Pharmac. 1986, 38: 335–343.
13. Zhang Y, Johnson KC. 1997. Effect of drug particle size on content uniformity of low-dose solid dosage forms. Int. J. Pharm. 154: 179–183.
14. Yalkowsky SH, Bolton S. 1990. Particle size and content uniformity. Pharm. Res. 7: 962–966.
15. Johnson MCR. 1972. Particle size distribution of the active ingredient for solid dosage forms of low dosage. Pharm. Acta Helv. 47: 546–559.
16. Rohrs BR, Amidon GE, Meury RH, Secreast PJ, King HM, Skoug CJ. 2006. Particle size limits to USP content uniformity criteria for tablets and capsules. J. Pharm. Sci. 95: 1049–1059.
17. Sallam E, Orr NA. 1986. Studies relating to the content uniformity of ethinyloestradiol tablets 10 μg: Effect of particle size of ethinyloestradiol. Drug Dev. Ind. Pharm. 12: 2015–2042.
18. Orr NA, Sallam EA. 1978. Content uniformity of potent drugs in tablets. J. Pharm. Pharmacol. 30: 741–747.
19. Midous NP, Hoek L, Pailleres J, Authelin R. 1999. Micronization of pharmaceutical substances in a spiral jet mill. Powder Technol. 104: 113–120.
20. ICH Q3B (R2). 2006. Guideline Note for guidance on impurities in new drug products. EMEA/CHMP/ICH/2738/99.
21. Sucker H. 1991. Theoretische Grundlagen der verfahrenstechnischen Grundoperationen. In: Sucker H, Fuchs P, Speiser P, editors. Pharmazeutische Technologie, 2nd ed. New York: Georg Thieme, pp. 39–41.
22. Kanneganti PPP, Wan LSC. 1987. Measurement of the particle size of tablet excipients with the aid of video recording. Pharm. Res. 4: 504–508.
23. Backensfeld T, Keitel S, Lipp R. 1997. Low-dose steroid tablets that contain gallic acid ester as an antioxidant, process for production and use. U.S. patent 6,156,341.
24. Cyclessa (desogestrel and ethinyl estradiol) Tablets. Physician's Desk Reference, 2006.
25. Hersey JA. 1975. Ordered mixing: A new concept in powder mixing practice. Powder Technol. 11: 41–44.
26. Yeung CC, Hersey JA. 1979. Ordered powder mixing of coarse and fine particulate systems. Powder Technol. 22: 127–131.
27. Backensfeld T, Heil W, Lipp R. 2005. Compositions of estrogen-cyclodextrin complexes. U.S. patent 6,958,326.
28. Wan L, Heng P, Muhuri G. 1992. Incorporation and distribution of low dose drug in granules. Int. J. Pharm. 88: 159–163.
29. Schaefer T, Wotis O. 1978. Control of fluidized bed granulation. Arch. Pharm. Chem. Sci. Ed. 6: 69–82.

30. Waldie B. 1991. Growth mechanism and the dependence of granule size on drop size in fluidized-bed granulation. Chem. Eng. Sci. 46(11): 2781–2785.

31. Crooks MJ, Schade HW. 1978. Fluidized bed granulation of a microdose pharmaceutical powder. Powder Technol. 19: 103–108.

32. Darton RC, LaNauze RD, Davidson JF, Harrison D. 1977. Bubble growth due to coalescence in fluidized beds. Trans. IChemE 55: 274–280.

33. Davidson JF, Harrison D. 1963. Fluidized particle. Cambridge: Cambridge University Press.

34. Hilligardt K, Werther JW. 1986. Local bubble gas hold-up and expansion of gas/solid fluidized beds. Germ. Chem. Engng 9: 215–221.

35. Ocone R, Sundaresan S, Jackson R. 1993. Gas–particle flow in a duct of arbitrary inclination with particle–particle interactions. AIChE J. 39: 1261–1271.

36. Lim KS, Gururajan VS, Agrawal PK. 1993. Mixing of homogeneous solid in bubbling fluidized beds theoretical modeling and experimental investigation using digital image analysis. Chem. Engng Sci. 48: 2251–2265.

37. Gao J, Motheram A, Hussain D. 2002. Fluid bed granulation of poorly water soluble, low density, micronized drug: comparison with high-shear granulation. Int. J. Pharm. 237: 1–14.

38. Davies W, Gloor W. 1971. Batch production of pharmaceutical granulation in a fluid bed: I: effects of process variables on physical properties of final granulation. J. Pharm. Sci. 60: 1869–1874.

CHAPTER 5

DEVELOPMENT OF LOW-DOSE SOLID ORAL FORMULATIONS USING WET GRANULATION

AHMAD ALMAYA
Pharmaceutical Sciences R&D, Lilly Research Laboratories, Eli Lilly and Company, Indianapolis, IN 46285

5.1 INTRODUCTION

Wet granulation is the most common granulation method in the pharmaceutical industry. It is the method that has been used for the longest time in the industrial production of tablets.[1] It can be defined as the process in which primary powder particles are made to adhere to form larger, multiple entities called granules.[2] These granules typically are in the range of 0.2–0.5 mm if they are intended to be compressed into tablets, or filled into capsules. Wet granulation is the process of choice for the manufacturing of dosage forms containing high-dosage drugs of poor flow and poor compressibility properties, as well as for dosage forms with very potent, low-dose drugs. Granulation typically starts with dry mixing of most or all of the ingredients, followed by granulation, drying and sizing of the dried granules.

There are different reasons for granulation, the most important of which are the following:[1–4]

- To prevent segregation of the constituents of the powder mix: Such segregation is mainly due to differences in the size or density of the components of the powder mix. Smaller and/or denser particles tend to segregate at the base of a container, with the larger and/or less dense particles concentrating at the top. So, an ideal granulation is one where all the components of the powder mix will be represented in the correct proportion in each granule. However, it is still important to control the particle size distribution of the granulation such that segregation of the individual granules themselves does not occur.

Formulation and Analytical Development for Low-Dose Oral Drug Products. Edited by Jack Zheng

This may lead to larger weight variation on a tablet press, or to a poor content uniformity within individual dosage units if the active ingredient is not distributed uniformly in small and large granules.

- To improve flow of the mix: Many powders, because of their size, shape, or surface properties, do not flow well. Granulation results in larger, denser granules leading to an improved flow. Moreover, granulation would ideally result in granules whose shape is closer to a sphere than starting materials, although this might not always be the case.
- To improve compaction properties of the powder mix: Granulation is known to improve the compaction properties of powders that otherwise do not readily lead to compactable mixes. This is linked to the use of some excipients (i.e., binders) whose distribution within the granules lead to easier compaction. Most binders facilitate compression by softening and deforming plastically under load.
- To reduce exposure to toxic/potent materials: Such materials are not appropriate to be handled in the powder form which leads to generation of dust. Dust generation is greatly reduced via granulation.
- To improve product content uniformity in low-dose formulation, which is the focus of this chapter.

In general, granulation can be achieved by either dry or wet methods.[4] In dry granulation, powders are compacted into granules by the use of high pressure. This can be achieved by either slugging (using specialized tablet presses that produce large tablets, or slugs), or by roller compaction by passing the powder mix between two rollers to produce ribbons. In each case, the compacted slugs or ribbons are then sieved to control the granule particle size, and then mixed with outside powders prior to tabletting. This method (i.e., dry granulation) may be more suitable for materials that are sensitive to moisture.

On the other hand, wet granulation is achieved by massing the powder mix with a granulation liquid. This granulation liquid consists of a solvent that can be dried off, in addition to other ingredients (binders, wetting agents). Such liquids can be aqueous, alcoholic, or hydro-alcoholic. Water is by far the most commonly used vehicle for wet granulation because it is more economical, nonflammable, and does not require the use of explosion-proof equipment. However, the use of water in wet granulation may impact the stability of the active ingredients if they are susceptible to hydrolysis. In addition, more energy is required to dry off water from wet granulations compared to alcohol.

The properties of the granulations, including granule size distribution and pore structure, are dependent on the method and conditions of the granulation. For example, granules produced by wet massing consist of drug particles held together in a sponge-like matrix of binder. Granules produced by fluidized bed granulations, on the other hand, possess higher porosity and the granule surface is covered by a film of binding agent.[2] This chapter is focued on development of low-dose solid oral formulations using high-shear wet granulation while the fluidized bed granulation is discussed in Chapter 4.

5.2 GRANULATION MECHANISMS

In order for granules to form, the forces working to hold the particles together in the granules must be strong enough to withstand subsequent processing steps. These forces may be divided into two groups—those that work to agglomerate individual particles into granules, and those that lead to granule progression.

5.2.1 Agglomeration of Particles into Granules

Forces that work to agglomerate individual particle into granules include five primary bonding mechanisms:[1–4]

- Adhesion and cohesion forces in the immobile liquid films between individual primary powder particles. These forces may not contribute significantly to the final granule strength once the granules have been dried. These forces arise from the thin liquid layers around particles that may be generated due to moisture uptake by the powders. This immobile liquid film tends to decrease the inter-particle distances leading to an increase in the van der Waals forces between particles.
- Interfacial forces and capillary pressure in mobile liquid films within the granules. During wet granulation, the amount of liquid used will exceed that needed to form an immobile film around the particles. This leads to a mobile liquid film that will be distributed around and in between the particles during wet massing, leading to the formation of liquid bridges. These liquid films are only temporary because they will cease to exist once the granules are dried. However, these liquid bridges are important since they are the prerequisite for the solid bridges. During granulation, these liquid films go through different states, depending on the amount of liquid added as well as the total amount of work exerted during the massing. At low moisture level, the *pendular* state exists where the particles are held together by liquid films via surface tension forces of the liquid–air interface and the hydrostatic suction pressure in the liquid bridge. Next is the *funicular* state, followed by the *capillary* state, in which most of the air from within the particles has been displaced, and the particles are held by the capillary attraction. The powder bed, during wet granulation, may move from the pendular state towards the capillary state via wet-massing, without additional liquid. This is because the work exerted during wet massing leads to densification of the granules, leading to replacement of the pore volume occupied by air by the liquid. Following the capillary state, a fourth state can be reached, though it is not desirable, which is the *droplet* or suspension state. In this state, particles are engulfed by a droplet of the liquid, and the strength of such a state relies on the surface tension of the liquid used in the granulation.
- Formation of solid bridges after solvent evaporation. These solid bridges are formed when the liquid films are dried leading to precipitation and

crystallization of the materials that were dissolved in the liquid films. These solid bridges certainly result from the deposition of soluble binders as well as the deposition of other soluble formulation components during drying. In addition, some materials in the powder blend may dissolve in the liquid films during wet granulation, leading to subsequent precipitation and crystallization of such materials upon drying in the solid bridges that hold the individual powder particles within the granules. The size and strength of the solid bridges depend on the quantity of the dissolved material as well as the processing conditions, massing duration and intensity, temperature rise during granulation, and amount of dissolved fraction in the granulation liquid. In addition, the size and strength of the solid bridges depend on crystallization rate. Shorter drying times lead to larger crystal size with subsequent increase in granule strength.

- Attractive forces between solid particles. These may be due to electrostatic forces or van der Waal forces. However, these forces are not dominant in granules produced by wet granulation. These forces are more relevant to granules manufactured by dry granulation.
- Mechanical interlocking. As expected, this will be affected by both shape and surface roughness of the individual particles.

5.2.2 Granule Progression

The second group of forces that work towards making the granules is the one that leads to granule progression. During wet granulations, particles agglomerate with addition of liquid to the powders that is being distributed among the powder particles via the mechanical agitation produced by the granulator. In general, the granulation process goes through three stages:

- *Nucleation*: This is where individual powder particles adhere to each other due to the liquid films. These particles will go through the different states discussed above from the pendular to the capillary state. These agglomerated particles in the capillary state will serve as nuclei for further granule growth.
- *Transition*: This is the stage where granules will grow either by addition of new powder particles to the already formed nuclei by pendular forces, or by the combination of individual nuclei. Such a transition will give rise to a wide size distribution of granules, which may be controlled by the combination of different factors, like the granulation parameters and binder solution properties.
- *Ball growth*: If massing continues, granule growth typically continues (assuming the mixing intensity is properly chosen), leading to large, over granulated spherical granules that may not be suitable for further processing. Such ball growth depends on the granulator and the powder bed properties, as well as on the properties of the granulation solution used.

In addition to the forces that work to hold the particles together (forces that work to agglomerate individual particles into granules, and those that lead to granule progression), other forces work towards granule breakage and attrition during the wet granulation process, especially in high intensity mixers. These forces affect the binder distribution and granule size in high intensity processes.[5]

5.3 GENERAL CONSIDERATIONS ON WET GRANULATION

5.3.1 Granulation Equipment

Wet granulators can be divided into three main types: low-shear granulators, high-shear granulators, and fluidized bed granulators.[1–4,6] The third type is the focus of another chapter in this book and will not be discussed in details here. Table 5.1 provides a summary of some of the different granulators that are commonly used in the pharmaceutical industry.

Low-Shear Granulators. These are the traditional granulators and are of the planetary type (e.g., Hobart, Collette) or the kneading type (Z-blade mixers). Another type of these low-shear granulators consists of a V-blender with an intensifier bar (e.g., Patterson–Kelley).

Low-shear granulators are lower speed and lower energy mixers. Here, the powders are added to the bowl and granulation liquid added, then the mixture is agitated by the paddle. The granulated mass is then usually passed through an oscillating granulator that forces the wet mass through the sieve screen. If the wet mass is overwetted, strings of material will form, and if the mass is too dry, granules will not form and the mass will be sieved to powder. In general, low-shear granulators suffer from

TABLE 5.1 Summary of Some Wet Granulation Equipment Commonly Used in the Pharmaceutical Industry

Granulation Type	Equipment Classification	Examples
High-shear wet granulators	Horizontal (side driven)	Lodige
	Vertical—bottom driven	Auromatic-Fielder (GEA-Niro Pharma Systems) Diosna Powrex–Glatt
	Vertical—top driven	Collete–Gral (GEA–Niro Pharma Systems)
Low shear wet granulators	Planetary	Collete (GEA–Niro Pharma Systems) Hobart
	Kneading (Z-blade mixers)	Morton Machines
Fluid bed granulators	Fluid bed	Aeromatic-Fielder (GEA–Niro Pharma Systems) Glatt

several disadvantages, including the use of several pieces of equipment, long duration, and high loss of materials.

High-Shear Granulators. Nowadays, high-shear granulators are extensively used in the pharmaceutical industry. Examples of these are the Diosna®, Powerex®, and the Fielder® granulators. Here, the granulators contain an impeller that turns generally at the speed of 100–500 rpm, and a chopper that turns generally in the speed range of 1000–3000 rpm. In general, high-shear granulators can be divided into horizontal or vertical granulators. In the horizontal type, the impeller shaft rotates in the horizontal plane. An example of this type is the Lödige® granulator, where the impeller arms are of a plough-like shape. This design was the first high-shear granulator widely used in the pharmaceutical industry. On the other hand, a vertical granulator is where the impeller shaft rotates in the vertical plane, and the impeller arms are bladelike. Vertical granulators can also be classified into bottom-driven (e.g., Diosna or Powrex granulators) or top-driven (e.g., Collete–Gral granulator). In the top-driven granulators, the granulation bowl is removable. Figure 5.1 shows an example of a vertical, bottom-driven, high-shear granulator (Diosna P-150).

In high-shear granulators, powders are added either premixed, or they can be mixed in the granulator, prior to wet granulation. Next, granulation fluid is added (poured, pumped, or atomized) and the bed mixed with both the impeller and the chopper. After the addition of the granulation fluid, the wet mass is usually mixed further (also called wet massing) in order to further distribute the granulation fluid, and to further increase the granule density and growth. Thus, both mixing and granulation can take place in the same equipment for high-shear granulators and can be achieved in a relatively short time (generally in less than 10 min). However, the process needs to be well controlled since over-granulation can take place quickly if the process is not well monitored.

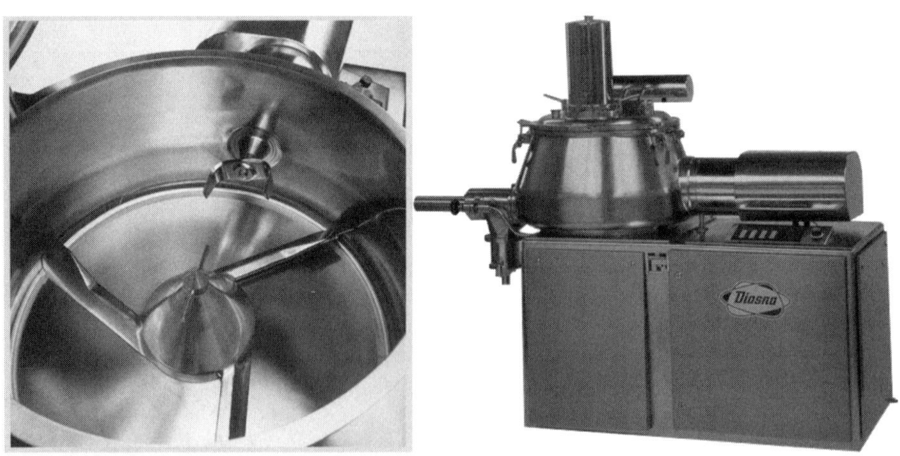

Figure 5.1 Diosna P-150 Granulator. The unit is shown on the right, and the inside of the granulator bowl on the left showing the impeller blade and the chopper.

The agglomeration behavior of granules may be different in the different types of high-shear granulators, and processes may not be directly transferable between different types of high-shear granulators. These differences between different granulators have been studied.[7–11] Granulations produced in high-shear granulators are generally denser than those made using low-speed mixers.[12] Moreover, because high-shear granulators utilize more energy than low-shear granulators, the amount of granulation liquid needed may be less than that for low-shear granulators, and consequently, high-shear granulations require shorter drying times.

The other commonly used granulators in the pharmaceutical industry are fluid bed granulators. In general, fluidized-bed granulators offer the advantage of performing mixing, granulation, and drying in one piece of equipment. However, there is a possibility of air pollution since air is blown into the atmosphere. Also, there is a higher risk of explosion in fluid air granulators since large amounts of oxygen are conveyed by the fluidizing air. Granulations produced by fluid beds are generally more porous and less dense than those produced in a high-shear granulator.[13]

5.3.2 Raw Materials

Raw materials used in wet granulations have different purposes and can be placed in different functional classes.[1–4] These materials may be part of the granules themselves (i.e., intragranular) or may be added externally to the granules (i.e., extragranular).

Drug Substance. Properties of the drug substance, that is, active pharmaceutical ingredient, may drive the selection of the other ingredients in the formulation. Thus, a thorough understanding of the physicochemical and biopharmaceutical properties of the drug is crucial to formulation development. These physicochemical properties as well as the stability characteristics of the API are also important in selection of the manufacturing platform of the dosage form. Thus, wet granulation is appropriate for some drugs while it may not be appropriate for others. In general, wet granulation processes are not suitable for drug substances that are sensitive to moisture and/or heat. In addition, a wet granulation process may not be suitable for drug substances that are very water-soluble and tend to form amorphous materials following wet granulation or for those prone to polymorph changes. The physical properties of the drug substance are important as well. For example, drug substance particle size may need to be controlled because of uniformity or dissolution reasons. This is very important for low-dose formulations in order to achieve appropriate content uniformity in the final dosage form.[14–17] The appropriate drug substance particle size needed to achieve acceptable content uniformity depends not only on the dosage strength, but also on the selected excipients, manufacturing platform, dose form weight/size, and the process parameters used to manufacture the drug product. The topic of drug substance particle size in relation to low-dose formulations will be discussed in a separate chapter in this book.

Some physical properties of drug substances are important to the selection of the manufacturing platform itself. For example, if the drug has low density or if it possesses poor compression characteristics, then wet granulation may be advantageous. There are several important properties of drug substances that must be considered when using a wet granulation manufacturing process. These include particle size, density, compressibility, polymorphism, solubility, ability to form amorphous content, dissolution rate, solid-state stability, hygroscopicity, ease of wetting with proposed granulation liquid, and solution stability. Table 5.2 lists some of the properties of the drug substance that are important for selection of the manufacturing platform.[1]

Diluents. In general, diluents make up most of the dosage form. The selection of diluents is very important, especially for low-dose formulations, since they may make up 85–95% of the granulation. These diluents may be soluble or insoluble. The most commonly used soluble fillers include lactose, mannitol and sucrose. Commonly used insoluble fillers include microcrystalline cellulose, starch, calcium sulfate, and dibasic calcium phosphate.

Disintegrants. These facilitate the breakup of tablets and granules, promoting dissolution. The traditional disintegrants include starch and microcrystalline cellulose. More recent disintegrants are called super-disintegrants because they are used in lower proportions and lead to faster disintegration. These include sodium starch glycolate, sodium carboxymethylcellulose cross-linked, and cross-linked polyvinylpyrrolidone.[18] Disintegrant performance may depend on the method of addition into the formulation.[19] Moreover, some disintegrants may be more efficient than others after incorporation into a wet granulation process.[20]

Binders. Binders are the materials that are responsible for granule formation. These may be dissolved in a granulating vehicle prior to granulation. Some binders may also be added dry and mixed with the rest of the powders and then granulated with the

TABLE 5.2 Drug Substance Properties that are Important in the Selection of Manufacturing Platforms

Importance to Platform Selection	Property
Low importance	Organoleptic properties
	pH in solution
Medium importance	Particle shape and crystal properties
	Particle size
High importance	Flowability
	Absolute and bulk densities
	Compressibility
	Polymorphism
	Solubility
	Solid-state stability
	Solution stability

granulation vehicle. Generally, binders are more effective when they are predissolved in the granulation solvent prior to addition. Binders are cohesive and adhesive, leading to the agglomeration of powder particles into granules. Properties of the granulations like particle size, density, hardness, disintegration and compressibility can be greatly influenced by the binder type and level. Highly viscous binders may lead to hard granules that are difficult to compress. On the other hand, insufficient amount of binder or an inefficient binder may lead to fragile granules leading to an excessive amount of fine powders in the granulation. In addition, even though binders may improve the dissolution rate of poorly soluble drugs, an excessive amount of binder may lead to slowing dissolution. Binders include starch, polyvinylpyrrolidone, methylcellulose, hydroxypropylcellulose, hydroxypropylmethylcellulose (hypromellose), sugars, and gelatin.

Granulation Liquids. The most commonly used solvent is water, although alcoholic or hydro-alcoholic mixtures may be used instead. Water is nonflammable, nontoxic and does not require the use of explosion-proof equipment. However, it requires more energy and longer time to dry off, and it may adversely affect stability of drugs that are susceptible to hydrolysis. Organic solvents on the other hand, may be used for moisture-sensitive drugs. Most also evaporate more readily than water. However, they are more expensive to use, require caution during use, require the use of special equipment, and may lead to generation of toxic vapors. In addition, it is important to monitor the residual amounts of solvents left in the granulations. The most commonly used organic solvents are alcohols.

5.3.3 Unit Operations in Wet Granulation Process

The steps utilized in a wet granulation process are summarized below and are outlined in Fig. 5.2.

Preparation of Granulation Liquid. The granulating liquid is prepared by dissolving or dispersing the binders in water or other solvents. Additionally, this granulation liquid may contain surfactants and drug substances. In the preparation of this granulation liquid, liquid temperature, order of component addition, rate of component addition, mixing speed, mixing time, de-aeration time, and allowable hold times should be considered.

Milling and Mixing of Powders. The dry powders should be well mixed for a successful granulation. Moreover, good mixing is crucial for drug content uniformity in the final dosage form. This step can be done prior to transfer to a granulator, or can be done within the granulator itself prior to addition of the granulation solution. Milling is an efficient way to break down aggregates for fine particles of drug substance. The milling or mixing operation prior to wet granulation can improve the containment for low-dose, potent drug substances and should be evaluated when a low-dose drug product is developed.

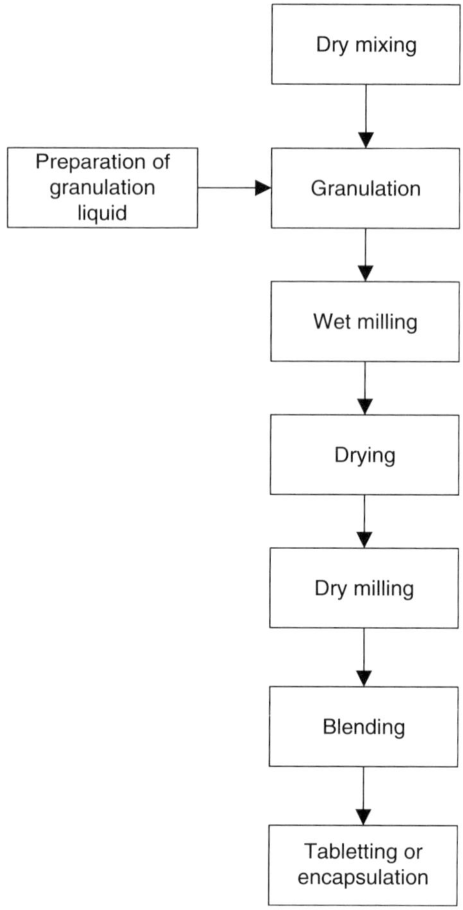

Figure 5.2 Scheme showing the steps in a wet granulation process.

Addition of Granulation Solution and Wet Massing of the Powders. This is when the granulation solution is added to the powder blend. Appropriate agitation is necessary to ensure an appropriate distribution of the granulation solution over the powder particles, especially if the granulation solution is viscous. The amount of granulation liquid needed to reach the capillary state depends on the wetting liquid (viscosity, surface tension, solid–liquid tension) as well as the powder components (particle size distribution, particle shape, surface area, solubility in the liquid and ability to absorb the liquid) and equipment properties. There are few guidelines in the literature for required amount of liquid for granulation, although this is strongly dependent on the materials and the granulation method.[3] For example, some reports advocate that high-shear granulators require two-thirds to three-fourths the amount of liquid needed by traditional low-shear granulators.[21] Surface tension of the granulation liquids is also an important factor. Liquids with lower surface tension wet better, but produce weaker wet agglomerates with slower growth.[22] The higher the surface tension of the granulation liquid, the higher the force of the liquid bridges, and the greater the cohesive forces pulling the particles together.

End Point of the Wet Massing. Granulation end point depends on the granulation equipment and the formulation characteristics. It may be determined manually; however, this requires sufficient experience. Other quantitative methods of assessing the granulation end point have been described. These may include measurements derived from probes like conductivity, capacity, resistance, or impact force; or measurements derived from the impeller motor or impeller shaft like power consumption, torque, and motor slip.[1–4,6,23–26] Such methods of monitoring the granulation end point are necessary in high-shear wet granulators since the transition from under-massed to over-granulated system can take place in a short time.

The most convenient and commonly used methods to study end points of wet massing are those that are based on the rheological properties of the mass like the torque on the motor shaft, or power consumption.[6,27] The torque measurements on the shaft provide a more accurate estimate of the resistance of the mass against the impeller; however, the signal is more complicated to obtain compared to power consumption. Power consumption measurement, on the other hand, is relatively easy to obtain, but it reflects the load on the motor rather than the load on the impeller. Moreover, the use of the power reading for the empty bowl or during dry mixing as a baseline value to account for the no-load losses may be confounded by a possible nonlinearity of friction losses with respect to the load.[27] Nonetheless, power consumption remains very popular and generally correlates with granule properties during wet massing, although this correlation may depend on several factors like the impeller design or the impeller speed.[28]

Wet Screening. Wet screening may be needed to break up the large granules in order to promote more uniform, and faster drying. It can be used to minimize thermal exposure of the formulation and to ensure complete drying. It may also be needed to aid in the control of the granule size distribution. However, it may not always be needed in the case of high-shear wet granulation since the chopper in the granulator can serve that function.

Drying. Drying the wet granules leads to formation of solid bridges, leading to strong granules that do not collapse back to the constituent powders. The target moisture content at the end of the drying should be selected based on the chemical stability of the drug product, the effect of the moisture content on the compressibility of the granulation, as well as on the equilibrium moisture content of the material at the relative humidity of the manufacturing plant. The effect of moisture content on the compressibility of the granulation is an important factor because the effect of binders is dependent on the residual moisture content in the granulations.[29] Drying can be carried out using tray dryers or using fluidized bed dryers. Tray drying is the more conventional process; however, it suffers from several drawbacks. The most important drawback is the long drying time. In addition, since drying takes place mainly from the upper surface of the bed on the tray, dissolved material migration to the top of the granule bed may become an issue. In addition, granule agglomeration can take place to a larger extent with tray dryers than fluid bed dryers since solid bridges can form between individual granules on the tray during drying. Fluidized bed drying process is faster than tray drying, which reduces the issue of aggregation and solute migration. However, drug loss through the filters may be an issue with fluidized bed dryers, especially with potent drugs (which are frequently micronized to ensure uniformity) and friable granulations.

Sizing. This step is important in order to reduce and control the particle size of the dried granules prior to further processing. Controlling the granulation particle size is important for maintaining an appropriate granulation flow and weight control during tabletting, as well as to minimize the likelihood of segregation. Different equipments are available for dry sizing of granules including conical screening mills (e.g., Quadro Comil®) and hammer mills (e.g., Fitzmill®). Several factors are important in controlling the granule particle size, including the mill speed, output screen size, and impeller/blade type.[30] It is very important to consider the contamination or health hazards due to dust generation during dry sizing of granulations, especially for low-dose, highly potent drug substances.

5.4 ADVANTAGES AND DISADVANTAGES OF WET GRANULATION

Wet granulation is one of the most commonly used manufacturing processes in the pharmaceutical industry because it provides several advantages. At the same time, it is one of the most complex processes, leading to some disadvantages.

5.4.1 Advantages

Wet granulation improves flow and sphericity of granules. It also improves compressibility of materials. Wet granulation also improves the content uniformity of low-dosage drugs. It prevents segregation of components. It also leads to an improved dissolution rate for hydrophobic drugs, and leads to low dust generation, resulting in lower cross contamination and airborne exposure.

5.4.2 Disadvantages

While wet granulation can be used to successfully manufacture moisture-sensitive drugs, this may require the use of nonaqueous granulation liquids. Alternative organic solvents are more costly and may pose hazards to the manufacturing personnel and the environment. Wet granulation may not be appropriate for heat-sensitive drugs since degradation of those may take place during drying. Solute migration during drying may be an issue, especially for soluble ingredients and drug substances. Incompatibility among formulation ingredients may be increased by bringing them closer by the granulation process. Moreover, wet granulation may be the manufacturing method for solid dosage forms that is most likely to be associated with process induced phase transformations of drug substances. However, the greatest disadvantage of wet granulation may be its complexity (because it involves several steps and many parameters to be controlled) and that it is expensive (equipment, energy, time).

5.5 USE OF WET GRANULATION FOR LOW-DOSE FORMULATIONS

In the last few sections, the basic principles of wet granulations were summarized. The focus of this section will be on the use of wet granulation as a manufacturing process in the production of low-dose formulations.

There are two main paths that can be followed to incorporate a low-dose active ingredient in a formulation via wet granulation:

- Addition of the potent active ingredient to the formulation ingredients in the dry state, prior to wet granulation. Here, the active ingredient is added to the dry powders via blending in a blender prior to charging into the granulator bowl, or by blending with the dry excipients directly in the granulation bowl. This is then followed by wet granulation, drying and sizing of the granulations.
- Addition of the potent active ingredient to the formulation ingredients via the use of a solution or a suspension. Here, the active ingredient is either dissolved or suspended in the granulation vehicle, which is then used to granulate the dry excipient blend.

Each of these two paths has advantages and disadvantages, and these will be discussed below.

5.5.1 Addition of Drug Substance in a Dry State

In this scenario, it is important to pay appropriate attention to the uniformity of the active ingredient in the powder mix prior to the wet granulation process. Even though the agitation during the wet granulation step itself may improve the uniformity of the active ingredient in the granulation, the uniformity of the active ingredient in the powder blend prior to wet granulation remains very important. The importance and the necessity of the blending step, some times called preblending, should be evaluated on a formulation-by-formulation basis, and may strongly depend on the intended drug load in the final formulation, excipient selection, and the process parameters. This blending step may be simple, involving blending of the active ingredient with all or most of the excipients in an appropriate blender (e.g., V-shell blender or a tumble bin). Alternatively, a geometrical dilution approach may be utilized, in which the active ingredient is mixed with part of the excipients (e.g., part of the diluent), and then subsequently diluted with equivalent portions of excipients until the desired final mix is achieved. The resultant blend may then be charged into the granulation bowl. The formulation scientist may evaluate the use of a tumble bin with an intensifier bar to improve the uniformity of the active ingredient in the powder blend. Alternatively, the preblend, containing the active ingredient with all or part of the diluents may be passed through a Comil®, in order to deaggregate any API lumps. This may be important since the active ingredient represents only a small fraction of the formulation and the effect of such lumps or aggregates on the final uniformity in the dosage form may be significant. Often, potent active ingredients are micronized in order to improve the uniformity in the dosage units, leading to higher surface area of the powders, thus resulting in a higher degree of aggregation. Also, if the active ingredients are oily, deaggregation of drug-rich nuclei will be more important prior to wet granulation.[31]

The formulation scientist may instead evaluate eliminating the preblending step prior to charging the powders into the granulation bowl. Such an approach should be evaluated carefully. On one hand, the elimination of the preblending step may minimize any potential loss of active ingredient during blending or during the transfer steps to the granulator bowl. This may be important in a number of occasions since the decrease in active ingredient particle size (e.g., by micronization) may increase the potential of active ingredient loss during transfer steps, especially if plastic bags are utilized in such transfer steps (e.g., polyethylene bags). Also, in addition to minimizing the transfer steps, mixing the powder blends in a granulation bowl, especially in high-shear granulators, may lend the advantage of decreasing the potential to operator exposure since the process may be contained. However, the process parameters during powder mixing in the granulator need to be studied. For example, is it necessary to use the chopper during powder blending? This may increase the chances of active ingredient loss; on the other hand, the chopper may aid in de-aggregation of active ingredient lumps prior to granulation. Additionally, an appropriate mixing time of the powder blend in the high-shear granulator needs to be studied for each formulation. Kornchankul et al.[32] studied the effect of process variables on the mixing uniformity of a powder blend for a low-dose formulation in a high-shear mixer and found that impeller speeds and mixing times had significant effect on the content uniformity of the powder blend. Table 5.3 lists some of the data in

TABLE 5.3 Mixing Uniformity of a Low-Dose, Dry Formulation as a Function of Impeller and Chopper Speeds

	Mixing Uniformity RSD, %	
Mixing Time, min	Impeller Speed: 261 rpm	Impeller Speed: 522 rpm
0.5	11.69	6.05
1	12.09	8.93
2	10.41	7.42
4	14.63	8.52
8	15.66	4.32
16	6.83	2.90
32	4.41	3.42

their work where the RSD values of mixing uniformity of a dry formulation containing 0.5% (w/w) active ingredient was studied using a high-shear granulator. At a low chopper speed (1800 rpm), increasing the impeller speed from 261 to 522 rpm led to lower mixing uniformity RSD values at all mixing time points (Table 5.3). This indicates the importance of using an appropriate impeller speed, even for dry mixing. The authors also indicated that de-mixing may be observed when high chopper speeds were utilized (3600 rpm).

The uniformity of the active ingredient in the powder blend prior to granulation can be assessed directly by taking samples of the powder blend from the granulator. This may be insightful during formulation development so that the impact of each of the unit operations on the uniformity of the finished granulations and the finished product can be clearly understood.

Following the powder blending operation, wet granulation can then be started. As described in the previous sections, the binder in the formulation may be dissolved in the granulation vehicle or may be added dry in the powder blend prior to wet granulation. Sometimes, only a portion of the binder can be dissolved in the granulation vehicle and the rest is added dry in order to maintain an appropriate viscosity of the granulation vehicle.

The parameters used during the wet granulation step should be evaluated very carefully since these can impact not only the properties of the granules (e.g., granulation particle size distribution, granulation density, and granulation compressibility),[33,34] but also the uniformity of the active ingredient in the granules and the finished product.[35–41] Such process parameters (e.g., impeller speed, granulation vehicle amount, method of addition of granulation vehicle, granulation time) may impact the uniformity of the active ingredient in the finished granules and may also impact the uniformity in the finished product. The effect of these process parameters cannot be generalized, since there may be a strong inter-play between the effect of these parameters and the properties of the materials used in the formulations (e.g., solubility, porosity, and particle size distribution of both the active ingredient and the excipients).

The study conducted by Vromans et al.[38] provides an excellent example of such an effect of process parameters on the uniformity of the active ingredient in the granules and the inter-play of the ingredient properties with the wet granulation process parameters. In their study, the uniformity of a micronized low-dose drug was found to be affected by the particle size of the excipients and the impeller speed during wet granulation in a high-shear granulator. High impeller speeds led to inhomogeneity of the drug in the granulations (large granules were superpotent) and lower impeller speeds improved granule uniformity. This was explained by the need for a balance between the impact pressure exerted by the impeller during wet granulation, and the shear resistance of the granulation nuclei. At high impeller speeds, the impact pressure is too high, leading to the breakage of the weak nuclei, resulting in particle rearrangement and poor homogeneity in the finished granules. On the other hand, smaller particle size of the diluent leads to stronger nuclei during wet granulation, resulting in good granule uniformity. The dependence of granule homogeneity on the impeller speed was influenced by the particle size of the filler. The authors concluded that high shear (i.e., high impeller speeds) should be avoided during granulation, especially if the particle size of the drug and the diluent are significantly different.[38] However, it is important to point out that, with the appropriate process parameters, a uniform drug distribution in the granules can be achieved even if the particle size of the drug substance and the excipients are significantly different.[41]

It is interesting to note that there are multiple examples in the literature where coarse granules were found to be super-potent in the low-dose, small particle size active ingredients, and fine granules were found to be subpotent.[37–43] For example, in one investigation, coarse granules were found to contain 150% of the target concentration while fine granules contained 50%, even though the powder blend prior to granulation was found to be homogenous with an RSD of less than 1%.[38] This phenomena has been explained by granule breakage and preferential layering[39] where granule breakage during wet granulation may lead to continuous exchange of primary particles, leading to a homogeneous granulation, whereas if granule breakage is minimal, there may be a preferential layering of the fine particles in the large granules. This layering of the large granules with the fine particles was found to take place regardless of whether the fine particles in the powder mix were those of the drug substance or of the diluent.[39] In addition, drug solubility was found to be an important factor in the homogeneity of drug in the granules.[37] The authors found that, depending on the drug solubility, the over-wetted regions in the initial stages of wet granulation may contain a significantly different drug concentration from the rest of the granules, leading to different drug concentrations in the different granule sizes. Miyamoto et al.[36] found that drug solubility, in addition to binder level, influenced the drug distribution in the different size granules. Drug distribution among coarse and fine granules was also found to be dependent on the water level used for the wet granulation, where less than optimal levels of water led to super-potent coarse granules and sub-potent fine granules.[35]

In addition to the process parameters during wet granulation, process parameters during the drying step may also be important for the drug uniformity in the granules and the finished drug product. For example, solute migration should be evaluated in case of soluble active ingredients, especially for tray drying, and active ingredient loss through the filters should be evaluated for fluidized bed drying. As granules dry, dissolved solutes migrate from the inside of the granules to the outer surfaces of the granules. This solute migration leads to the precipitation of the dissolved ingredients (including drug) on the surface of the granules. Upon sizing of the dry granules, fines will be enriched with the drug due to the abrasion of this drug rich surface layer.[44,45]

The above discussion illustrates that for a wet granulation process to be used for a low-dose formulation, the effect of process parameters on active ingredient uniformity and potential loss during the manufacturing steps should be evaluated, in addition to the study of the effect of such process parameters on the commonly studied drug product properties (e.g., effect of granulation end point on granule particle size distribution, density, and porosity, effect of granulation vehicle amount and granulation time on compressibility of granulation, and effect of granulation end point on dissolution of the finished product).

The process described in this path (i.e., addition of active ingredient in the dry state to the excipient blend prior to granulation) may be utilized to produce a concentrated granulation. For example, if the drug load in the finished drug product is 0.1%, a concentrated granulation containing 1% of drug may be manufactured, followed by dilution of this concentrated active granulation with excipients or with a placebo granulation. Such an approach has the obvious advantage of improving the uniformity of the active ingredient in the concentrated granulation because a higher drug load is utilized. In addition, there may be a lower risk of drug loss during the manufacturing steps or transfer steps due to the higher drug load in the concentrated granulation. This approach may also be very useful because multiple tablet/capsule strengths may be manufactured using a common active granulation. However, mixing of the concentrated active granulation with the extragranular excipients or placebo granules becomes important and should be well evaluated. Even though wet granulation lowers the risk of segregation because the active ingredient particles are "fixed" within the granule structure, segregation among active and nonactive granules may take place if their properties are not matched properly. Thus, the physical properties of both the concentrated active granulation as well as the extragranular materials are important such that appropriate uniformity is achieved following the dilution step to reach the desired strength without any significant segregation.

5.5.2 Addition of Drug Substance to the Granulation Vehicle

In this scenario, the active ingredient is either dissolved or suspended in the granulation vehicle and then used to granulate the dry excipient blend. Such an approach may have two main advantages. First, uniformity of the active ingredient in the granulation may be improved, especially if the active ingredient is dissolved in the granulation vehicle. This is because the active ingredient is mixed at the molecular level with the excipient powder particles. Second, such an approach should improve the containment of the potent, low-dose drug product since the active ingredient is not utilized in the dry state in the manufacturing operations that often lead to higher operator exposure (e.g., blending, de-agglomeration by use of a Comil®).

In this process, a solution or a suspension of the active ingredient is prepared in the granulation vehicle. If a solution of both the active ingredient and the binder is used, the order of component addition to the granulation vehicle may be important. The formulation scientist may want to consider dissolving the active ingredient in the vehicle first, the binder is then dissolved in the active ingredient solution. Alternatively, if the binder is dissolved first, followed by addition of the active ingredient to the viscous solution, longer mixing times may be needed to achieve uniformity of the active ingredient in the viscous binder solution. Another approach may be to prepare two separate solutions of the binder and the active ingredient, and then to mix the two solutions together.

In case of drug suspensions, the formulation scientist will need to evaluate the need for a homogenization step in order to improve the uniformity of the suspension prior to wet granulation. In addition, appropriate measures should be used to prevent settling of the drug particles from the suspension prior to and during the wet granulation process. The use of binders in the granulation vehicle may lower the risk of drug particle settling from the suspension because of the higher viscosity. However, mechanical agitation may still be needed to ensure uniformity of the suspension throughout the process.

A critical factor that should be evaluated here is the chemical and physical stability of the active ingredient in the granulation vehicle, regardless of whether a solution or a suspension of the drug substance is used. The active ingredient should have appropriate chemical stability in the granulation vehicle. If the active ingredient is dissolved in the granulation solution, the active ingredient should be chemically stable in such a vehicle for an appropriate amount of time in order to minimize any degradation prior to and during the granulation and drying processes. The active ingredient may be in solution for hours prior to granulation, in addition to the time between the wet granulation step and drying of the granules. In addition, the granules may be exposed to higher than ambient temperatures during the granulation step in addition to the high temperatures utilized during the drying step. Understanding the mechanisms of drug degradation pathways in solution becomes very important if the active ingredient is to be dissolved in the granulation vehicle, and the effect of solution components and solution properties (e.g., use of cosolvents or alcohols in the granulation vehicle, solution pH, presence of co-solutes, ionic strength) should be studied thoroughly. In particular, solution pH and solution temperature effects should be studied appropriately. Generation of pH-stability profiles may prove very advantageous. For example, the use of pH-modifiers in the granulation vehicle or in the excipient blend may improve the chemical stability of the active ingredient.[46]

As expected, the use of active ingredient suspensions instead of solutions may limit the impact of any potential chemical stability issues.[47] This is because only the portion of the active ingredient that is dissolved will be subjected to the chemical degradation pathways in solution (e.g., hydrolysis). The use of active ingredient suspensions in the granulation vehicle instead of an active ingredient solution may be forced onto the formulation scientist due to the poor solubility of the active ingredient. However, the granulation vehicle may be designed by the formulation scientist such that the solubility of the active ingredient is minimized. This may be achieved by the appropriate selection of active ingredient salt (or the use of the free acid or base form of the active ingredient),[48] or by the appropriate selection of solution components, cosolutes, pH, or ionic strength.[49] In this approach, the use of active ingredient suspensions to alleviate issues with chemical stability of dissolved active ingredient should be beneficial. However, this approach generates other challenges to the formulation scientist like the selection of an appropriate active ingredient particle size, de-agglomeration or homogenization process, and agitation of the suspension to minimize settling of the active ingredient particles.

Physical stability of the active ingredient is an important factor that should not be overlooked. The effect of polymorphism on properties of both the active ingredient (e.g., chemical stability, solubility, dissolution rate) and the drug product (e.g., bioavailability) have been extensively studied. Polymorphs or amorphous states of the active ingredient may impact chemical stability as well as dissolution rates, solubility, and bioavailability. This should be studied appropriately. This is discussed further in the sections below.

5.5.3 Impact of Particle Size of API and Excipients on Product Uniformity

The particle size of the starting materials in wet granulation can impact granulation agglomeration and granule properties[50,51] as well as the uniformity.[38,41,42] It is well known that particle size of the active ingredient is very important for low-dose formulations, and should be controlled for each formulation in order to attain an acceptable product uniformity.[17] However, the particle size of the excipients may also be an important factor that may influence the uniformity of the finished granules as well as the uniformity of the finished drug product. As discussed earlier, there may be a strong interplay between the properties of the materials in the formulation (e.g., physical properties of the active ingredient as well as the excipients like particle size, solubility, and surface area), and the process parameters used during preparation of the wet granulation. Thus, it may be hard to generalize any rules; however, there may be some general themes that can be extracted from published investigations. It is also important to note that the majority of the published investigations focused on the homogeneity within granules (e.g., in coarse vs fine granules) rather than focusing on the uniformity of the finished drug product. While an inhomogeneity in the drug content within the different granule size fractions may potentially lead to uniformity problems in the finished drug product, this inhomogeneity in granule drug content will not necessarily lead to a nonuniform drug product in the absence of segregation among the different granules.

One example of the effect of excipient particle size is provided by Egermann et al.[42] Salicylic acid was granulated with lactose at a level of 0.5%. Micronized or crystalline salicylic acid was granulated with crystalline or micronized lactose in a planetary mixer. When the drug was smaller in particle size than the diluent, the granule fines were subpotent, and coarse granules were superpotent. On the other hand, when the drug particle size was larger than that of the diluent, the granule fines were superpotent and the coarse granules showed appreciable variation in drug content. The best uniformity was attained when micronized salicylic acid was granulated with micronized lactose.

The effect of particle size of active ingredients and excipients was also studied by Vromans et al.,[38] where the impact of the granulation process parameters was different depending on the particle sizes of the active ingredient and the excipients. Using a steroid hormone at a level of 0.01%, the authors found that drug content in the granules ranged between 50% and 150% when micronized hormone was granulated with unmicronized lactose. The uniformity was worse when an unmicronized hormone was used for the granulation where variation in the drug content in the granules was found to range between 40% and 225%. On the other hand, the authors found that the best uniformity in the drug content in the different granule sizes was found when a micronized hormone was granulated with micronized lactose.[38]

Van den Dries and Vromans[41] studied three different particle sizes of lactose with a low-dose formulation containing micronized estradiol at a drug load of 0.1%. A "demixing potential" was calculated which related to the nonuniform distribution of the drug in the different sized granules. It was found that a large demixing potential was always associated with an increase in the drug concentration in the large granules and a decrease in the drug concentration in the small granules. The authors also found that the effect of the particle size of the diluent was clear. A low demixing potential, relating to a good uniformity, was found when there was a small difference in the particle size between the diluent and the drug substance (23 and 5 μm, respectively). However, a good uniformity was also obtained when a larger diluent particle size was used (~141 μm) while the worst uniformity was obtained with an intermediate diluent particle size (50 μm). In that study, the effect of process parameters (wet massing time) was also studied and showed that the effect of the wet massing time on the uniformity of granule drug content was least important when the diluent particle size was closer to that of the active ingredient.

5.5.4 Case Studies

Even though a large number of publications focus on various aspects of wet granulations (e.g., effect of starting material properties on final granules, effect of process conditions, and effect of granulation equipment), only a few examples can be found in the literature that focus on low-dose formulations and the effect of material properties or process conditions on the uniformity of the finished product. One such example is a study that compared low-shear, high-shear, and fluidized bed granulations on the uniformity of a low-dose tablet formulation at a drug load of 0.1%.[52] The formulation consisted of the drug, lactose monohydrate, microcrystalline cellulose (Avicel® PH102), povidone, crospovidone, and magnesium stearate. In this study, the drug was either dissolved or suspended in the granulating fluid in order to improve the uniformity in the finished product. The low-shear granulation was done in a V-blender with an intensifier bar (Patterson-Kelly), the high-shear granulation was done in a GRAL 25 (Collette), and the fluidized bed granulation was done in a GPCG-5 (Glatt). In addition, a Diosna VAC20 (Servolift) and a Quadro comil were used.

TABLE 5.4 Process Parameters and Uniformity Data for Tablets Manufactured Using Different Granulation Methods

Process	Powder Blending	Liquid Addition Rate, mL/min	Granulation Time, min	Minimum Mean Tablet Assay (%)	Maximum Mean Tablet Assay (%)	%RSD
Low-shear wet granulation (V-blender)	5 min with I-bar on	60–150	10–15	96.8	97.8	2.2–2.6
High-shear wet granulation (GRAL)	3 min	300	3–7	97.5	100.8	0.7–1.6
High-shear wet granulation (Diosna)	Not available	300	7	99.1	106.1	0.6–1.9

Table 5.4 lists some of the process parameters used to manufacture the granulations along with the uniformity data for the resultant tablets.[52] The authors also tested methanol as a granulation fluid instead of water. In all cases, the uniformity of the finished tablets was acceptable with small RSD values regardless of the process used (low-shear, high-shear, or fluid bed), even though the properties of the granules were slightly different depending on the granulating fluid or the manufacturing process used. This example shows the utility of dissolving the API in the granulation fluid where the API will be added to the formulation at the molecular level, leading to excellent uniformity.

5.6 PROCESS-INDUCED FORM CHANGES IN WET GRANULATION

The appropriate selection of the active ingredient polymorphic form or the use of an amorphous active ingredient in drug products is an important decision that preformulation and formulation scientists evaluate for each drug product.[53] In addition, any process-induced form changes should be studied thoroughly during product development. This is true for any drug product, and for any manufacturing platform, and wet granulation is no exception. As a matter of fact, wet granulation may be the most likely oral dosage form manufacturing process to result in phase changes.[54] This is due to the conditions used in wet granulation that may exacerbate phase transformations and, thus, a thorough evaluation of any process-induced form changes due to the wet conditions during granulation, as well as the use of high temperatures during drying, should be considered. These transformations often take place through solution or solution-mediated mechanisms. Solution-mediated transformations to a more stable polymorphic form or the formation of a hydrated form are possible.[55] Also, a portion of the active ingredient may dissolve in the granulation vehicle during wet granulation, especially for soluble active ingredients. This portion of active ingredient that dissolves during wet granulation may precipitate out of solution as an amorphous content, or may crystallize into the same or a different polymorphic form than what was used in the formulation. The final form(s) in the formulation is thus not only affected by the wet granulation process only, but also by the drying conditions. Drying conditions (temperature, humidity, speed) may be determining factors in any potential phase transformations, especially when the dissolved portion of the drug substance precipitates as an amorphous content or when enantiotropic forms of the drug substance exist whose transition temperature approaches the drying temperature.[56]

Studying such phase transformations by conventional techniques (e.g., X-ray powder diffraction) may not be feasible for potent drugs that are present in the formulation at low levels. Other methods may be more appropriate for such cases, like solid-state NMR techniques.[57] The different analytical techniques used to study potential phase transformations will not be discussed here, because this is the focus of another chapter in this book.

A good understanding of these potential API phase transformations is very important if the active ingredient is dissolved or suspended in the granulation vehicle prior to wet granulation. The advantages of the use of a solution or a suspension of the active ingredient are outlined in the section above. However, the possibility of process-induced form changes should be investigated in such cases, especially if a drug solution is utilized.[58] If a drug solution is used, the drug may form a metastable or an amorphous form after drying.[55] Even if the drug is added dry to the formulation blend and was not intentionally dissolved in the granulation vehicle, some drug dissolution during the wet granulation process is inevitable depending on the drug solubility, the amount of granulation solution added, granulation time, and the method of addition of the granulation solution.

If an amorphous form is generated in the finished granules, the dissolution rate will be fastest immediately after the drug product is manufactured. If this amorphous form crystallizes slowly upon storage, the dissolution rate may become slower on storage. This may or may not have implications on the in vivo performance of the drug product, depending on the solubility and the permeability of the drug substance, and the intended use of the drug product. Thus, for highly soluble, stable, and bioavailable drug substances, the impact of phase transformation on product stability and bioavailability is low.

The kinetics of the possible phase changes are important in determining whether such changes will be complete during the manufacturing process, or on storage.[55] The extent of conversion will depend on the amount of drug substance dissolved during the wet granulation process, which depends on the solubility, dissolution rate, amount of granulation vehicle used, the amount of time used during the wet granulation and drying processes, and the temperatures achieved during the drying process.

There are several examples in the literature of drug physical form changes during wet granulation. Williams et al.[59] studied the effect of wet granulation on physical form stability. Wet conditions (aqueous granulation fluids, manufacturing delays between granulation and drying steps) led to dissociation of a highly crystalline hydrochloride form to an amorphous free base. This dissociation/transformation was studied by *in-situ* Fourier transform (FT) Raman spectroscopy. In another example, wet granulation led to a chemical instability and that was associated with a solution-mediated transformation of an anhydrate form to an amorphous form.[54,60] Because of the low drug load used in these formulations, the authors utilized a formulation containing a 30% drug load to study this solution-mediated transformation and concluded that a wet granulation method was not appropriate for that active ingredient. Their investigation revealed that during wet granulation there was a conversion from the anhydrous to the monohydrate form, which later transformed to the amorphous forms during drying with other excipients. These excipients inhibited the crystallization of the amorphous form in the formulation, leading to poor chemical stability of the tablets.[54] The authors also promoted the use of polarized light microscopy to qualitatively evaluate process-induced transformations in low-dose formulations because it may be difficult to identify the drug form in low-dose formulations using typical techniques [e.g., differential scanning calorimetry

(DSC), X-ray powder diffraction (XRPD)].[60] These literature examples and others indicate that, for low-dose formulations, the formulation scientist may be forced to use qualitative techniques, and may have to study higher drug loads in order to evaluate the potential of drug form changes due to the wet granulation process. Also, the formulation scientist should evaluate other indirect methods of assessment of drug solid form changes in the formulations (e.g., dissolution testing, chemical stability).

It is noteworthy to mention here that there are examples in the literature, indicating that the observed process-induced transformations following a wet granulation process may be influenced by the excipient selection in the formulation. This has been reported for theophylline and nitrofurantoin.[61,62] This effect was attributed to either the water absorbing ability or the crystallinity of the filler. Data indicated that the potential for drug substance form changes was lower if the formulation contained amorphous fillers or fillers with a higher water absorbing ability. Moreover, the effect of drug loading in the formulation and the amount of granulating fluid on phase transformation has been investigated[63] and the potential for phase transformations has been found to be higher for lower drug loads. This clearly indicates that phase transformations during wet granulations may be more critical for low-dose formulations.

5.7 CONCLUDING REMARKS

Wet granulation is the most commonly used manufacturing process for oral dosage forms. It is the manufacturing method that has been used the longest in the pharmaceutical industry. Different pharmaceutical companies have different preferences with regard to the selection of the manufacturing process for tablets or capsules and some companies may prefer dry manufacturing methods instead (direct compression or roller compaction). However, wet granulation remains the most robust manufacturing method. It is the method that has the best ability to mask the variability in the properties of the incoming raw materials (particle size, density, porosity, compressibility, surface area), thus ensuring a robust and predictable performance.

The manufacture of low-dose formulations is challenging to the formulation scientists regardless of the method used for the drug product manufacture. Often, the selection of one manufacturing process over another is driven by the properties of the drug substance itself. Wet granulation may not be feasible for moisture- or heat-sensitive compounds or for compounds that have a high tendency to undergo phase transformation in wet conditions, leading to poor chemical stability or to unpredictable drug product performance. However, wet granulation is the most studied drug product manufacturing method and is the method that is the most established across the pharmaceutical industry. The complexity of the wet granulation method may be viewed as a disadvantage. However, this method, through its multiple manufacturing processes, provides the formulation scientist with numerous steps that can be taken advantage of in order to influence and control the drug product, so that the quality of the finished drug product is built through multiple steps, as opposed to utilizing a simpler process (e.g., blend and compress) which may be more risky.

REFERENCES

1. Torres-Suarez AI, Gil-Alegre ME. 1997. Wet granulation. In: Swarbrick J and Boylan JC, editors. Encyclopedia of pharmaceutical technology, volume 16. New York: Marcel Dekker.
2. Summers M, Aulton M. 2002. Granulations. In: Aulton M, editor. Pharmaceutics: science of dosage form design. London: Churchill Livingstone.
3. Kristensen HG, Schaefer T. 1987. A review on pharmaceutical wet-granulations. Drug Dev. Ind. Pharm. 13(4–5): 803–872.
4. Kristensen HG, Schaefer T. 1992. Granulations. In: Swarbrick J and Boylan JC, editors. Encyclopedia of pharmaceutical technology, volume 7. New York: Marcel Dekker.
5. Iveson SM, Litster JD, Hapgood K, Ennis BJ. 2001. Nucleation, growth and breakage phenomena in agitated wet granulation processes: a review. Powder Technol. 117: 3–39.
6. Holm P, Lundbeck H. 1997. High shear mixer granulators. In: Parikh DM, editor. Handbook of pharmaceutical granulation technology. New York: Marcel Dekker.
7. Holm P, Jungersen O, Schaefer T, Kristensen HG. 1983. Granulation in high speed mixers. Part 1: Effects of process variables during kneading. Pharm. Ind. 45: 806.
8. Holm P, Jungersen O, Schaefer T, Kristensen HG. 1984. Granulation in high speed mixers. Part 2: Effects of process variables during kneading. Pharm. Ind. 46: 97.
9. Holm P, Schaefer T, Kristensen HG. 1985. Granulation in high-speed mixers. Part VI. Effects of process conditions on powder consumptions and granule growth. Powder Technol. 43: 225–233.
10. Holm P, Schaefer T, Kristensen HG. 1985. Granulation in high-speed mixers. Part V. Power consumption and temperature changes during granulation. Powder Technol. 43: 213–223.
11. Schaefer T, Bak HH, Jaegerskou A, Kristensen A, Svensson JR, Holm P, Kristensen HG. 1986. Granulation in different types of high speed mixers. Part 1: effects of process variables and up-scaling. Pharm. Ind. 48: 1083.
12. Hunter BM and Ganderton D. 1973. The influence on pharmaceutical granulation of the type and capacity of mixers. J. Pharm. Pharmac. 25(suppl.): 71P–78P.
13. Gao JZH, Jain A, Motheram R, Gray DB, Hussain MA. 2002. Fluid bed granulation of a poorly water soluble, low density, micronized drug: comparison with high shear granulation. Int. J. Pharm. 237: 1–14.
14. Johnson MCR. 1972. Particle size distribution of the active ingredient for solid dosage forms of low dosage. Pharm. Acta Helv. 47: 546–559.
15. Yalkowsky SH, Bolton S. 1990. Particle size and content uniformity. Pharm. Res. 7: 962–966.
16. Egermann H. 1991. Comments on "Particle size and content uniformity," by Yalkowsky and Bolton. Pharm. Res. 8: 1076–1077.
17. Rohrs BR, Amidon GE, Meury RH, Secreast PJ, King HM, Skoug CJ. 2006. Particle size limits to meet USP content uniformity criteria for tablets and capsules. J. Pharm. Sci. 95: 1049–1059.
18. Augsburger LL, Hahm HA, Brzeczko AW, Shah U. 2007. Super disintegrants: characterization and function. In: Encyclopedia of pharmaceutical technology. New York: Marcel Dekker; 3553–3567.

19. Gordon MS, Rudraraju VS, Dani K, Chowhan ZT. 1993. Effect of the mode of super disintegrant incorporation on dissolution in wet granulated tablets. J. Pharm. Sci. 82(2): 220–226.
20. Zhao N, Augsburger LL. 2006. The influence of granulation on super disintegrant performance. Pharm. Dev. Technol. 11(1): 47–53.
21. Record PC. 1980. A review of pharmaceutical granulation technology. Int. J. Pharm. Technol. Prod. Manuf. 1: 32–39.
22. Rohera BD, Zahir A. 1993. Granulation in a fluidized-bed: effect of binders and their concentration on granule growth and modeling the relationship between granule size and binder concentration. Drug Dev. Ind. Pharm. 19: 773–792.
23. Sirois PJ, Craig GD. 2000. Scale-up of a high-shear granulation process using a normalized impeller work parameter. Pharm. Dev. Technol. 5(3): 365–374.
24. Faure A, Grimsey IM, Rowe RC, York P, Cliff MJ. 1999. Process control in a high shear mixer-granulator using wet mass consistency: the effect of formulation variables. J. Pharm. Sci. 88(2): 191–195.
25. Faure A, York P, Rowe RC. 2001. Process control and scale-up of pharmaceutical wet granulation processes: a review. Eur. J. Pharm. Biopharm. 52(3): 269–277.
26. Faure A. Grimsey IM, Rowe RC, York P, Cliff MJ. 1999. Applicability of a scale-up methodology for wet granulation processes in Collette Gral high shear mixer-granulators. Eur. J. Pharm. Sci. 8: 85–93.
27. Levin M. 2006. Wet granulation: end-point determination and scale-up. In: Encyclopedia of pharmaceutical technology. New York: Marcel Dekker; 4078–4098.
28. Holm P, Schaefer T, Larsen C. 2001. End-point detection in wet granulation process. Pharm. Dev. Technol. 6(2): 181–192.
29. Ridgway K and Rubinstein MH. 1971. Solute migration during granule drying. J. Pharm. Pharmac. 23(suppl.): 11S–17S.
30. Motzi JJ, Anderson NR. 1984. The quantitative evaluation of a granulation milling process II. Effect of output screen size, mill speed and impeller shape. Drug Dev. Ind. Pharm. 10(5): 713–728.
31. Kato Y, Namiki T, Kawamura M. 2004. Effects of oily drug rheology on content uniformity in granules obtained by wet granulation with a high-shear mixer. Drug Dev. Ind. Pharm. 30(6): 649–655.
32. Kornchankul W, Parikh NH, Sakr A. 2000. Effect of process variables on the content uniformity of a low dose drug in a high shear mixer. Pharm. Ind. 62(4): 305–311.
33. Zoglio MA, Huber HE, Koehne G, Chan PL, Carstensen JT. 1976. Physical aspects of wet granulation II: factors involved in prolonged and excessive mixing. J. Pharm. Sci. 65(8): 1205–1208.
34. Badawy SF, Gray DB, Hussain MA. 2006. A study of the effect of wet granulation on microcrystalline cellulose particle structure and performance. Pharm. Res. 23(3): 634–640.
35. Kato Y, Moroshima K, Hashizume M, Ando H, Furukawa M. 2001. Further observation of content uniformity of d-alpha-tocopheryl acetate as an oily drug in granules obtained by wet granulation with a high-shear mixer. Drug Dev. Ind. Pharm. 27: 781–787.
36. Miyamoto Y, Ryu A, Sugawara S, Miyajima M, Ogawa S, Matsui M, Takayama K, Nagai T. 1998. Simultaneous optimization of wet granulation process involving

factor of drug content dependency on granule size. Drug Dev. Ind. Pharm. 24(11): 1055–1065.

37. Ojile JE, Macfarlane CB, Selkirk AB. 1982. Drug distribution during massing and its effect on dose uniformity in granules. Int. J. Pharm. 10: 99–107.
38. Vromans H, Poels-Janssen HGM, Egermann H. 1999. Effects of high-shear granulation on granulate homogeneity. Pharm. Dev. Technol. 4(3): 297–303.
39. Van den Dries K and Vromans H. 2003. Experimental and modelistic approach to explain granulate inhomogeneity through preferential growth. Eur. J. Pharm. Sci. 20: 409–417.
40. Van den Dries K, de Vegt O, Girard V, Vromans H. 2003. Granule breakage phenomena in a high shear mixer; influence of process and formulation variables and consequences on granule homogeneity. Powder Technol. 133: 228–236.
41. Van den Dries K, Vromans H. 2002. Relationship between inhomogeneity phenomena and granule growth mechanisms in a high-shear mixer. Int. J. Pharm. 247: 167–177.
42. Egermann H, Reiss W. 1988. Effect of particle size of drug and diluent on drug distribution in granule size fractions. Acta Pharm. Technol. 34: 5S.
43. Scott AC, Hounslow MJ, Instone T. 2000. Direct evidence of heterogeneity during high-shear granulation. Powder Technol. 113: 205–213.
44. Selkirk AB. 1976. The effect of solute migration on the distribution of borax throughout a batch of granules. J. Pharm. Pharmac. 28: 512–515.
45. Warren JW and Price JC. 1977. Drug migration during drying of tablet granulations. II. Effect of binder solution viscosity and drying temperature. J. Pharm. Sci. 66: 1409–1412.
46. Badawy S, Vickery R, Shah K, Hussain M. 2004. Effect of processing and formulation variables on the stability of a salt of a weakly basic drug candidate. Pharm. Dev. Technol. 9(3): 239–245.
47. Martin A, Bustamante P, Chun AH. 1993. Physical pharmacy, 4th ed. Baltimore, MD: Williams and Wilkins.
48. Gould PL. 1986. Salt selection of basic drugs. Int. J. Pharm. 33: 201–217.
49. Yalkowsky SH. 1999. Solubility and solubilization in aqueous media. Washington, DC: American Chemical Society/New York: Oxford University Press.
50. Badawy SF, Hussain MA. 2004. Effect of starting material particle size on its agglomeration behavior in high shear wet granulation. AAPS PharmSciTech. 5(3): Article 38.
51. Badawy SF, Lee TJ, Menning MM. 2004. Effect of drug substance particle size on the characteristics of granulation manufactured in a high-shear mixer. AAPS PharmSciTech. 1(4): Article 33.
52. Hausman DS. 2004. Comparison of low shear, high shear, and fluid bed granulation during low dose tablet process development. Drug Dev. Ind. Pharm. 30(3): 259–266.
53. Haleblian J, McCrone W. 1969. Pharmaceutical applications of polymorphism. J. Pharm. Sci. 58: 911–929.
54. Zhang GZ, Law D, Schmitt EA, Qiu Y. 2004. Phase transformation considerations during process development and manufacture of solid oral dosage forms. Adv. Drug Delivery Rev. 56: 371–390.
55. Morris KR, Griesser UJ, Eckhardt CJ, Stowell JG. 2001. Theoretical approaches to physical transformations of active pharmaceutical ingredients during manufacturing processes. Adv. Drug Deliv. Rev. 48: 91–114.

56. Grunenberg A, Henck JO, Siesler HW. 1996. Theoretical derivation and practical application of energy/temperature diagrams as an instrument in preformulation studies of polymorphic drug substances. Int. J. Pharm. 129: 147–158.
57. Stephenson GA, Forbes RA, Reutzel-Edens SM. 2001. Characterization of the solid state: quantitative issues. Adv. Drug Delivery Rev. 48: 67–90.
58. Wostheinrich K, Schmidt PC. 2001. Polymorphic changes of thiamine hydrochloride during granulation and tabletting. Drug Dev. Ind. Pharm. 27: 481–489.
59. Williams AC, Cooper VB, Thomas L, Griffith LJ, Petts CR, Booth SW. 2004. Evaluation of drug physical form during granulation, tabletting and storage. Int. J. Pharm. 275: 29–39.
60. Wardrop J, Law D, Qiu Y, Engh K, Faitsch L, Ling C. 2006. Influence of solid phase and formulation processing on stability of Abbott-232 tablet formulation. J. Pharm. Sci. 95(11): 2380–2392.
61. Airaksinen S, Karjalainen M, Kivikero N, Westrmarck S, Shevchenko A, Rantanen J, Yliruusi J. 2005. Excipient selection can significantly affect solid-state phase transformation in formulation during wet granulation. AAPS PharmSciTech. 6(2): Article 41.
62. Airaksinen S, Luukkonen P, Jorgensen A, Karjalainen M, Rantanen J, Yiliruusi J. 2003. Effects of excipients on hydrate formation in wet masses containing theophylline. J. Pharm. Sci. 92(3): 516–528.
63. Herman J, Remon JP, Visavarungroj N, Schwartz JB, Klinger GH. 1988. Formation of theophylline monohydrate during the pelletization of microcrystalline cellulose–anhydrous theophylline blends. Int. J. Pharm. 42: 15–18.

CHAPTER 6

CHALLENGES IN DEVELOPMENT AND SCALE-UP OF LOW-DOSE DRUG PRODUCTS BY DRY GRANULATION: A CASE STUDY

MARY T. AM ENDE, DANIEL O. BLACKWOOD, DANIEL S. GIERER, and CHRISTOPHER P. NEU

Pfizer Global Research & Development, Oral Products Center of Emphasis, Pfizer, Inc., Eastern Point Road, MS 8156-01; and Groton, CT 06340

6.1 INTRODUCTION

The design and development of low-dose solid drug products present a unique set of challenges for the formulator and process scientist. Low dosage strengths are generally considered for drug loadings of less than 1% by U.S. standards or less than 2% by European standards, where such dosage forms are considered specialized and potentially categorized as nonstandard.[1,2] Since the issues associated with low dosage strength products are exaggerated with greater dilution, this chapter focuses on the higher-dilution situation (<1%), although the designation of "standard" or "specialized" formulation will be case-specific.

The currently preferred drug product processing method selected for low-dose (high-dilution) drugs is wet granulation. Other manufacturing platforms, such as dry granulation and direct compression, have been also used for the manufacture of low-dose drug products. In this chapter, the specific formulation and process challenges resulting from dry granulation development are discussed, including agglomeration, content uniformity, segregation, loss of drug, and sampling technique. The authors demonstrate that the issues associated with dry granulation for low-dose drugs can be overcome by proper design and control of the formulation and process. Moreover, dry granulation offers significant advantages over wet granulation approaches, especially in terms of stability and process efficiency, such that in many cases it may be the preferred granulation technique. To illustrate how the challenges

Formulation and Analytical Development for Low-Dose Oral Drug Products. Edited by Jack Zheng

can be overcome while maintaining the advantages of dry granulation, two case studies with 0.25–1.0% drug loading are examined in details.

In developing these case studies, an overview of the dry granulation equipment, dividing it into three physical operations including (i) the feed system; (ii) the roller compaction system; and (iii) the granulator or mill system, is provided. The technology transfer strategy in scale-up and equipment design type changes is also discussed. The formulation challenges for successfully producing these dry granulated dilute products are described, including agglomeration of the API, excipient selection, propensity for segregation, enhancement of chemical degradation due to excipient—API interaction, film coating ingredient—API interactions, and sampling issues for the blends compared to tablets. Specifically, the two case studies are compared with regard to the target API particle size specification in relation to the final tablet potency uniformity. The process challenges are described considering their impact on blend content uniformity, tablet content uniformity, and subsequent compression properties. A comparison of blending equipment types and approaches is described (high-shear dry blending, tumble blending, and serial dilution blending). The optimization of the dry granulation process to minimize segregation potential was determined to impact subsequent compression during tableting. Therefore, the optimization strategy was considered over multiple process steps to ensure performance with a balanced view. The case studies presented in this chapter demonstrate that dry granulation is a viable option worthy of serious consideration as the lead for new low-dose drug products being developed.

6.2 DRY GRANULATION PROCESS—PROS AND CONS

Commercial products with less than 1 mg active ingredient(s) are readily available in tablet and capsule forms. There are more than 24 products listed in the *Physician's Desk Reference*,[3] with dosage strengths as low as 25 μg. The two most common treatment classes utilizing low dosage strengths are for hypothyroidism and birth control/hormone replacement therapies. However, low-dose products are available across multiple treatment classes and a cross-section of commercially available products has been tabulated in Chapter 1 of this book. Based on ingredients listed, an experienced formulator would conclude these products were processed predominantly by wet granulation.

Dry granulation processing offers improved chemical and physical compatibility compared to wet granulation, while being comparable with direct compression. Granulation (wet or dry) lowers the potential for segregation as compared to direct compression. Dry granulation also requires fewer variables for scale-up and technology transfer to a commercial site when compared to wet granulation, which requires an additional drying operation to remove the granulating agent.

The major disadvantages of dry granulation are the reduction in tablet compressibility, formulation-dependent process optimization, and inconsistency of equipment types with respect to the process parameters being measured (e.g., roll force vs roll pressure), thus complicating transfer between equipment types. In spite of these challenges, dry granulation should be considered as a viable, and even preferred, process option in many cases.

6.3 OVERVIEW OF DRY GRANULATION PROCESSES AND EQUIPMENT DESIGN

For solid oral dosage forms, the manufacturing process for high potency compounds is nearly identical to the manufacturing process for "standard" (nonlow-dose) products. Generally, the same equipment is utilized and the same regulatory guidances apply for both low and standard dose products. However, in the case of powder blend uniformity guidance, increased sampling intensity may be expected for low-dose products to detect any content uniformity issues in the final drug product to ensure that uniformity is not lost during subsequent material transfer and processing operations.[4,5]

Blending is a key unit operation used to achieve adequate uniformity prior to granulation, and prior to tableting or encapsulating. Low-dose formulations may require more mixing energy to uniformly blend the material compared to a standard formulation with traditional blending techniques (e.g., bin blending). Other approaches can be investigated in lieu of blending for a longer time and include blend–mill–blend processing, where the material is passed through a screening mill between blends to reduce agglomeration and aid in mixing, or high-shear granulation in a dry blending mode. Table 6.1 presents these two examples for manufacturing processes of low-dose products. The option for an additional blend step after dry granulation is included in the process flow diagrams to account for the addition of extragranular excipients (e.g., lubricant), but is not required.

Dry granulation is a common and well precedented method of processing in the pharmaceutical industry. Through this technology the particle size and density of an active blend can be specified and controlled, and a polydisperse blend can be transformed into more uniform granules. Particle size and density play a large part in the segregation potential, flow, and compressibility for subsequent processing steps.

With low-dose products, flow and compressibility are relatively minor issues since formulations are essentially placebos. The low percentage of active loading allows for the addition of ample amounts of excipient(s) that possess good flow

TABLE 6.1 Dry Granulation Manufacturing Process Approaches: (1) Blend Mill and (2) High Shear-Dry Blend

Blend Mill for Drug A	High-Shear Dry Blend for Drug B
Blend	Dry blend in high-shear granulator
Mill	
Blend	Blend
Dry granulation	Dry granulation
Blend	Blend
Tablet compression/capsule filling	Tablet compression/capsule filling
Tablet coating	Tablet coating

and compression properties. The key concern for a low-dose product is achieving and then maintaining content uniformity (i.e., minimizing segregation potential). Dry granulation will not improve the uniformity of an up-stream blend, but it will generally aid in maintaining the uniformity during down-stream processing. For this reason, ordered mixing is used to improve uniformity in the blend prior to feeding the dry granulator (see Section 6.5.2).

One of the major flaws in dry granulation for low-dose products is the granulation efficiency is lower than wet granulation. The material that bypasses the rolls, referred to as bypass, is the source of the incomplete granulation by roller compaction. Equipment factors that affect bypass in the feed system, roller compaction system and mill system are the focus of the discussion below.

The most common form of dry granulation is roller compaction. A roller compaction system consists of a feed system which conveys powder between two counter-rotating rolls. The powder is drawn between the rolls where a specified force is applied causing the powder to compact into a briquette or a continuous "ribbon." The compacted material can then be milled in-line or collected and milled off-line in a separate processing step (i.e., screening mill).

Quality attributes of the compact formed during roller compaction are a function of the blend properties and the roller compaction equipment design and operating parameters. Similarly, the final granulate properties are related to the compact properties and the selected milling equipment design and operating properties. The operating parameters will be specific to the attributes of the in-going blend; however, the focus of this section is on the equipment design aspects. This section provides an overview of the design of various marketed roller compactors by breaking the units into their functional sections described in the Table 6.2. For the granulator/mill system, only in-line mills are discussed.

6.3.1 Feed System Designs

The feed system of a roller compactor generally consists of a connection point for a blender, an intermediate hopper, and a screw auger conveyance system. Screw feeders convey powder by use of a slowly rotating screw or screws depending on the hopper and roll arrangement. Since the powder conveyance is slow, there is little opportunity for segregation in the direction of transport. A schematic of four typical feed system arrangements located above the roller compaction region can be found in Fig. 6.1, depicted with an intermediate hopper.

TABLE 6.2 Functional Sections of a Dry Granulator

Section	System	Function
A	Feed system	Convey loose powder to rolls
B	Roller compaction system	Densify/compact loose powder into ribbons or briquettes
C	Granulator/mill system	Mill ribbons or briquettes into granules

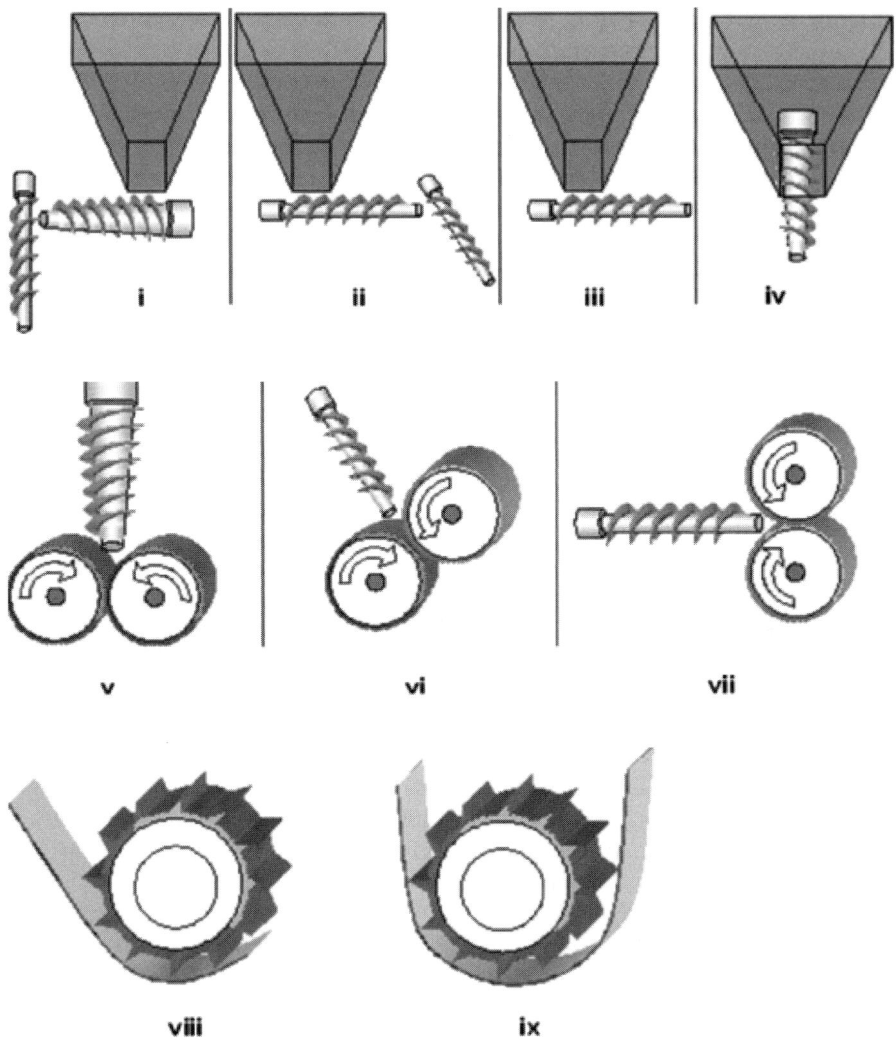

Figure 6.1 Schematic diagrams depicting different dry granulation designs (four typical feed systems with intermediate hoppers; three typical roller compaction systems; and two typical granulator systems).

In the case of low-dose formulations, it is important that the feed system convey material without allowing the material to segregate. All of the feed system arrangements shown in Fig. 6.1 rely on gravity feed for the powder to reach the force feeding screws. Feed systems i, ii, and iii can be outfitted with an agitator in the intermediate hopper which will aid in powder flow and delumping.

Feed systems i and iv detail an auger that is tapered. Bates[6] has shown that tapered augers, compared to nontapered augers, have improved feeding for powder conveyance. Figure 6.1 presents the "off the shelf" unit arrangements. Each unit can be customized with various augers and other add-ons depending on the blend properties and desired granulation properties.

The pitch of the screw can also have a major impact on the feeding properties of powders. A uniform pitch flight construction empties the contents of one end of the hopper, leaving the remaining level of material undisturbed until the extraction has worked its way along the screw.[6] This cascading effect can cause segregation issues if the hopper is not well agitated. Any new material dispensed to the intermediate hopper will find its way into the drawdown channel and discharge before the original load. The best screw design to avoid this issue is one where the screw pitch offers a continuously increasing capacity along its length. Additionally, if the intermediate hopper is agitated then the powder can be forced into the screw flights thereby negating this effect.

Ultimately, the feed system is not only responsible for conveying powder to the rolls, but also aiding in an initial deaeration of the blend. Weggel[7] found that the torque on the feed system screw(s) is directly related to the precompaction pressure. He concluded that by maintaining a constant back pressure, the resulting compact quality can be better controlled.

The ungranulated material bypassing the rolls is a source of potential segregation concern, since the particle size and bulk density are not being altered. Bypass is mostly a function of the equipment design, specifically attributed to the feed system, roll surface, and roll orientation. The feed system will cause bypass if excessive pulsing and/or any uneven feed of powder is experienced by the roller compaction system. This can cause fluctuations in the gap width, which if not controlled by a properly tuned controller, can cause fluctuations in ribbon or briquette properties. Fluctuations from the feed system occur most often for poorly flowing and/or highly cohesive blends. For low-dose drug products designed using cohesive blends to facilitate ordered mixing, the feed system fluctuations are an important factor to consider during development and commercialization.

6.3.2 Compaction Roll Designs

The compaction system consists of two, counter-rotating rolls at equivalent speeds. One roll is normally fixed while the other is allowed to "float." The floating roll was implemented to control the roll gap. The roll force is applied to the floating roll by hydraulic pressure, which is counteracted by the normal force of the fixed rolls. This force is subsequently applied to the blend in the gap. A schematic of three typical roller compaction system arrangements with a feed screw can be found in Fig. 6.1.

Through this technology, a powder blend is consolidated into a continuous ribbon or briquette. Figure 6.2 details two roll designs, one briquetting and the other continuous ribbon-forming. The designs can take a blend with a wide distribution in particle size and create a more uniform ribbon or briquette that can then be milled toward a target granulation particle size distribution. A compaction roller also has the effect of improving and equalizing the final blend density. Although granulation and densification are achieved by roller compaction, the factors affecting bypass must be

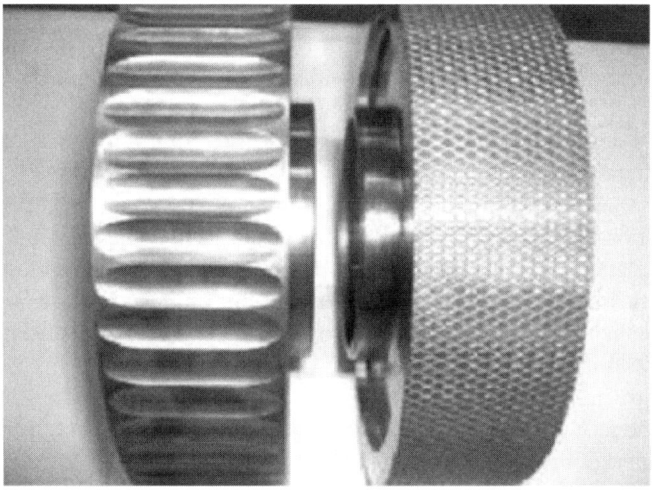

Figure 6.2 Dry granulation roll design options: briquetting (left) and continuous ribbon (right).

understood and controlled to minimize the impact on content uniformity in the final product. Equipment factors that affect bypass in the roller compaction system include roll surface roughness, roll orientation, and vacuum deaeration.

Bypass is ungranulated material that circumvents the rolls completely, or passes between the rolls without being sufficiently compacted. This material has neither been densified nor sized, and poses a possible risk for segregation. In most pharmaceutical applications, and low dosage strength tablets specifically, the component of the blend with the smallest particle size is the API. If the API is not "adsorbed" onto the excipients, this can become a critical problem for low-dose formulations since the material that bypasses compaction is often the material with the smallest particle size.

The roll surface is important in maintaining a back pressure on the powder flow so powder does not pass through the nip region faster than the rolls are turning.[8] This is one of the most common causes of bypass and its impact is magnified for low-dose formulations. Fortunately, it can be corrected easily by using rolls with a greater surface roughness or textured surfaces (i.e., knurled rolls). There are three different types of continuous ribbon rolls with different surface designs intended to maintain this back pressure, including knurled roll, serrated roll, and smooth roll.

The roll orientation can also play a large role in generating bypass. Roller compaction orientation v, shown in Fig. 6.1, is susceptible to significantly more bypass than vi or vii. In orientation v, powder is flowing with gravity unless there is sufficient back pressure (from rolls with a rough surface), and therefore material can pass through without being compacted. In orientations vi and vii, direct bypass through vertical rolls is minimized since the powder rides on the rolls and therefore would be preferred for low-dose products.

One means of mitigating the amount of bypass due to the selected roll surface and roll orientation is the use of side seals on one roller when available. Side seals create interlocking rolls which almost completely eliminate the ability for powder to bypass perpendicular to the roll. A small amount of powder may still bypass due to the high pressures in the compaction zone if the side seals and rolls do not have a precision machine fit. Side seals can significantly reduce the overall material bypass; however, this does not reduce the risk of material passing through the rolls without being sufficiently compacted.

An additional general method to reduce bypass is through vacuum deaeration. Miller[9] performed experiments on a low-density active blend with and without vacuum deaeration, while holding all other parameters constant, and quantified the bypass for each trial. With the vacuum deaeration engaged, the bypass rate was ~2% as compared to the control rate of over 20%. He also observed that the powder feed was uneven and the compact quality was not uniform. Most units are equipped with this capability and it should be considered to minimize bypass for low-dose products. However, vacuum deaeration can cause potency loss, unless the collected material is recirculated to the feed system.

The overall recommendation for the roller compaction system design that minimizes bypass is to employ a higher surface roughness or textured surface on the rolls, rolls oriented similar to vi or vii, and to conduct an assessment of vacuum deaeration.

6.3.3 Granulator/Mill System Designs

The product from the roller compaction system is a ribbon or briquette, and therefore a mill must be used to convert these compacts into a granulation with reasonable flow properties. As depicted in Fig. 6.1, most designs of roller compactors employ an in-line oscillating mill where the main difference between granulator viii and ix is the orientation of the mill screen. The differences in mill screen orientation do not impact the final particle size. The only purpose is to allow for more material to be held in the mill while it is in operation (mill orientation viii). More material in the mill will generally increase the throughput slightly due to more mass holding the material against the screen.

The mill rotor design can also be changed to impart more or less energy (through contact surface area). Utilizing a mill rotor with more surface area may increase the throughput of the mill, thus reducing the residence time in the mill. A long residence time in the mill may overprocess the material and reduce its available compressibility for downstream processing (i.e., compression). There are two mill rotor designs with significantly different surface areas, that is, star design or pocket design. The pocket-designed rotor provides more contact area between the rotor, ribbon or briquette, and the mill screen thereby imparting more energy into the material to aid in granulation. However, the star or pocket-designed rotor may be used since both generally produce a granulation with a similar particle size distribution.

Mill screens come in many sizes and types. The mill screen size should be selected based on the desired particle size of the granulation. In situations when the granulation is blended with extragranular excipients, the preferred strategy is to target similar particle size distributions for the granulation and extragranular component to minimize segregation.

The two main types of mill screens are wire mesh and rasping plates. Wire screens allow milling in both directions (clockwise and counter-clockwise), while the rasping screens mill in one direction. Rasping screens can generate a slightly denser granulation compared to a wire screen due to the shearing action inherent to the design, though they both generate comparable particle size distributions for a given screen size.

The overall recommendation for the roller compaction mill system design that minimizes bypass or fines is to utilize an efficient rotor design (e.g., pocket) and a rasping screen.

6.4 CHALLENGES FOR LOW-DOSE PRODUCT DEVELOPMENT AND THEIR ASSESSMENT METHODS

The active pharmaceutical ingredient in a low-dose formulation is typically a small molecule, designed to meet a small particle size requirement for uniformity purposes, and can be susceptible to effects of static charge and segregation. The impact of static charge on the accuracy of blend uniformity measurements (i.e., sampling bias) is discussed in the next section.

6.4.1 Segregation

Segregation is mainly caused by particle size and/or particle density difference between materials in a bulk blend. Particle shape and surface roughness impact the segregation potential, but to a lesser degree. There are two main types of segregation in pharmaceutically relevant processing,[10] which are due to intraparticle interactions and to external forces (i.e., unconfined flow). Therefore, segregation can occur whenever bulk materials are in motion, which includes handling, transport, conveying, or vibrating operations.

Sifting Segregation. Sifting segregation occurs when particles in a blend have different particle sizes or a broad particle size distribution, and when the blend is moving, as defined by Prescott and Hossfeld.[10] The sifting segregation potential can be tested by following ASTM: D 6940-03.[11] This ASTM covers the required apparatus and the method for testing a bulk powder or blend for its sifting segregation potential.

The movement of the blend allows gaps to occur between the larger particles that can be filled by the smaller particles. By this segregation mechanism, a blend that is well mixed at the top of a dynamic region may become significantly segregated near the end of the dynamic region. Differences in particle density will magnify the impact of sifting segregation. If sifting segregation is an issue for a bulk powder or blend, it is important to control uniformity for the final granulation particle size distribution and particle density through process optimization.

Fluidization Segregation. In order for fluidization segregation to occur, particles in a blend must have different particle sizes and/or a broad particle size distribution as well as different particle densities. This type of segregation may occur when a bulk powder or blend is pneumatically conveyed, filled or discharged at high rates, or if counter-current gas flow is present. A counter-current gas flow can develop if a pipe or unit operation is not properly vented and a vacuum occurs. The potential for this type of segregation can be tested by following ASTM: D 6941-03.[12] This ASTM covers the required apparatus and the method for testing a bulk powder or blend for its fluidization segregation potential.

Fine particles (mean particle size $<100\ \mu m$) generally have a lower permeability than coarse particles and therefore tend to be retained in the air longer. Thus on filling a hopper, the coarse particles are driven into the bed while the fine particles remain fluidized near the top surface. This can also occur after tumble blending if the material is fluidized during blending.

If fluidization segregation is an issue in a bulk powder or blend, it is more important to normalize the blend particle size distribution and particle density. Again, this can be achieved through milling or through a granulation technology unit operation (i.e., roller compaction). Additionally, minimizing drop heights and reducing blender speeds may help avoid fluidizing the bulk powder or blend, thereby further reducing the risk of fluidization segregation.

Sieve Cut Potency. An additional method to assess the segregation potential of a blend or granulation is sieve cut potency. Through sieve cut potency, the potency distribution of the blend or granulation can be determined as a function of the particle size distribution. Ideally, the potency distribution is spread equally over the range of particle sizes. This is rarely the case in blends unless a particle size operation (i.e., milling) has been implemented to narrow the particle size distribution. Granulation techniques will aid in improving sieve cut potency if the correct process parameters are selected.

The sieve analysis is carried out in order to determine the geometric mean granule size and sieve cut potency variability, or sieve cut potency %RSD. The sieving is performed at conditions that are previously determined to cause no detrimental effect on the particle size distribution. The samples collected from each sieve are analyzed for potency using the appropriate analytical method. Individual sieve cut samples for these case studies ranged from 0.5 to 2 g, and were analyzed in their entirety, allowing for a more accurate assessment of the amount of drug present in each sieve cut sample. The variability in drug potency as a function of particle size is assessed by calculating the percentage relative standard deviation (%RSD) of the sieve cut potency samples for each run.

For low-dose drug products, the dry granulation processing should be optimized to minimize the segregation potential or tendency, although the impact of the resulting granulation properties should be thoroughly investigated on subsequent manufacturing processes.

6.4.2 Blend Uniformity and Sampling Issues

With dilute formulations, segregation can result in unacceptable variations in tablet or capsule potencies. While one approach to achieving API content uniformity is to eliminate the driving force for segregation by matching particle sizes and densities of major diluents with the API, for low dosage strength applications, the small API particle size needed based on distribution statistics makes this approach impractical due to its detrimental impact on blend flow and electrostatic charge. A preferred approach for low-dose products is to promote strong interactions between small particle API and large particle excipient(s) both by the choice of excipients and the granulation technology.

Once the formulation and manufacturing process for a new chemical entity is defined by the formulator, the next challenge is identifying an acceptable technique for achieving representative blend sampling. The sampling technique must be able to take a nonbiased, representative blend sample capable of assessing the true content uniformity of the powder blend. Regulatory agencies generally expect blend content uniformity testing, in fact industry guidance states that such sampling should be a routine in-process control test.[4,5] This can pose quite a few challenges, particularly for low-dose formulations.

Sampling biases can occur from differences in particle size distribution, particle density, particle shape, and particle electrostatic charge. Minimizing these particle property differences will increase the likelihood that the blend content uniformity is a true representation of the batch.[13,14] It also aids in the reduction of sampling bias which will improve the experimental blend content uniformity.

Garcia et al.[15] discussed the greatest challenge for their low-dose product as developing a nonbiased technique to sample blends that is representative of the true content uniformity. Their product formulation is similar to the formulation developed for model Drug B at an active loading of 2%. Their studies demonstrated that the blend was uniform when (i) the bin blender was grounded for at least 4 days prior to sampling, or (ii) the sample size was increased from 2× to 20× the unit dose weight (i.e., 200 mg to 2.0 g). The latter eliminated the preferential API filling into the sampling thief. That work was performed on a powder that was mixed in a low-shear blender and then compressed. A granulation technology will generally reduce the segregation potential of the blend as well as improve the flow, thereby reducing the sampling bias due to thief type.

Kornchanbul et al.[16] determined that mixing of low-dose products was a challenge because the mixer was unable to break up agglomerates for their product. Their work also demonstrated that longer mix times were required to achieve the target uniformity for low-dose blends comparing a 10-fold difference in drug loading (0.5 vs 5.0% API loading).

The stratified tablet sampling methodology specifically targets problematic areas during a compression run to increase the probability of detecting an aberrant content uniformity result. The key is to concentrate sample points in problematic areas of the batch (i.e., start-up, bin change-over if applicable, and shutdown) as opposed to evenly spacing the sample locations throughout the batch. The key to effective stratified sampling is balancing the number of samples and sample locations such that accurate data is obtained without making analytical testing the rate limiting step.

6.5 CASE STUDY: FORMULATION CHALLENGES FOR LOW-DOSE PRODUCTS

Dry granulation processing has been implemented for low-dose products, but has not traditionally been the first choice. In fact, it is not currently possible to predict from molecular properties of the API that dry granulation processing will be suitable to ensure stability and manufacturing performance. At present, there are empirical methods, such as tableting indices measurements and compaction simulator experiments, to predict the dry granulation properties. Scientific advancements are necessary to transform the level of fundamental understanding. A few examples of opportunities in this field include measuring particle-particle interactions between API and excipients, measuring interactions between particles and equipment surfaces, and predicting their impact on flow, manufacturability, and potency losses to equipment. However, when dry granulation processing works, the advantages of continuous operation with reduced unit operations make it a highly desirable process from a commercial perspective. As an illustration, two model drugs have been developed using dry granulation processing with the details discussed in this chapter.

In the case studies discussed here, dry granulation was selected for the solid dosage form manufacturing process. These formulations were developed relying on the concept of ordered mixing.[17,18] The theory behind ordered mixing, also referred to as carrier-mediated or interactive mixing, is that small drug particles will adhere to the surface of excipients with sufficiently larger particle size. A mixing study conducted by Orr and Sallam compared the random and ordered mixing concepts.[19] Their findings revealed that tablet potency results were skewed in distribution and were attributed to the cohesive properties of small API particles not disrupted from their agglomerated state. Kornchankul et al.[16] discussed targeting API-to-excipient particle sizes to be similar for random mixing and to be small-to-large to achieve ordered mixing, respectively. In addition, they determined that certain particle shapes, such as that of microcrystalline cellulose, affected flow and caused bridging. Poor flow of the blend was detrimental to uniform die filling, and therefore resulted in higher variability for tablet potency content uniformity. These interactive mixing methods rely on API interacting more favorably with excipients than other API particles, balancing API agglomerate formation with cohesive interaction.

The cohesive and adhesive properties of an API promote interactions with excipients or other API particles to form agglomerates. Loosely bound API agglomerations break down readily through mechanical methods vs interaction with diluents. In 2006, am Ende and Rose reviewed methods of achieving the target API particle size to fit the needs of the dosage form.[20] The extent of API—excipient interaction is a function of the mixing process and diluent flow properties.[21,22] Generally, more free-flowing diluents facilitate faster mixing, which is attributed to their abrasive properties acting mechanically to disperse the agglomerated API. API tensile strength and flow properties may also indicate the magnitude of energy to disperse agglomerates. Cheng[23] developed a theory for the tensile strength of powders being a function of density, particle size distribution, and interparticulate forces. These concepts support the formulation rationale for the drugs employed in the case studies presented in this chapter. For instance, granular forms of lactose, microcrystalline cellulose, and dicalcium phosphate dibasic anhydrous were selected for their particle size, cohesive and abrasive properties. The case studies presented in this chapter demonstrate methods for overcoming challenges for dry granulation products, including achieving good content uniformity, minimizing segregation, blend sampling, and loss of drug to equipment surfaces. Dry granulation is a viable commercial manufacturing process, and it is important to consideration as a preferred process for new chemical entities being developed.

Oral drug product formulation and manufacturing process development can use a hierarchical approach to meeting three conditions based on, in order of importance, bioavailability, stability, and manufacturability. The bioavailability of a drug product is the most critical condition and must meet established criteria or the product is not viable. Drug substance properties such as salt form, solubility, and particle size can significantly affect pharmacokinetic and pharmacodynamic performance of a product. The dosage form platform, formulation design, and manufacturing process can also affect the PK/PD profile of a product. Therefore, all selections must maintain the required pharmacokinetic/pharmacodynamic outcome and work within these confines to achieve a stable and robust product/process.

While the bioavailability target of the drug is being defined, the drug product is also often under development with stability as the primary quality attribute. A stable dosage form target can be more challenging for a low-dose product. Adequate chemical and physical stability is often considered to be at least a two year shelf-life for a commercially viable product. Formulation design can aid in assuring drug product stability by selection of nonreactive excipients or by indicating additives that counter degradation reactions; however, other factors can be implemented to assist in stabilizing the drug product. For example, packaging and storage controls, such as the addition of a desiccant for moisture control, a foil blister for light and moisture control, antioxidants (e.g., oxygen scavengers, peroxide quenchers and chain terminators) for oxygen control, or refrigeration for temperature control, are routinely utilized to enhance product stability.[24]

Manufacturability and product performance/robustness are important conditions; however, the solutions to these challenges often have more flexibility in achieving acceptability and are rarely rate-limiting conditions. For example, content uniformity is a manufacturing challenge for low-dose drug products that can be addressed by multiple pathways. Content uniformity of the dosage form can be achieved and maintained through formulation design (i.e., API particle size, physical and mechanical properties, as well as excipient selection), manufacturing selection (e.g., wet granulation, dry granulation process), and equipment/engineering controls (e.g., mass flow bins/hoppers, control feed systems). Figure 6.3 is a flow diagram summarizing the formulation development process based on the three conditions described above and has been applied to the development of Drugs A and B. Although bioavailability remains the most critical factor in the initial formulation design, for the purpose of this discussion, it is assumed that the bioavailability is independent of the formulation and process.

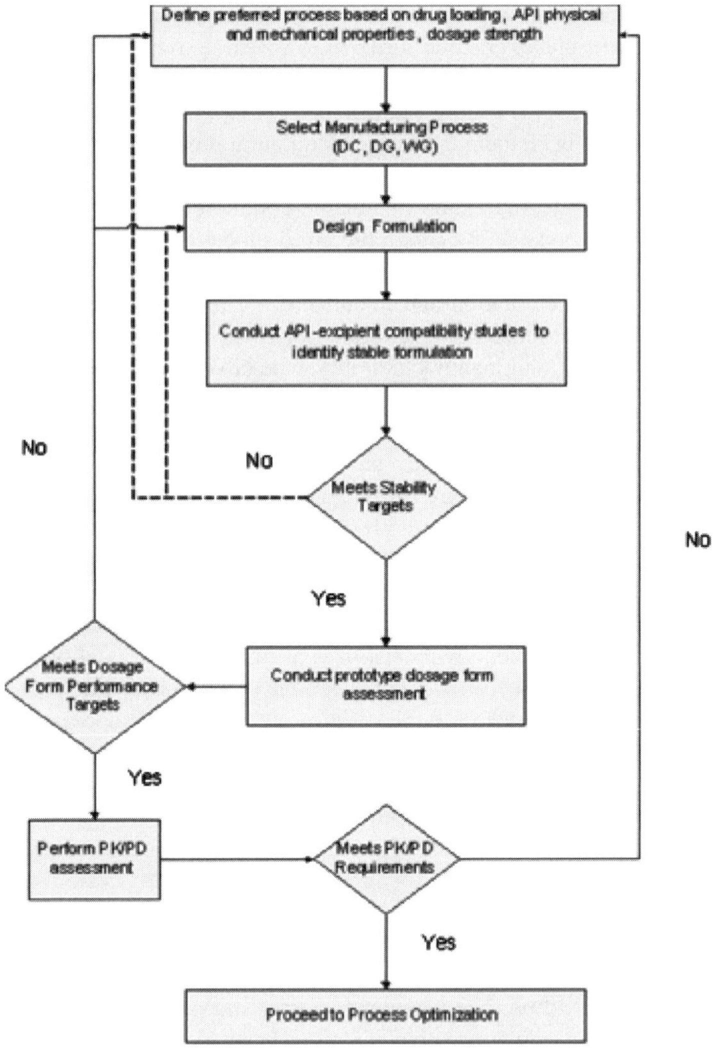

Figure 6.3 Formulation flow chart for designing and developing drug products.

6.5.1 Chemical Stability Challenge in Designing Formulation

The challenges of developing a high potency solid drug product ($\leq$1 mg dose) largely are due to low drug loading of 1% or less. To ensure homogeneity, wet granulation processes are commonly preferred in the pharmaceutical industry; however, the benefits achieved from utilizing a wet granulation process can be offset by the increased occurrence of chemical instability of the active drug substances sensitive to water or solvents (e.g., hydrolysis and/or polymorph conversion). Therefore, an alternative approach is the use of a dry granulation process to achieve a robust product which can maintain homogeneity and potentially improve chemical stability. In this chapter, case studies of Drugs A and B are discussed and shown to demonstrate the successful application of dry granulation processing in conjunction with formulation design to develop low-dose immediate-release film-coated tablets.

Dry granulation can be a preferred process approach with respect to ensuring physical and chemical stability as compared to wet granulation, in which the drug substance is exposed to solvent and elevated temperatures for a short period of time. However, low-dose tablets produced by dry granulation may also exhibit stability issues from film coating, which exposes the dosage form to solvent, elevated temperatures and additional excipients. Table 6.3 provides basic general pharmaceutics background on model drug candidates, Drugs A and B. Although both compounds were considered stable drug substances, manufacturing process selection and formulation design were critical in developing a robust commercial drug product.

Excipient compatibility studies are considered to be an important assessment tool during early dosage form development. Binary and/or ternary excipient blend mixtures with Drug A or B were prepared and stored at elevated temperature and humidity conditions. The excipient compatibility results presented in Table 6.4 indicate that, at elevated temperature and humidity, sodium starch glycolate and a film-coating plasticizer, polyethylene glycol, are reactive with Drug B. The purity profiles from excipient compatibility studies of Drug A suggest that lactose is not a preferred excipient for tablet core or film coating, unlike the results from Drug B. In addition, these stability results for Drug A were used to identify croscarmellose sodium as the preferred disintegrant, similar to the findings for Drug B. These results suggest the two main degradation mechanisms affecting the formulations of Drugs A and B are oxidation and the Maillard reaction.

Oxidation is a common degradative pathway concern for pharmaceutical dosage forms.[25] Oxidation is generally described as the loss of one or more electrons. Oxidative mechanisms include autoxidation, electron transfer, peroxide, catalysis, acidity, and pH effects. Amines are known to be susceptible to oxidation, resulting in the formation of N-oxides. Additionally, the two most common groups of excipients associated with peroxide impurities are the polymeric ethers; examples include polyethylene glycols, polysorbates and polyethylene oxides, and polyvinylpyrrolidone-based excipients. It is also important to consider any ingoing raw material or excipient manufacturing process that incorporates a bleaching operation, using peroxide or hypochlorite, which can contain residual impurities as exemplified by some cellulosics.[25]

TABLE 6.3 Summary of General Pharmaceutics for Model Drugs A and B

Property	Drug A	Drug B
Structure	Secondary amine	Tertiary amine
Solubility	>10 mg/mL in pH buffer 8	0.66 mg/mL in unbuffered water (pH 3.8)
Hygroscopicity	Not applicable	Not applicable
Formulation drug loading	≤1% w/w	≤1% w/w

TABLE 6.4 Total Percentage Impurities for Excipient Compatibility Studies with Drug A or B Stored for 6 Weeks at 40°C/75% Relative Humidity

Excipient(s)	Drug A	Drug B
MCC	—	ND
MCC/DCP	0.1	—
Mannitol/DCP	0.1	—
Lactose anhydrous	—	ND
Lactose hydrate	—	ND
Lactose/DCP	2.6	—
Pregelatinized starch	—	ND
Croscarmellose sodium	ND	0.1
Sodium starch glycolate	0.6	3.2
Polyvinylpyrrolidone	0.3	0.3
Polyethylene glycol	—	1.7 (12 weeks)
Triacetin	—	0.2 (6 months)
Hypromellose, titanium dioxide, PEG	1.2[a]	—
Hypromellose, titanium dioxide, triacetin	1.6[a]	—
Hypromellose, lactose, titanium dioxide, triacetin	3.9[a]	—
Polyvinyl alcohol, titanium dioxide, PEG	3.3[a]	—

MCC, microcrystalline cellulose; DCP, dicalcium phosphate, anhydrous; ND, not detected.
[a]Accelerated stability condition was 70°C/75% RH for 1 week.

Based on this knowledge, oxidation is the probable explanation for the destabilizing effects of sodium starch glycolate, polyvinylpyrrolidone, and polyethylene glycol on Drug B. Data also support oxidation as the primary degradation pathway for Drug A, which is consistent with N-oxide being identified as the most prevalent degradant. Hartauer et al.[26] reported a similar occurrence with raloxifene hydrochloride. Raloxifene hydrochloride, as a tertiary amine, generated an N-oxide degradant in the presence of povidone and crospovidone.

Another well-known degradation pathway for solid oral drug products is the Maillard reaction. The Maillard reaction is a chemical reaction between an amino acid and a reducing sugar and is a form of nonenzymatic browning. Qiu et al.[27] break down the Maillard reaction into three stages. The first stage is the condensation of the amine and reducing sugar, forming water and a ketoseamine, and the second stage is the degradation of the unstable ketoseamine. The third stage is the formation of the color and flavor compounds. The Maillard reaction is known to occur more readily with primary and secondary amines.[27] This is consistent with the degradation pathways for model Drugs A and B, and provides supporting evidence for the increased reactivity of the secondary amine containing Drug A with the reducing sugar, lactose, as compared to the tertiary amine of Drug B. To further investigate the excipient reactivity of Drug A, film-coated tablets were studied following an accelerated stability challenge. The excipient compatibility results for some commonly used film coating systems is shown in Table 6.4. The results indicate destabilization of Drug A when in the film coating contained lactose. HPLC analysis revealed the primary degradant peak associated with the lactose-containing film coating eluted at the same relative retention time as that identified in the drug–lactose excipient compatibility studies.

In addition to the thermal and humidity challenge that must be met in developing a stable drug product, for wet granulation processing, solvent exposure can increase the occurrence of drug instability. The most common granulating solvent used in a wet granulation process is water and the addition of a binder is typically required. Commonly used binders include the polyvinylpyrrolidone-based excipients (e.g., povidone), and cellulose-based excipients (e.g., hydroxypropyl and hydroxypropylmethyl celluloses).[28] Water may serve a key role in destabilizing an active compound. The use of water during the granulation process can lead to the generation of amorphous drug or interaction with the existing amorphous portion of the drug substance that results from increased mobility and reactivity of the material.[29] Drugs A and B were wet granulated and assessed for chemical stability. The formulations for each compound contained components previously determined to be stable in a dry granulation process, except for the use of water as the granulating solvent and the addition of a binder. A binder solution was added to an active dry blend and granulated for Drugs A and B. An additional trial of dissolving Drug B in the binder solution was also assessed. As reported in Table 6.5, a wet granulation process destabilized Drugs A and B. The total impurities and/or the primary oxidative degradant levels significantly increased in the presence of water. Thus, wet granulation is not an appropriate manufacture process for this compound.

A common approach to offset oxidative degradation is through the addition of antioxidants to the formulation. Akers[30] generally classified antioxidants as delaying the formation of free radicals (e.g., metal sequestering agents—ethylenediaminetetraacetic acid, EDTA), preventing the free radical chain reaction (e.g., water insoluble antioxidants—butylated hydroxyl toluene, BHT), and preferred substitute compounds (e.g., water-soluble antioxidants—ascorbic acid). However, antioxidants are frequently unable to completely prevent oxidation for an extended period of time without additional controls such as suitable packaging. The use of antioxidants was not fully evaluated for these products because the dry granulation process was selected considering the preferred chemical stability and faster development timelines.

TABLE 6.5 Chemical Stability of Granules for Model Drugs A and B Made by Wet Granulation and Stored in HDPE Bottles

	5% w/w Povidone	5% w/w Hydroxypropyl Cellulose	5% w/w Povidone	1% w/w Hydroxypropyl Cellulose
Drug	B	B	B	A
API addition	Dry	Dry	Solution	Dry
Granulating solvent	Water	Water	Water	Water
Storage condition	Total percentage impurities at 6 weeks' storage			Percentage *N*-formamide
40°C/75% RH	2.6	4.3	7.5	0.1
50°C/20% RH	2.2	5.3	10.2	0.2

Through appropriate formulation and manufacturing selection, Drugs A and B were designed into dry granulated formulations that achieved chemical and physical stability. The formulations were designed as stable, commercially viable drug products, and therefore did not require additional external controls.

6.5.2 Formulation Design and Development for Low-Dose Products

Designing a drug product formulation is dependent on the process selected, as denoted in the formulation flowchart (Fig. 6.3). In these two case studies, dry granulation processing was selected over wet granulation or direct compression based on meeting the target stability, commercially viable processing with no additional need for external controls to assure stability. The formulation scientists developing these two drug products set additional design criteria that favored interactive mixing to accentuate blend uniformity prior to granulation. Furthermore, the formulations and process operations were designed to ensure manufacturing and bioavailability performance. For these reasons, the major diluents of microcrystalline cellulose, lactose and dicalcium phosphate, were selected for their (i) chemical compatibility with API, (ii) large particle size for interactive mixing and flow, and (iii) mechanical properties. The diluent component levels (listed in Table 6.6) were utilized at precedented levels for the ingredient function.[31]

The physical and mechanical properties of excipients were important variables in achieving performance of the final products as well. The preferred formulation strategy for a low-dose product using dry granulation is to design a cohesive blend to

TABLE 6.6 Physical and Mechanical Properties of the Drug and Diluents Used in the Low-Dose Dry Granulation Formulations

Physical or Mechanical Property	Model Drugs	Diluent 1	Diluent 2	Diluent 3
Component	Drug A or B	Microcrystalline cellulose	Lactose anhydrous	Dibasic calcium phosphate anhydrous
Primary deformation mechanism	Ductile	Ductile	Brittle fracture	Brittle fracture
Percentage in formulation	0.25–1.0%	25–63%	0–70%	0–33%
True density (g/cm^3)	1.8	1.6	1.6	2.8–2.9
Bulk density (g/cm^3)	0.7	0.3–0.4	0.5	0.7–0.8
Geometric mean Diameter (μm)	<35	100–180	~100	180
Cohesivity (s)	—	5.0 (low)	6.0 (moderate)	3.7 (very low)
Tensile strength (MPa)	—	2.8–6.9 (high)	1.8 (moderate)	1.3 (moderate)
Flow category	—	Good	Good	Good

minimize segregation.[10] In the case of Drug B tablets, the formulation contains lactose to produce a cohesive blend and it was found to be less prone to segregation (see "Process Challenges during Dry Granulation Optimization for Low-dose Products" Section 6.6). However, Drug A was chemically incompatible with the cyclic sugar, and therefore the major brittle diluent selected for this dosage form was anhydrous dicalcium phosphate. Important manufacturing benefits were realized for the latter formula in terms of providing a wide operating region for tablet compression force–hardness profile.

In this section, two case studies are compared with regard to the target API particle size specification in relation to the final tablet potency uniformity. The process challenges are described considering their impact on blend content uniformity, tablet content uniformity, and subsequent compression properties. A comparison of blending equipment types and approaches is described (high-shear dry blending, tumble blending, and serial dilution blending). The optimization of the dry granulation process to minimize segregation potential was determined to impact subsequent compression during tableting. Therefore, the optimization strategy was considered over multiple process steps to ensure performance with a balanced view.

6.5.3 Development of Target API Particle Size Specification

The target drug substance particle size specifications for Drugs A and B were set based on a theoretical model and experimental data generated from studies performed to determine the effect of drug substance particle size distribution on the content uniformity of the tablets.

A theoretical model was used during early development to estimate the effect of drug substance particle size on content uniformity.[32] This computer model simulates the number, size, and mass of the drug particles in the batch and distributes them evenly across all unit doses. The input data included the lowest dosage strength of 0.25 mg for Drug B and 0.5 mg for Drug A, the drug substance density of 1.4 and 1.3 g/cm^3, respectively, and the geometric standard deviation of 1.8 based on batch history at that time. Based on achieving content uniformity in each dosage form (i.e., setting conservatively at 100% potencies between 97% and 103%), this computational method predicted a geometric mean particle size of 29 μm and a D95 of 75 μm for the drug substance. The model assumptions include ideal mixing and a log–normal function for the particle size distribution, and therefore the model output is considered as a preliminary target and supportive information to the experimental results.

Drug A is characterized as a highly soluble and highly permeable drug substance. Therefore, the particle size of the drug substance (over the range studied) had no impact on the in vitro performance (i.e., dissolution or disintegration) of the drug product. Content uniformity of the drug product was the primary attribute in the setting of the particle size specification.

Segregation of drug substance from its excipients during transfer and processing is a main concern for low-dose formulations; therefore the stratified core tablet content uniformity results, which should be a more discriminating test than content

TABLE 6.7 Analytical Results for Stratified Tablet Samples

Number of Locations	Mean Potency (% Target)	Potency Range (% Target)	RSD (%)
10	97.1	93.0–102.7	2.73
31	96.8	93.0–102.7	1.89

uniformity of film-coated tablets, were used to support the establishment of the drug substance particle size specification.

A prototype formulation for model Drug A on a commercial scale was manufactured and two stratified sampling location plans were utilized: one plan for 31 sampling locations and the other plan for a 10 sampling locations. Table 6.7 summarizes the stratified sampling locations (as a function of the percentage of the batch compressed). As can be seen, the formulation showed no major segregation at the beginning and the end of compression. For the 10-location stratified sampling scheme, 60% of the stratified samples were taken within 7% of startup or shutdown (targeted for two events where segregation is most likely to be seen). Only 40% of the samples were taken over the remainder of the compression run where there is the most confidence in the potency of tablets being on target. For the 31-location stratified sampling scheme, 45% of the stratified samples (14 of 31 tablets) were taken within 7% of startup or the end of compression, with the remaining 55% of the samples being taken during the portion of the run where the chance of finding an aberrant tablet is minimal. The %RSD data demonstrate that fewer locations resulted in a higher value (2.7 vs 1.9% for 10 vs 31 locations, respectively). Both sampling schemes provide comparable potency means and ranges (Table 6.7). Additionally, both sampling schemes pass the FDA stratified sampling criteria. The benefit of the 10-location sampling scheme is that it requires approximately one-third the analytical testing of the 31-location sampling scheme while producing results that are less biased by the portion of the run where the chance of finding an aberrant tablet is minimal.

The stratified tablet core content uniformity is presented by manufacturing facility and scale in Tables 6.8 and 6.9 as a function of mean drug substance particle size $D[4,3]$ for Drugs A and B, respectively. The development batches produced at laboratory scale ranged from 1 to 3 kg batch size and employed a broad range of mean drug substance particle size ($D[4,3]$) ranging from 13 to 60 μm. These development batches demonstrated tablet content uniformity with %RSD $<1.5\%$. The pilot and commercial-scale batches (50–150 kg) employed drug substance with mean particle size ($D[4,3]$) of 6.5 to 33 μm for Drug A. The particle size distribution of Drug B was determined by a light scattering technique and was represented by two parameters: $D[4,3]$ or VMD (volume mean diameter), and $D(v,0.9)$. Low-dose tablets (0.25 mg) have been successfully manufactured at two manufacturing sites with acceptable uniformity using drug substance lots with VMD values less than or equal to 34 μm, and $D(v,0.9)$ values less than or equal to 68 μm.

The results shown in Tables 6.8 and 6.9 demonstrate that the stratified tablet core content uniformity %RSD values for these batches were $\leq 5\%$. Film-coated tablet

TABLE 6.8 Effect of Mean Size of Drug A on Stratified Tablet Core Content Uniformity at Different Scales and Manufacturing Sites

	Stratified Tablet Content Uniformity (%RSD)		
D[4,3] (μm)	Laboratory Scale	Pilot Scale	Commercial Scale
6.5	—	1.6	—
11	—	0.8	—
13	0.8	1.8; 3.0	—
16	—	2.7	1.0; 1.2
17	—	1.3; 1.6	0.8
18	—	—	1.1; 1.2
19	—	—	1.3
25	—	1.8	—
26	—	1.4; 2.0	1.1; 4.1
29	—	1.4; 2.3	1.2; 1.2; 1.3; 1.4
29	—	—	1.4; 1.4; 2.0
33	—	2.2; 2.2	0.9; 1.2; 1.9; 2.1
60	1.2	—	—

content uniformity %RSD values for these large-scale batches were <2.5%, well below the acceptable limit of 5.0%. These results further support the demonstration that stratified tablet content uniformity is a more sensitive method for detecting potency and uniformity issues as compared to film-coated tablet content uniformity.

Based on the supporting theoretical model, and the experimental results on tablet content uniformity, the API particle size specifications can be established. For model Drug A, *D*[4,3] and *D*(*v*,0.9) were ≤35 and ≤100 μm, respectively, while particle sizes *D*[4,3] and *D*(*v*,0.9) for Drug B were ≤20 and ≤50 μm, respectively.

TABLE 6.9 Effect of the Particle Size of Drug B on Stratified Tablet Core Content Uniformity at Pilot and Commercial Scales

	Stratified Tablet Content Uniformity (%RSD)	
D[4,3] (μm)	Pilot Scale	Commercial Scale
4	0.9	1.1
4	1.4	—
4	2.0	—
5	—	1.6
6	—	1.1
6	—	1.3
15	—	2.0
34	—	2.8

6.5.4 Agglomerates of API and Accelerated Agglomeration Studies

One of the greatest challenges in meeting the desired API particle size for a low-dose, oral drug product is in overcoming the formation of particle assemblages. These assemblages may be in the form of easily dispersed particles of API, referred to as soft agglomerates.[33] These assemblages may also be in the form of rigidly bound particles, referred to as hard agglomerates, or previously known as aggregates.[34]

A laser light scattering method was used to characterize the particle size distribution of agglomerates and primary particles of Drug A using 0 and 30 s sonication times, respectively. As shown in Fig. 6.4, agglomerates are detectable when tested

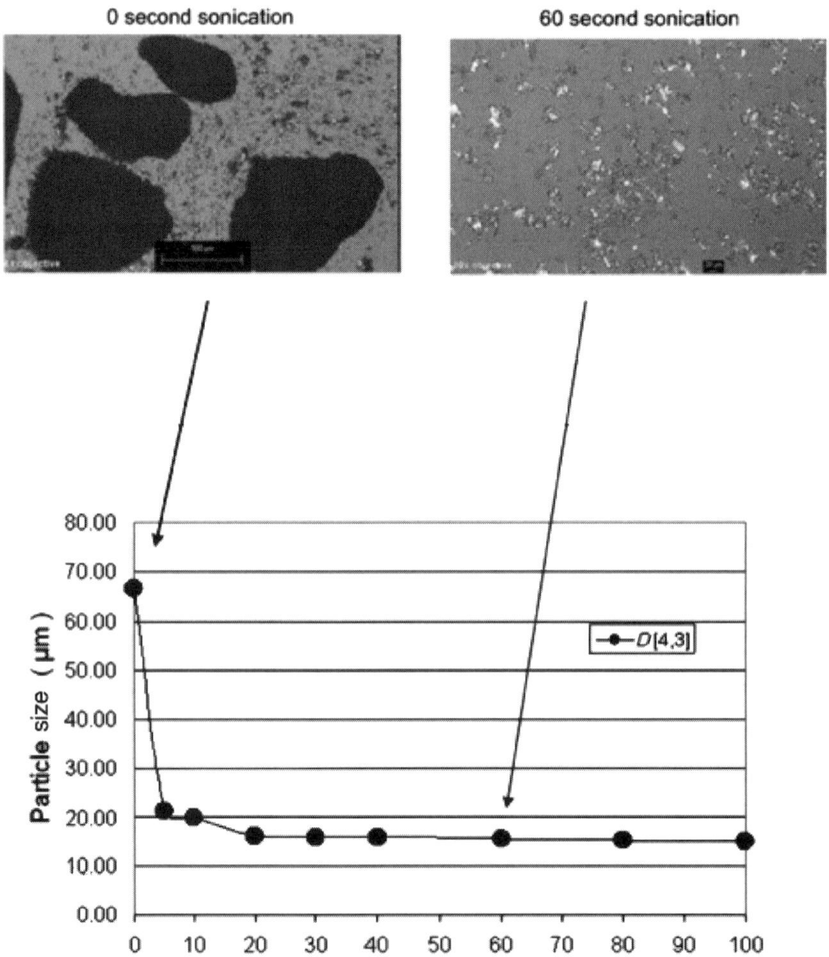

Figure 6.4 Effect of sonication time on API particle size in terms of *D*[4,3]. (See color insert.)

initially with no sonication during sample preparation. These results also demonstrate that sonication time exceeding 30 s is effective at breaking up Drug A agglomerates into primary particles. These particle assemblages are categorized as "soft" agglomerates because the loose clusters are easily broken apart with mild application of pressure or energy. For this reason, the process development and optimization assessed the need for a delump milling process to ensure uniformity of the blend prior to dry granulating.

The type of agglomerate (soft vs hard) resulting after shipping the bulk API to the DP facility was a potential concern early in development. This was addressed by conducting an accelerated agglomeration study to assess the impact on drug product quality. This study was designed to evaluate whether the recommended drug product processing was capable of handling the API agglomerates.

The study was conducted using two different treatment approaches to induce formation of agglomerates: thermal cycling and 4 months' exposure to 40°C/75% relative humidity (RH) as compared with the initial control sample. The thermal cycle samples were exposed to 2 days at −20°C and 2 days at 40°C/75% RH for six cycles. The samples were then analyzed for particle size using the method described above. Photomicrographs of the original samples after 0 and 60 s sonication utilized a polarized light microscope (Fig. 6.4). These samples depict the large agglomerates detected with no sonication, and the reduction in size to primary particles after sonication. The agglomerates initially present in the sample were loose in consistency and readily dispersed in suspension.

The sonication study for the samples exposed to thermal cycling resulted in the largest initial agglomerates that were not easily dispersed (Table 6.10). Product experience with multiple lots of API revealed the agglomerates continued to exist as "soft" agglomerates. Therefore, the thermally cycled study that resulted in hard agglomerates was not consistent with the API properties.

In these case studies, the two model drug compounds formed loosely bound agglomerates that were readily dispersed to their primary particle sizes through the use of sonication during preparation for particle size analysis.

TABLE 6.10 Effect of Sonication Time on the Agglomerated API Particle Size After Exposure to Thermal Cycling[a]

Sonication Time (s)	$D(v,0.1)$ (μm)	$D[4,3]$ (μm)	$D(v,0.9)$ (μm)
0	8	180	513
5	6	156	510
10	5	115	414
20	4	83	346
30	4	100	429
40	4	49	53
60	3	26	39
100	3	24	36

[a]Thermal cycle defined as 2 days at −20°C and 2 days at 40°C/75% RH, repeated for six cycles.

TABLE 6.11 Effect of API Particle Size on Stratified Tablet Content Uniformity for Drug Product Batches Produced at Commercial Scale

Drug Substance Milling Method	Drug Substance Particle Size Distribution (μm)			Final Blending Uniformity (%RSD)	Stratified Tablet Content Uniformity (%RSD)
	$D(v,0.1)$	$D[4,3]$	$D(v,0.9)$		
Jet-milled	1	6.5	13	0.8	1.6
Fitz-milled	3	16	34	4.0	2.7
Wet-milled	4	25	54	2.2	1.8

6.5.5 API Milling Considerations

The desired API particle size distribution is primarily achieved by controlling the conditions used to crystallize the drug substance. In the case of Drug A, milling steps were incorporated into both the drug substance and drug product manufacturing processes to break up agglomerates that may be present. A different tact was pursued to meet the target particle size specification for Drug B, which utilized jet milling. The jet-milling approach may have incurred more challenges in terms of blend sampling accuracy due to formation of agglomerates by electrostatic charge. However, the final tablet content uniformity met the stratified sampling acceptance criteria.

The effect of significantly reducing the drug substance particle size using jet milling on content uniformity was explored on a large-scale drug product batch for Drug A. This study was conducted in campaign with three alternative drug substance milling methods (Table 6.11) including jet-milled, Fitz-milled and wet-milled. The jet-milled drug substance particle size distribution was characterized as 1 μm for $D(v,0.1)$, 6.5 μm for $D[4,3]$, and 13 μm for $D(v,0.9)$. Final blend and stratified tablet content uniformity results demonstrated that significantly reducing the drug substance particle size distribution through jet milling had no detrimental affect when compared with Fitz milling or wet milling. Both methods of achieving the target API particle size distribution used for these products assured acceptable quality products.

6.6 PROCESS CHALLENGES DURING DRY GRANULATION OPTIMIZATION FOR LOW-DOSE PRODUCTS

Following formulation selection activities, a successful technology transfer and optimization of a low-dose dry granulation process is typically centered around balancing competing factors that define a formulation's quality attributes, such as tablet content uniformity or potency, and factors that define a formulation's manufacturability, such as dry granulation throughput (mass per unit time) or compression speed (tablets per hour). In general, eight major process challenges drive the optimization of the dry granulation process parameters, from a product quality attribute and manufacturability perspective. These eight process challenges are summarized in

TABLE 6.12 Process Challenges for Optimizing a Low-Dose Dry Granulation Process

Process Challenges	Driver	Method of Assessment	Attribute
(1) Achieve a homogeneously distributed API within the initial blend, prior to dry granulation	Quality	Blend sampling or stratified tablet core sampling	Blend uniformity or tablet content uniformity
(2) Evaluate dry granulation process parameters to achieve a desired target throughput	Manufacturability	Mass per unit time	Mass flow rate (kg/h)
(3) Evaluate granulation particle size distribution	Manufacturability	Particle size analysis or powder flow assessment	Powder flow
(4) Achieve a homogeneously distributed API within the range of granulation particle sizes	Quality	Granulation sieve cut potency	Tablet content uniformity
(5) Reduce the mobility of the API, by mechanically binding the API to the formulation excipients	Quality	Granulation fluidization and sifting segregation potential	Tablet content uniformity
(6) Achieve homogeneous final blending process, prior to compression	Quality	Blend sampling or stratified tablet core sampling	Blend uniformity or tablet content uniformity
(7) Minimize the compression force required to achieve target tablet hardness	Manufacturability	Compaction simulator or tablet press	Compression force
(8) Evaluate tablet physical properties	Manufacturability	Mass per unit time	Mass flow rate (kg/h)

Table 6.12 and a decision tree of optimization activities is summarized in Fig. 6.5. Two model low-dose drug candidates, Drugs A and B, serve as case studies for evaluating the process selection and optimization.

6.6.1 Initial Blend Process Selection and Evaluation of Initial Blend Uniformity

In general, the process selection is primarily driven by a desire to impart significant mixing energy into the initial blend to achieve a uniform, homogenous blend. As described previously, this increased mixing energy into the blending process

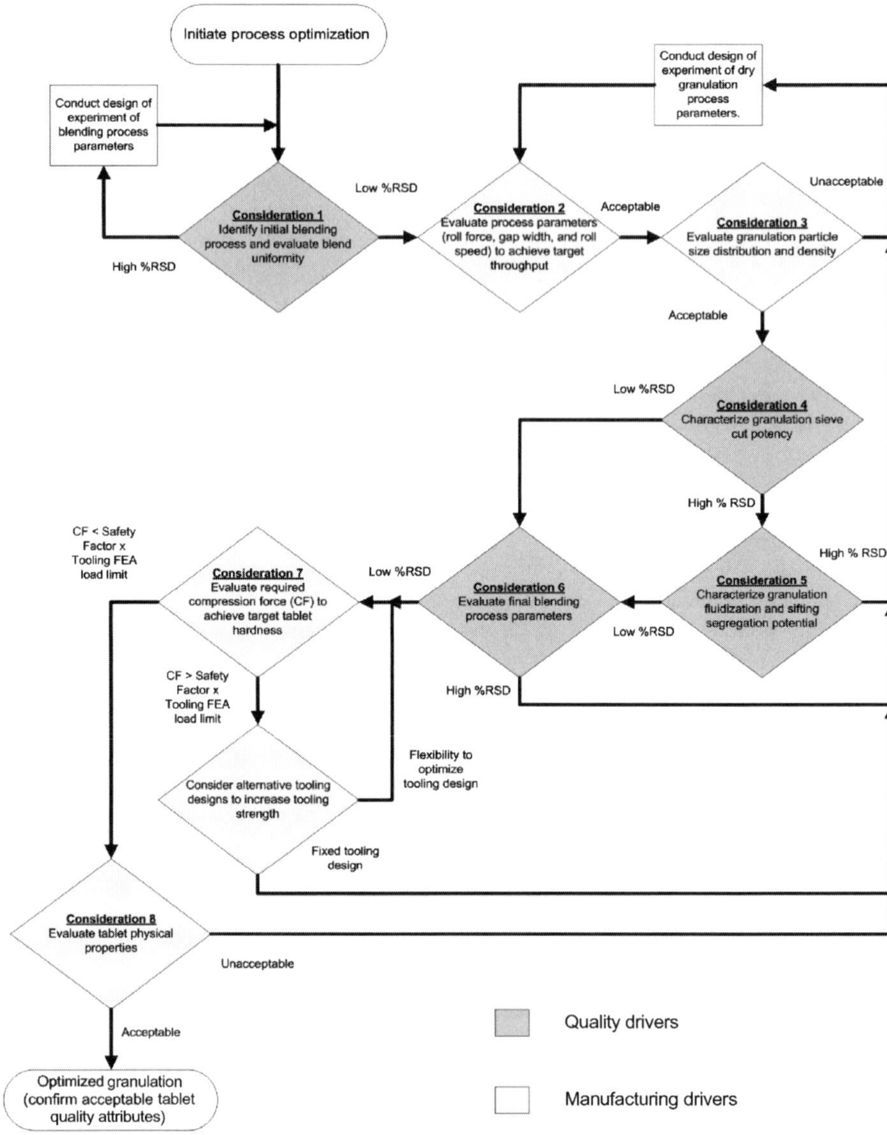

Figure 6.5 Low-dose dry granulation process optimization decision tree.

enables the deagglomeration of loosely bound API particles within the initial blend, through the use of high-shear blending forces. Two mixing processes, blend-mill (Drug A) and high-shear dry blending (Drug B), have been successfully demonstrated to achieve a homogeneous initial blend for these two case study formulations.

Table 6.13 provides a comparison of the significant attributes of the high-shear dry blending process and the blend-mill process. Each of these two initial blending processes offers comparable mixing times to achieve the desired blend homogeneity, and

TABLE 6.13 Comparison of Attributes of a High-Shear Dry Blending (HSDB) Process and a Blend-Mill (BM) Process

Attribute	BM Process	HSDB Process	Rationale
Blending vessels	Portable	Fixed	BM: Portable blending vessels (e.g., intermediate bulk container)
Powder discharge process	Gravity-assisted	Impeller assisted	BM: Gravity-assisted discharge process HSDB: Impeller required to discharge material from high-shear mixing vessel
Residual powder remaining within mixing vessel	Lower	Higher	HSDB: Powder can remain within the clearance between the rotating impeller and the bottom surface of the bowl. Additionally, this powder can reflect the potency of smaller and less mobile particles
High-intensity mixing—deagglomerate API	Additional milling unit operation required	Utilize high-shear mixer chopper element	BM: Separate milling step required for blend-mill process HSDB: Chopper can be used to impart mixing energy during blending step
Overall equipment surface area	Higher	Lower	BM: Required separate in-line milling process introduces greater equipment surface area

they are viable alternatives for establishing the initial blending process. The ultimate process selection decision, therefore, must be based on a series of secondary considerations, and represents a calculated trade-off between the relative benefits of a blend-mill process vs those of a high-shear dry mixing process.

Blend-Mill Advantages. A blend-mill mixing process offers the advantage of completion of the blending activities within a portable container (e.g., intermediate bulk container or IBC), designed for efficient transport of materials from one location to another. In contrast, commercial-scale high-shear blending vessels are often installed in a fixed location within the manufacturing plant. Additionally the blend-mill process offers a gravity-assisted discharging of materials from containers design with mass-flow characteristics.

In contrast, the high-shear dry blending vessels are discharged by utilizing the impeller to sweep material out of the vessel. Additionally, due to the clearance between the rotating impeller and the bottom surface of the high-shear mixer bowl, residual powder can remain within the high-shear mixer following the discharge process, resulting in a potential yield loss or potential potency loss to the process.

High-Shear Dry Blending Advantages. In general, a high-shear dry blending process offers the advantage of completing high-intensity mixing, to distribute and deagglomerate API particles, within the same unit operation. In contrast, due to the lower-shear mechanism of blending, a blend-mill process requires the addition of a separate milling unit operation to achieve this same mixing intensity. This process advantage serves to reduce the number of processing steps, resulting in a simplified manufacturing process for a high-shear dry mixing process. Additionally, this advantage decreases the overall process train equipment surface area, and therefore minimizes the potential of API potencies losses, through adherence, to equipment stainless steel surfaces.

A study has been conducted to compare the impact of the initial blending time on the resulting initial blend uniformity for Drugs A and B. The higher blend uniformity and variability with longer blend times is evidence that the blend electrostatic charge is playing a role in sampling bias. Electrostatic charge was shown to be the issue through further studies not presented here, and corroborated by uniformity of tablet potency throughout the compression. For both Drug A (15–45 min, B-M mixing process) and Drug B (10–20 min, HSDB process), acceptable initial blend uniformity ($\%\text{RSD} < 5.0\%$) was achieved for each formulation at multiples scales and sites of manufacture. Following initial blending, dry granulation, milling and final bin blending activities were performed. The final blend uniformity was also assessed for both Drug A and Drug B. The results of (%RSD) values are $<4.0\%$, which is smaller than that of corresponding initial blend value, for all but one comparison. The lower final blend %RSD values are typically a result of additional blending energy imparted into the formulation during subsequent dry granulation, milling and the final blending process, and a reduction in sampling bias due to sampling granulation powders vs un-granulated powders.

In these case studies, the two model drug compounds formed loosely bound agglomerates that were readily dispersed in the drug product processing operations through the use of milling or high-shear blending.

6.6.2 Dry Granulation Throughput

The dry granulation throughput (mass per unit time) is defined by the following two equations, assuming a no-slip condition at the interface between the roller and the ribbon at the compaction zone, and negligible compaction zone bypass.

$$\text{Roll tangential velocity (mm/s)} = \text{roll speed (RPM)} \times \text{roll diameter (mm)} \times \Pi \times 1\ \text{min}/60\ \text{s} \quad (6.1)$$

$$\begin{aligned}\text{Throughput (kg/h)} &= \text{roll width (mm)} \times \text{ribbon thickness (mm)}\\ &\quad \times \text{roll tangential velocity (mm/s)}\\ &\quad \times \text{ribbon density (g/cm}^3\text{)}\\ &\quad \times (1\ \text{cm}/10\ \text{mm})^3 \times 1\ \text{kg}/1000\ \text{g}\end{aligned} \tag{6.2}$$

Recognizing that the roll diameter from Eq. (6.1) and roll width from Eq. (6.2) are noncontrollable process parameters for a given dry granulation process equipment, the remaining process parameters identified within these two equations, roll speed, ribbon thickness, and ribbon density, serve to define the dry granulation throughput.

Increases to roll speed, ribbon thickness (i.e., increasing the gap width between rollers), and/or ribbon density (i.e., increasing the roll force applied during compaction) increase the corresponding dry granulation throughput. From solely a business perspective, it is highly desirable to maximize each of these three process parameters, to achieve a corresponding increase in dry granulation throughput. However, as described in subsequent sections, it must be recognized that each of these process parameters, has the potential to influence quality attribute(s) of the granulation or the final tablet. And ultimately, the optimization of these parameters must be tempered to include both their impact on business drivers, such as dry granulation throughput, and impact on tablet quality attributes.

6.6.3 Evaluation of Granulation Particle Size Distribution and Density

A primary goal of dry granulation processing is to densify and build particle size in the resulting granulation. These two goals serve to increase the powder flow characteristics of the granulation, during the subsequent compression process, and maximize the quantity of material that can be charged into a given blending vessel volume (e.g., 2000 L IBC).

Figure 6.6 depicts the granulation particle size distribution for Drugs A and B. The granulation particle size distribution of Drug A shows a significant increase in the weight percent of material remaining in the 40 and 60 mesh screen sizes (23.8–36.4%), following the dry granulation activities. Due to the brittle characteristics of this formulation, an increase in the weight percent of the material remaining in the range of 200 mesh to pan (29.7–33.1%) is observed, due to a combination of particle fracture during the milling step and the contribution of ungranulated roller by-pass. As described in the next two sections, this increase in small, mobile particles results in additional processing challenges. The granulation tapped density significantly increases from 0.59 to 0.74 g/mL. The greatest increase in granulation mean particle size is obtained when roll force and granulator screen size are increased simultaneously.[35]

Similarly, the granulation particle size distribution of Drug B shows a significant increase in the weight percent of material remaining in the 20, 40, and 60 mesh screen

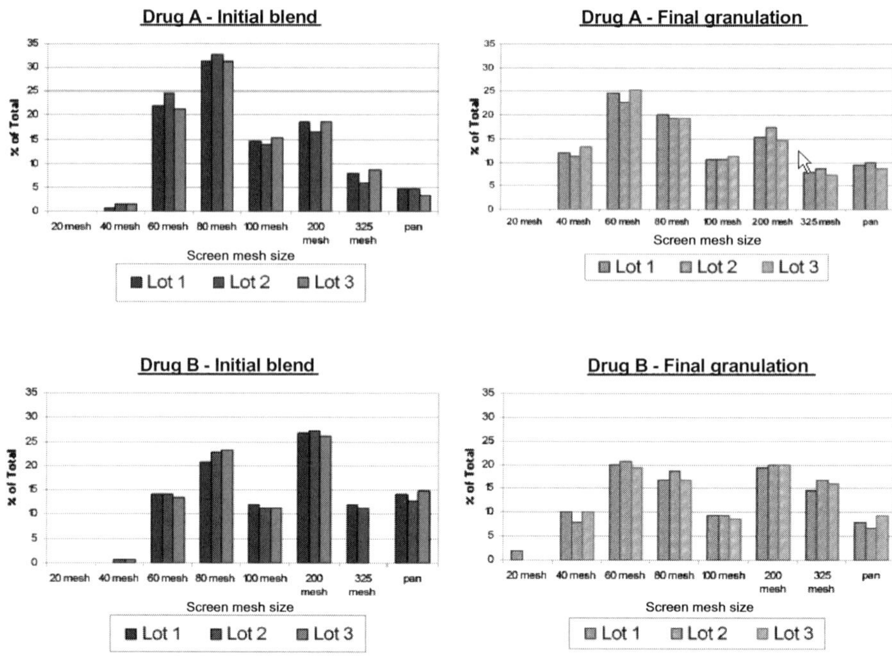

Figure 6.6 Comparison of initial blend and final granulation particle size distribution—Drugs A and B.

sizes (14.2–30.0%), following the dry granulation activities. Additionally, due to the cohesive properties of this formulation, there is a slight decrease in the weight percent of the material remaining in the 200 and 325 mesh and pan (48.2–43.6%), as fines are not generated during the milling process. The granulation tapped density remains relatively unchanged from 0.80 to 0.82 g/mL.

6.6.4 Variability in Granulation Sieve Cut Potency

A fourth process challenge in the optimization of a dry granulation process is to achieve a uniform distribution of API within each of the granulation sieve cut particle sizes. This uniform distribution ensures (1) that both smaller and larger granulation particle sizes have the same proportionate weight percentage of API within their respective particle sizes, (2) the resulting variability in granulation sieve cut potency is minimized, and (3) the influence of segregation forces on tablet quality attributes, such as potency or content uniformity, is minimized.

In general, increasing roll force reduces the variability of granulation sieve cut potency by increasing the density of the compacted ribbon or briquette. This densification process results in the physical binding of the API to carrier excipient particles, leading to an increase in overall granulation particle size. Additionally, higher roll forces minimize the initial blend passing through the compaction zone ungranulated. Together, these two factors serve to shift the concentration of API from the smaller to larger particles, thereby improving the uniformity.

In contrast, increasing the gap width between the dry granulator rollers decreases the density of the compacted ribbon or briquette (also possible when other factors, such as feed rate or roll force, are changed). This reduced densification process results in a weaker binding of API to carrier excipients, and reduced overall granulation particle size distribution and increased bypass.

A granulation optimization study on model Drug A targeted the least variability in sieve cut potency.[35] The highest percentage bypass levels were concentrated in the region of minimal roll force values and maximal gap width values.

The variability of sieve cut potencies for Drugs A and B as a function of various roll force levels and dry granulation equipment manufacturers is tabulated in Table 6.14. The change in equipment type had no significant affect on sieve cut potency variability for Drug B. The increased roll force using the same equipment type did impact the variability of sieve cut potencies for Drug A in terms of RSD.

During process development, an initial granulation of Drug A was manufactured at 5 kN/cm roll force, and 3.8 mm gap width. The resulting variability (RSD) in sieve cut potency was 35.2% while the RSD of corresponding tablet content uniformity was 2.4%. In an effort to improve the tablet content uniformity, an additional granulation was manufactured at 9 kN/cm roll force, and the mill gap width was reduced to 2.3 mm. Due to these process changes, the percentage of bypass was reduced from ~10 to ~1.5%.[35] Correspondingly, the RSD value of the sieve cut potencies was reduced to 13.8%, and the RSD value of the corresponding tablet content uniformity was reduced to 1.8%.

In contrast, Drug B was manufactured at two different blend strengths, on dry granulators from two different equipment manufacturers. The RSD value of sieve cut potencies ranged from 74.2 to 43.1%. However, in contrast to Drug A, the reduction in sieve cut potency for Drug B does not significantly reduce the corresponding tablet content uniformity (1.4–1.5%RSD). This observation is consistent with the low segregation potential observed for Drug B formulation (cohesive), as shown in Table 6.15, or the influence of electrostatic forces created during the sieving process, exaggerating the true blend uniformity, or a combination of both factors.

6.6.5 Granulation Sifting and Fluidization Segregation

A fifth process challenge in the optimization of a dry granulation process is to achieve a granulation that is resistant to fluidization and sifting segregation forces. In general, process parameters that influence segregation potential are similar to those that influence variability in sieve cut potency.

As shown in Table 6.15, for Drug A, increasing roll force and decreasing gap width reduced the fluidization and sifting segregation potentials for this granulation, and resulted in a corresponding decrease in tablet content uniformity. The intentional formulation design of Drug B with excipients possessing cohesive properties was found to be more resistant to segregation, as demonstrated by the segregation test that RSD values are <1%. Therefore, no further optimization to mitigate the risk

TABLE 6.14 Variability in Sieve Cut Potency as a Function of Roll Force

Sample	Drug A		Drug B			
Batch no.	1	2	1	2	3	4
Manufacturing site	Site 1	Site 1	Site 2	Site 2	Site 3	Site 3
Theoretical blend potency (%)	0.5	0.5	0.25	0.5	0.25	0.5
Dry granulator manufacturer	Gerteis	Gerteis	Freund	Freund	Bepex	Bepex
Roll force	5 kN/cm	9 kN/cm	30 kg/cm^2	30 kg/cm^2	35 kN	35 kN
Sieve size (μm)	Potency (% of theory)					
<45	131.5	106.2	205.6	233.0	150.8	133.8
45	63.2	72.2	63.6	67.4	72.8	97.4
75	51.6	83.7	61.6	53.8	43.2	42.8
150	69.9	87.5	60.4	51.8	50.0	55.4
180	66.3	91.8	64.8	51.0	53.2	50.2
250	79.8	100.9	79.2	66.6	64.8	63.2
425	111.8	107.0	98.4	95.4	98.8	98.6
%RSD	35.2	13.8	58.0	74.2	49.4	43.1
Tablet content uniformity (%RSD)	2.4	1.8	1.5	1.5	1.4	1.5

TABLE 6.15 Variability in Segregation Potential as a Function of Formulation and Roll Force

	Potency (% Theoretical)		
	Drug A		Drug B
Sample	Batch 1 5 kN Roll Force	Batch 2 9 kN Roll Force	Batch 1
	Fluidization Segregation Test		
Top sample	90.7%	92.3%	93.0%
Middle sample	88.9%	97.4%	91.7%
Bottom sample	65.6%	104.4%	92.8%
Reference	98.2%	98.6%	—
%RSD (TMB)	17.1	6.2	0.8
Span (max–min)	25.1%	12.1%	1.3%
Tablet content uniformity (%RSD)	2.4%	1.8%	Not tested
	Sifting Segregation Test		
First sample	92.6%	97.6%	92.9
Middle sample	91.6%	98.3%	93.2
Last sample	70.5%	101.6%	93.8
Span (max–min)	22.1%	4.0%	0.9
Reference	98.2%	98.6%	Not tested
Tablet content uniformity (%RSD)	2.4%	1.8%	Not tested

of segregation was warranted, despite the higher variability in sieve cut potency observed for this formulation (Table 6.14).

6.6.6 Evaluation of Final Blending Process Parameters

For a low-dose dry granulation process, the final blending process is typically employed to incorporate a lubricant (e.g., magnesium stearate) as an extragranular excipient. The lubricant typically serves as a compression aid, to reduce the occurrence of sticking of the granulation to the tablet tooling, during the compression process. However, due to the lubricating properties of these materials, the use of excessive blending forces (high-shear or extended blending times) can result in tablets with lower crushing strength (i.e., tablet hardness). Additionally, due to the hydrophobic properties of lubricants, excessive blending time can also slow down the disintegration time or dissolution rate of the resulting tablets. Again, the optimization of the final blending process seeks to find a balance between distributing the lubricant throughout the formulation, without "over-lubing" the granulation, resulting in tablets with lower strength or longer disintegration or dissolution times.

Since the properties that influence granulation blend uniformity (variability in sieve cut potency, segregation potential) have already been established during the dry granulation process, a minor secondary function of the final blending process

TABLE 6.16 Impact of Lubrication Time for Drug A Final Blend on Tablet Physical Properties

Lot No.	Lube Blend Time (min)	Compression Force (kN)	Average Hardness (kp)	Disintegration Time	Dissolution (%) (Mean of Six Tablets) (Range of Values)	
				min : s	5 min	15 min
Lot 1	2	3.3	6.3	00 : 11	98 (95–101)	100 (98–102)
Lot 2	2	6.1	10.1	00 : 21	101 (100–103)	100 (98–102)
Lot 3	3	3.0	5.9	00 : 13	98 (95–102)	98 (94–102)
Lot 4	3	6.5	10.4	00 : 24	101 (99–103)	101 (97–103)
Lot 5	5	2.9	5.7	00 : 11	97 (95–98)	97 (96–98)
Lot 6	5	6.5	10.4	00 : 28	100 (97–101)	101 (99–103)

is to overcome any segregation forces that act upon the granulation during charging into the blending container. Table 6.16 lists the impact of final blending time and compression force on mean tablet hardness, disintegration time, and dissolution profiles. Acceptable tablet compression operation was observed for each of the granulations prepared, and therefore the range of final lubrication blending times was limited to between 2 and 5 min. Additionally, as shown in this table, tablet hardness and dissolution profiles were not impacted by the range of final lubrication blending times and compression forces studied. Although the lubrication time had no significant affect on disintegration time, compression force had a detectable, but unimportant, effect on disintegration time. In this case, the disintegration test was found to be the most sensitive method for detecting process changes.

6.6.7 Minimization of the Compression Force Required to Achieve Target Tablet Hardness

Tablets manufactured for low-dose formulations are frequently small in size, due to their low drug loading levels. These smaller tablet sizes, for example, 100 mg, present significant challenges from a tablet compression optimization perspective. The tablet size and strength of the compression tooling punch tip is also proportionately smaller and weaker, respectively. Additionally, the tablet compression process is designed to ensure that the compression forces during routine manufacture remain sufficiently below the yield or failure limit of the tooling steel by a conservative factor of safety. Together, these two factors significantly limit the overall compression force that can be applied to a granulation to achieve a desired tablet hardness, and therefore can represent a significant process challenge constraint.

The use of brittle excipients vs ductile excipients influences the overall compressibility of the formulation, with brittle formulations maintaining greater overall compressibility. However, it is recognized that there is a loss of compressibility for a powder previously compressed and milled, that is, by dry granulation.[36,37] Secondarily, increasing roller compaction force during the dry granulation process requires a corresponding increase in compression force during the compression process to achieve a desired tablet hardness. From this perspective, it is desirable to minimize the roller compaction force used during the dry granulation process, to ensure sufficient compressibility remains during tableting. In contrast, increasing the gap width during the dry granulation process enables a corresponding decrease in compression force during the compression process to achieve the desired tablet hardness.

Therefore, for a given formulation (brittle vs ductile), a balance in the level of applied compaction force and roller gap width must be identified to control factors that influence tablet content uniformity (variability in sieve cut potency, sifting, and fluidization segregation) without sacrificing factors that influence manufacturability (compression force required to achieve target tablet hardness).

As shown in Table 6.17, the hardness—compression force profile for Drug A tablets is linear across the range of compression forces studied. This linear profile is attributed to the properties inherent in the brittle and ductile excipients chosen for this formulation. In contrast, the hardness—compression force profile for Drug B shows a plateau in tablet hardness at higher compression forces ($>\sim$11 kN), as listed in Table 6.18.

The relationship between compression force and tablet hardness as a function of gap width and compaction roll force for Drug A tablets was developed.[35] Lower compaction roll force combined with higher gap widths resulted in reduced tablet compression forces. Increasing compaction roll forces translated into corresponding increases in tablet compression forces, with higher gap widths serving to moderate tablet compression forces. Finally, Table 6.19 identifies the relationship between compression force at target tablet hardness as a function of roll force and mill screen size for Drug A.

As a secondary measure, the design of the commercial tablet shape can be modified to increase the overall tooling strength, to overcome deficiencies in granulation compressibility. Table 6.20 provides a summary of maximum allowable compression forces for round compression tooling: shallow concave, standard concave and deep concave, for a range of tooling diameters.[38] For this tooling shape, tablet tooling

TABLE 6.17 Effect of Tableting Speed on Compression Profile for Drug A Formulation

Press Speed (Tablets/h)	Compression Force (kN)	Tablet Hardness (N)
250,000	7.0	89.8
250,000	10.4	141.0
250,000	12.9	170.4
275,000	7.1	89.0
275,000	9.6	130.6
275,000	9.8	122.1
275,000	13.1	159.8
300,000	7.3	95.6
300,000	9.7	134.7
300,000	13.3	155.3

TABLE 6.18 Effect of the Compression Speed and Main Compression Force on Physical Properties of Drug B Tablets

Press Speed (Tablets/h)	Compression Force (kN)	Tablet Hardness (N)	Tablet Weight Variation (%RSD)	Mean Tablet Friability at 4 rpm (%)	Mean Tablet Friability at 15 rpm (%)
140,000	9.0	108.9	1.1	0.2	0.3
160,000	6.2	80.0	0.8	0.2	0.3
160,000	11.8	122.4	0.8	0.3	0.5
210,000	5.0	58.0	0.5	0.2	0.3
210,000	9.0	106.8	0.6	0.2	0.3
210,000	9.0	107.2	0.6	0.3	0.4
210,000	9.0	106.0	0.8	0.2	0.4
210,000	13.0	120.8	0.5	0.3	0.4
260,000	6.2	69.9	0.6	0.2	0.3
260,000	11.8	120.0	0.8	0.3	0.4
280,000	9.0	105.8	0.3	0.2	0.4

TABLE 6.19 Effect of the Roll Force, Roll Gap, and Mill Screen Size on Main Compression Force at Target Tablet Hardness

Roll Force (kN)	Gap Width (mm)	Sieve Size (mm)	Compression Force at 7 kPa Crushing Strength
4	1.7	0.8	5.1
4	1.7	0.8	5.3
4	2.6	0.8	4.9
4	3.5	0.8	4.8
4	3.5	0.8	4.7
8	3.5	0.8	6.3
12	1.7	0.8	9.7
12	1.7	0.8	10.5
12	1.7	0.8	9.8
12	3.5	0.8	8.3
12	3.5	0.8	8.0
4	3.5	1.0	4.5
8	2.6	1.0	6.7
12	3.5	1.0	8.1
4	1.7	1.5	5.1
4	1.7	1.5	4.4
4	3.5	1.5	4.5
8	3.5	1.5	6.7
12	1.7	1.5	11.0
12	1.7	1.5	9.5
12	2.6	1.5	8.1
12	3.5	1.5	7.7
12	3.5	1.5	7.8

TABLE 6.20 Tablet Tooling Strength as a Function of Tablet Size and Fill Weight (Adapted from Ref. 38)

	Maximum Tooling Strength (kN)		
Tooling Diameter (mm)	Round Shallow Concave	Round Standard Concave	Round Deep Concave
3.175	12.5	4.4	2.7
3.970	18.0	7.0	4.2
4.763	27.0	9.6	6.1
5.555	37.0	14.0	8.3
6.350	49.0	20.0	12.5

strength can be significantly increased by utilizing shallow tooling cup depths, for a given tooling diameter.

Similarly, this logic can be applied to complex tablet geometries to increase the strength of the compression tooling. Therefore, the tooling strength can be improved by optimization of the tip curvature of the compression tooling from a deep cup, single radius (DCSR), to a deep cup, dual radius (DCDR), to a shallow cup, dual radius (SCDR) for a capsular shaped tablet (Fig. 6.7, Table 6.21).

6.6.8 Tablet Physical Properties

A final process challenge in the optimization of a dry granulation process is to evaluate tablet physical properties during the compression process. As shown in Table 6.22, mean hardness, hardness variability, mean weight, weight variability, friability, and disintegration of tablets should be evaluated, as a function of the optimized granulation, to ensure that the dosage form is established with appropriate quality attributes.

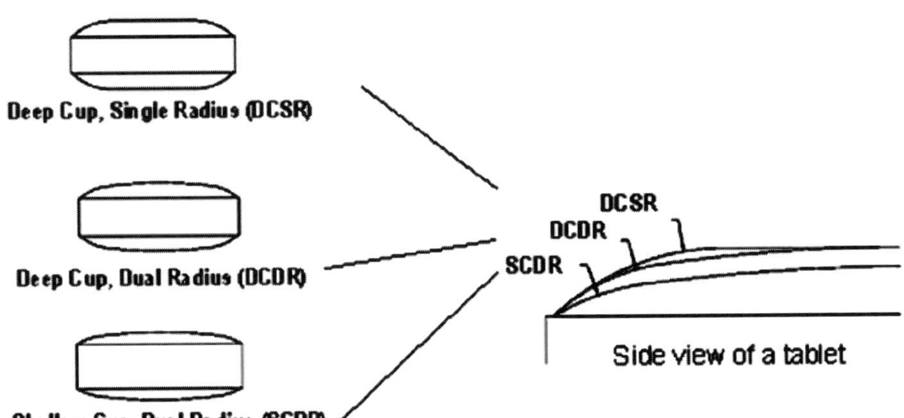

Figure 6.7 Influence of tooling design on tooling strength.

TABLE 6.21 Influence of Tooling Design on Tooling Strength with Tablet Shapes Depicted in Fig. 6.7

Tooling Type	Tooling Maximum Allowable Force (kN)[a]	Force Required for Target Crushing Strength (kN)	Percentage of Maximum Tooling Force (%)
DCSR	13.0	11.4	88%
DCDR	13.0	9.3	72%
SCDR	21.0	10.2	49%

[a]By finite element analysis.

TABLE 6.22 Influence of Tablet Physical Properties on Tablet Quality Attributes

Tablet Physical Property		Tablet Quality Attribute
Mean hardness and hardness variability	→	Dissolution profile
		Disintegration
		Appearance
Mean weight and weight variability	→	Tablet assay
		Tablet content uniformity
Tablet friability	→	Appearance

Mean tablet hardness and hardness variability may influence the resulting dissolution profile, disintegration times, and tablet appearance. As shown in Table 6.16, the compression force strongly influences mean tablet hardness, while the dissolution profile and disintegration times are largely unaffected.

A study was conducted to understand the effect of press speed on tablet weight variability for Drug B formulations. As seen in Table 6.18, tablet weight variability is inversely related to tablet press speed. This trend was repeatedly demonstrated that improved tablet weight control was achieved at higher press speeds. Another aspect of this study was to assess the impact of tablet compression force on friability. Tablet friability slightly increases with increasing compression forces (Table 6.18). Moderating the tablet compression force may minimize the potential for tablet visual defects, particularly for tablets debossed with logo or alpha-numeric identification codes, which are prone to erosion forces present during subsequent processing steps (i.e., film coating).

In summary, the process challenges that impacted quality considerations included 1, 4, 5, and 6, whereas 2, 3, 7, and 8 affected manufacturing considerations during drug product development for these low-dose products.

6.7 CONCLUSIONS

The formulation and process challenges encountered in the development of low-dose drug products using dry granulation have been thoroughly discussed. In addition, ways of addressing and overcoming these challenges were described through the use of two case studies.

For low-dose, immediate-release drug products, the formulation should be designed with cohesive diluents, such as lactose, to enhance ordered mixing prior to the dry granulation process. Based on the two case studies reported here, it was also demonstrated that this formulation approach reduced the propensity for the powder blend to segregate.

In the case where stability issues prevent the pursuit of the preferred formulation, then it becomes more important to optimize the dry granulation process to achieve an improved uniformity of drug as a function of particle size. For these cases, it is important to consider the impact of the optimized granulation on tableting performance. Although it is important to consider the commercial manufacturing efficiency, the process challenges that impact quality are of primary importance.

Finally, these two case studies have demonstrated that dry granulation is a viable process option worthy of consideration as the lead preference, even for low-dose drug products.

ACKNOWLEDGMENTS

The authors extend their gratitude to the following for their valuable contributions: William Arikpo, Robert Ball, Deborah Booth-Schindler, Stephane Caron, Xiaoping Cao, Anthony Carella, Mikalina Efros, Alanya Engtrakul, Rashmi Gadkari, Thomas Garcia, Timothy Graul, Douglas Kremer, Bruno Hancock, Barbara Johnson, Anja Kruse, Lana Liem-McDonnell, Ralph Moessner, Sara Moses, Kenneth Norris, Cynthia Oksanen, Angel Otano, Kirsten Reinheimmer, Eveline Reininger, Dana Settell, Eric C. Shen, Daryl Simmons, Dharam Singhal, Robert Timpano, Thomas Vendola, Kim Vukovinsky, Ken Waterman, Weili Yu, Holger Weyhers, and Carl Ziegler. A special note of gratitude goes to Tom J. Baxter and James Prescott of Jenike & Johanson for their technical expertise in segregation and powder flow.

REFERENCES

1. CPMP/QWP/848/96. 2001. Note for guidance on process validation. London: The European Agency for the Evaluation of Medicinal Products; 1 March 2001.
2. CPMP/QWP/2054/03. 2004. Note for guidance on process validation. Annex II. Non-standard processes. London: The European Agency for the Evaluation of Medicinal Products; 10 August 2004.
3. Physician's Desk Reference, vol. 60. 2006. Montvale, NJ: Thomson PDR.
4. FDA. 2003. Draft guidance for industry. Powder blend and finished dosage units—stratified in-process dosage unit sampling and assessment. Rockville, MD.
5. FDA. 2003. Draft guidance for industry. Powder blend and finished dosage units—stratified in-process dosage unit sampling and assessment: revised attachments. Rockville, MD.

6. Bates L. 2000. Guide to the design, selection, and application of screw feeders. London: Professional Engineering Publishing.
7. Weggel RW. 1982. The basics of force feed roll briquetting. Manuf. Engng 88(3): 107–109.
8. Johnson JR. 1965. A rolling theory for granular solids. J. Appl. Mech. 32(4): 842–848.
9. Miller RW. 1994. Advances in pharmaceutical roller compactor feed system designs. Pharm. Technol. 18(3): 154–162.
10. Prescott, JK, Hossfeld RJ. 1994. Maintaining product uniformity and uninterrupted flow to direct-compression tableting presses. Pharm. Technol. 18: 99–114.
11. ASTM D 6940-03. 2003. Standard practice for measuring sifting segregation tendencies of bulk solids. In: Annual book of ASTM standards, vol. 04.08.
12. ASTM D 6941-03. 2003. Standard practice for measuring fluidization segregation tendencies of powders. In: Annual book of ASTM standards, vol. 04.08.
13. Egermann H. 1978. Dosage accuracy of single dose, solid drug forms with a low active principle content. Part 3. Effects of active principle grain size on dosage accuracy. Sci. Pharm. 46(3): 188–193.
14. Egermann H. 1982. Problems in assessing actual content uniformity by spot sample assays. Int. J. Pharm. Technol. Product Manuf. 3(2): 59–66.
15. Garcia T, Wilkinson S, Scott JF. 2001. The development of a blend-sampling technique to assess the uniformity of a powder mixture. Drug Dev. Ind. Pharm. 27(4): 297–307.
16. Kornchankul W, Hamed E, Parikh NH, Sakr A. 2002. Effect of drug proportion and mixing time on the content uniformity of a low-dose drug in a high shear mixer. Pharmazie 57(1): 49–53.
17. Hersey JA. 1974. Powder mixing by frictional pressure. Specific example of use of ordered mixing. J. Pharm. Sci. 63(12): 1960–1961.
18. Hersey JA. 1997. Ordered mixing: a new concept in powder mixing practice. Powder Technol. 11: 41–44.
19. Orr NA, Sallam EA. 1978. Content uniformity of potent drugs in tablets. J. Pharm. Pharmac. 30: 741–747.
20. am Ende DJ, Rose PR. 2006. Strategies to achieve particle size of active pharmaceutical ingredients. In: Abdel-Magid AF, Caron S, editors. Fundamentals of early clinical drug development: from synthesis design to formulation. John Wiley & Sons, Inc.; 247–267.
21. Orr NA, Shotton E. 1973. Mixing of cohesive powders. Chem. Engrs (UK) 269: 12–19.
22. Egermann H. 1974. Dosage accuracy of singly dosed, stable drug forms with a small content of active substance. II. Influence of particle size on the homogeneity of the distribution of the active substance. Sci. Pharm. 42(1): 1–19.
23. Cheng DCH. 1968. The tensile strength of powders. Chem. Engng Sci. 23: 1405–1420.
24. Waterman KC, Roy MC. 2002. Use of oxygen scavenger to stabilize solid pharmaceutical dosage forms: a case study. Pharm. Dev. Technol. 7(2): 227–234.
25. Waterman KC, Adami RC, Alsante KM, Hong J, Landis MS, Lombardo F, Roberts CJ. 2002. Stabilization of pharmaceuticals to oxidative degradation. Pharm. Dev. Technol. 7(1): 1–32.
26. Hartauer KJ, Arbuthnot GN, Baertschi SW, Johnson RA, Luke WD, Pearson NG, Rickard EC, Tingle CA, Tsang P, Wiens RE. 2000. Influence of peroxide impurities in povidone

and crospovidone on the stability of raloxifene hydrochloride in tablets. Identification and control of an oxidative degradation product. Pharm. Dev. Technol. 5(3): 303–310.

27. Qiu Z, Stowell JG, Cao W, Morris KR, Byrn S, Carvajal MT. 2005. Effect of milling and compression on the solid state Maillard reaction. J. Pharm. Sci. 94(11): 2568–2580.
28. Kibbe AH. 2000. Handbook of pharmaceutical excipients, 3rd ed. Washington, DC: American Pharmaceutical Association.
29. Byrn SR, Xu W, Neuman AW. 2001. Chemical reactivity in solid-state pharmaceuticals: formulation implications. Adv. Drug Del. Rev. 48: 115–136.
30. Akers MJ. 1982. Antioxidants in pharmaceutical products. J. Parent. Sci. Technol. 36(5): 222–228.
31. Rowe RC, Sheskey PJ, Weller PJ, editors. Handbook of pharmaceutical excipients, 4th ed. Chicago, IL: Pharmaceutical Press.
32. Zhang Y, Johnson KC. 1997. Effect of drug particle size on content uniformity of low-dose solid dosage forms. Int. J. Pharm. 154(20): 179–183.
33. Nichols G, Byard S, Bloxham MJ, Botterill J, Dwason NJ, Dennis A, Diart V, North NC, Sherwood JD. 2002. A review of the terms agglomerate and aggregate with a recommendation for nomenclature used in powder and particle characterization. J. Pharm. Sci. 91(10): 2103–2109.
34. Gerstner W. 1966. Crystal form and particle size of organic pigments in printing inks and paints. J. Oil Col. Chem. Assoc. 49: 954–973.
35. am Ende MT, Moses SK, Carella AJ, Gadkari RA, Graul TW, Otano AL, Timpano RJ. 2007. Improving the content uniformity of a low-dose tablet formulation through roller compaction optimization. Pharm. Dev. Technol. 12(4): 391–404.
36. Miller RW. 1997. Roller compaction technology. In: Parikh DM, editor. Handbook of pharmaceutical granulation technology. New York: Marcel Dekker.
37. Gereg GW, Cappola ML. 2002. Roller compaction feasibility for new drug candidates: Laboratory to production scale. Pharm. Tech. suppl.: 14–23.
38. Young LL. 2003. Tablet specification manual, 6th ed. Washington, DC: American Pharmaceutical Association; 80.

CHAPTER 7

DEVELOPMENT OF LOW-DOSE SOLID ORAL TABLETS USING DIRECT COMPRESSION

JACK Y. ZHENG and ROBERT L. TERNIK
Pharmaceutical Sciences R&D, Lilly Research Laboratories, Eli Lilly and Company, Indianapolis, IN 40285

7.1 INTRODUCTION

The global pharmaceutical industry manufactures most tablets by a process of wet or dry granulation before compression into tablets. Granulation produces a mixture of API and excipients that has acceptable flow, compressibility, and compactibility for tableting. Wet granulation methods include high-shear, low-shear, and fluid-bed granulation; dry granulation methods use roller compaction and slugging processes. Both wet and dry granulation methods of tablet manufacture are multistep processes, and thus are time-consuming, complex, and expensive.

Direct compression is a simpler alternative tablet manufacturing method. With direct compression, tablets are compressed directly from a powder mixture of an API and appropriate excipients. Like granulation methods, this approach is also based on the required flow, compressibility, and compactibility of a formulation. Direct compression offers both time and economic advantages by eliminating intermediate granulating and drying steps.

The first direct compression excipient, spray-dried lactose, was introduced in the early 1960s as a filler specifically designed for direct compression processes. Over many years, more direct compression API and excipients, especially diluents and binders, were developed. Since these are now commercially available, design of direct compression formulations is readily possible. However, despite the simplicity of the direct compression process, the pharmaceutical industry still produces most tablets by wet granulation methods.[1]

Formulation and Analytical Development for Low-Dose Oral Drug Products. Edited by Jack Zheng

To a large extent, the physical and chemical properties of the API, as well as the performance criteria of the drug product, determine the manufacturing platform selection. Different manufacturing platforms present different technical challenges for formulation and process development scientists. The direct compression manufacturing process simply requires mixing the API and excipients together. The resultant mix is lubricated and then compressed into tablets. The critical process prior to tableting (or capsule filling) is mixing, which produces a homogeneous blend for compression into tablets. A direct compression manufacturing platform presents obvious challenges for product content uniformity, as well as for obtaining and maintaining a homogenous blend. Therefore, this platform requires a critical approach to excipient selection, powder blending, and in-process control. The process should not simply be considered another form of making tablets or capsules. Without careful evaluation, failures are very likely, especially in low-dose drug product manufacture.

This chapter discusses key considerations in excipient selection; formulation and process design and control; and blending and content uniformity during development of a low-dose direct compression formulation.

7.2 ADVANTAGES OF DIRECT COMPRESSION

Compared to wet granulation and roller compaction, the direct compression platform allows tablet manufacture with fewer unit operations, as listed in Table 7.1. The sections that follow discuss several advantages and disadvantages of using direct compression for tablet manufacture.

TABLE 7.1 Comparative Unit Operations in Tablet Manufacture Using Wet Granulation, Roller Compaction, and Direct Compression

Wet Granulation	Roller Compaction	Direct Compression
1. Weighing and dispersing	1. Weighing and dispersing	1. Weighing and dispersing
2. Pre-mixing	2. Pre-mixing and/or milling	2. Mixing
3. Preparing granulation solution	3. Roll compaction	
4. Wet massing		
5. Wet screening		
6. Drying		
7. Sizing/milling	4. Milling	
8. Admixing (disintegrant, glidant, lubricant)	5. Admixing (flow aid, disintegrant, glidant, lubricant)	3. Admixing (disintegrant, glidant, lubricant)
9. Compressing	6. Compressing	4. Compressing

7.2.1 Cost-Effective

Direct compression is cost-effective when compared with wet granulation and roller compaction processes. Cost savings are realized in a number of areas. As seen in Table 7.1, fewer unit operations translate to a reduction in manufacturing equipment and associated process rooms. Several pieces of equipment required for wet granulation, such as granulators and fluid bed driers, are not needed to produce tablets by direct compression. This reduces capital investment in equipment and facility expansion. Also, fewer unit operations can reduce manufacturing cycle time and lower labor costs so that manufacturing efficiency and productivity can be improved. Last but not least, fewer unit operations decrease the costs associated with development and process validation before product launch. Of course, interest in the direct compression process would decrease in the absence of these economic advantages.

7.2.2 Advantages for High-Volume Products

A direct compression manufacturing platform for a tablet product has fewer unit operations in comparison with wet granulation or dry granulation. This significantly reduces the manufacturing cycle time and allows production of more tablets in a specified time. Thus, direct compression provides great advantages for a high volume drug product.

7.2.3 A Dry Process Suitable for Labile Compounds

Direct compression tablet manufacture does not require the steps of liquid addition and subsequent removal by drying, as required in wet granulation processes. Liquids such as water and organic solvents can facilitate chemical degradation of drug substances and can also act as a medium to partially dissolve drug substance. This can lead to polymorphic transition, amorphous crystallization, and hydration (e.g., physical form change). Drying at a high temperature for a period of time may facilitate some chemical reactions and may result in degradation of the drug substance. The direct compression platform minimizes the chance of change in the polymorphic form of a drug substance and chemical degradation during the manufacturing process. Additionally, liquid and high temperature may cause chemical degradation of excipients and may form new impurities, such as peroxides or aldehydes, which are incompatible with many drug substances. Therefore, the direct compression platform provides an advantage for a drug substance that has physical and chemical stability problems when exposed to moisture and high temperature.

7.2.4 Product Quality Attributes Maintained Over Time

For drugs that must be dissolved in gastrointestinal fluid and absorbed into the blood stream, tablet disintegration is one of most important product quality attributes. Directly compressed tablets disintegrate into primary particles, rather than granules. This eliminates the need for granule disintegration prior to dissolution of the drug substance. With wet or dry granulation, small particles with a large surface area agglomerate with the aid of a binder to form a large particle. This results in decreased surface area and potentially slows dissolution. Granulated particles also may harden over time, which further increases disintegration of granules and dissolution of drug substance. Changes in dissolution profiles are less likely to occur in tablets made by direct compression than in those made from granulation.

On the other hand, the direct compression process has its limitations. Generally, the physical and mechanical properties of drug substances and excipients used in direct compression need better characterization and control than the materials used in wet granulation. Without careful consideration, the simplicity of the manufacturing platform could lead to failures in developing direct compression tablets, especially for a low-dose drug product. Due to differences in density, particle size, and shape between drug substance and excipients, a homogenous powder blend may be difficult to achieve. Direct compression blends may have a greater tendency to segregate during transfer steps from the mixer to drums, tote bins, and hoppers. Drug substances for low-dose drug products may be micronized to obtain acceptable blend uniformity, but this could worsen the issues in blend uniformity and segregation.

7.3 CHALLENGES IN LOW-DOSE TABLET DEVELOPMENT USING DIRECT COMPRESSION

Direct compression is an attractive platform for manufacturing tablet drug products. However, developing a low-dose drug product using direct compression poses great challenges to consistently producing high product quality. These challenges may range from control of raw materials (e.g., drug substance, excipients, and packaging components) to design of formulation and manufacturing process. Major challenges discussed in the following sections include control of the physical properties of drug substance, mixing homogeneity, segregation, and lubricity.

7.3.1 Control of Particle Size of Drug Substance

If a low-dose drug (<1 mg per dose unit) is formulated as tablets or capsules, it can be very difficult to uniformly distribute a trace amount of drug substance into a single unit dose, especially when direct compression is selected as the manufacturing platform. Major factors controlling the degree of homogeneity of the final blend are the mean particle size and the size distribution of drug substance. It is often difficult to determine whether these factors are suitable for preparation of a low-dose drug product.[2] Generally, reduction of drug substance particle size by milling or micronization is essential for a low-dose drug product to meet the USP content uniformity criteria for tablets and capsules.[3]

Several publications in the literature address the particle size of the drug substance and USP content uniformity from a theoretical and statistical basis. In 1972, Johnson[2] established an equation that predicts the expected variation in a unit dose when the particle size distribution of drug substance is analyzed. This theoretical calculation was validated by measurement of content uniformity of a well-mixed powder blend.[4,5] It is particularly useful to evaluate whether the particle size distribution, rather than inadequate mixing and segregation, could be the root cause for the content uniformity problem.

Later, Yalkowsky and Bolton[6] derived an equation with an attempt to calculate the minimum number of particles and maximum mean particle size required to ensure a 99% probability of passing the USP content uniformity test. The calculation was based on assumptions that the particles of drug substance are spherical with a log–normal distribution, and the number of particles in a tablet is distributed by the Poisson distribution. They also recommended that particle size specifications for low-dose drug products include a requirement for a size distribution limit besides mean particle size. However, this method requires a sophisticated understanding of statistics and no experimental data were provided to test the given analysis. To simplify the method, Zhang and Johnson[7] developed a simple computer program to understand the relationship between the particle size distribution of drug substance and content uniformity under ideal mixing conditions. More recently, Rohrs et al.[3] modified the equation by converting the suggested limits to metrics commonly used to describe a particle size distribution, the median diameter on a weight basis (d_{50}), and geometric standard deviation (σ_g) as the descriptor of the distribution width (Fig. 7.1). That relationship, expressed in terms of the coefficient of variation (e.g., RSD), is:

$$\mathrm{CV} = 100 \times \left(\frac{\pi \cdot \rho}{6 \cdot D}\right)^{1/2} \cdot \left((d'g) \cdot e^{4.5 \ln^2 \sigma g}\right)^{1/2} \times 10^{-9/2} \qquad (7.1)$$

where CV = coefficient of variation (RSD) of the dose (%), D = dose (mg), ρ = density of the drug substance (g/cm^3), d'_g = geometric mean particle diameter on a weight (or volume) basis (d_{50}, μm) and σ_g = geometric standard deviation.

Figure 7.1 provides a means for a quick estimate of the maximum volume median diameter (d_{50}) on a weight basis. For instance, to pass USP stage I content uniformity criteria at a p-value ≥ 0.99, a 1 mg dose would have a d_{50} upper limit of 70 μm for $\sigma_g = 2$. Figure 7.1 also demonstrates that, by just reducing the width of the particle size distribution, one gains a significant increase in the maximum acceptable d_{50}.[3] The geometric standard deviation, σ_g, is a descriptor of the particle size distribution, and its value is typically estimated by the ratio $(d_{84.1}/d_{15.9})^{0.5}$ or $(d_{97.7}/d_{50})^{0.5}$.

The theoretical method can provide initial guidance in setting particle size specifications to avoid poor content uniformity of low-dose drug products. These new modifications have made the theoretical model easier to use. However, those theoretical models do not take into account the particle size and size distribution of excipients used in a unit formula. Chapter 3 presents more detailed discussions of the theoretical consideration of the relationship between the drug particle size and product content uniformity.

Besides particle size and drug concentration, particle shape and density of powders are also important factors for achieving a homogenous mixture. Powders with nearly spherical particles are easier to mix than those with irregularly shaped particles. Micronized, needle, or flat particles require longer blending time due to aggregate

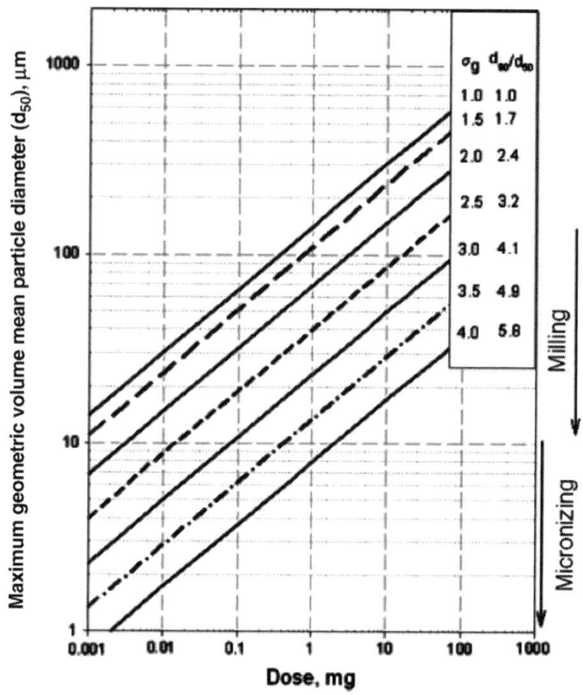

Figure 7.1 Relationship between drug particle size and dose to pass USP Stage I content uniformity criteria with 99% confidence. (Adapted from Rohrs et al.[3])

formation,[10] although these particles have less tendency to segregate once blended than spherical powders. In addition, expect various problems when the density of drug substance is significantly different from the excipients. Gravitational forces pull more dense particles to the bottom, leaving the less dense particles on top, resulting in segregation. Vibration of the blend can accelerate this segregation process.[10] Therefore, carefully consider physical properties of drug substance such as particle size, shape, and density when developing a low-dose drug product.

7.3.2 Powder Mixing and Mixing Homogeneity

Powder mixing is the most important unit operation in the manufacture of oral solid dosage forms using direct compression. Mixing ensures that the powder blend and the final product are homogeneous in drug content. Three principal mechanisms—diffusion, convection, and shear—accomplish the mixing of solid particles.[8] Diffusion (i.e., micromixing), is a process of redistribution of particles by the random movement of particles relative one to the other. Convection (i.e., macromixing), is the movement of groups of adjacent particles from one place to another within the mixture. Shear is mediated by the change in the configuration of ingredients through the formation of slip planes in the mixture.

A chess board, which may be regarded as a two-dimensional mixture of equal quantities of black and white squares, can be considered a perfect mixture, that is, one in which a sample containing two adjacent squares will always consist of one white and one black square. With solid powders, an ideal or perfect mixture—in which any sample removed from the mixture will have exactly the same composition as all other samples taken from the mixture—is virtually unattainable. In low-dose drug products, the excipient-to-drug ratio is often large to huge (e.g., 500–50,000), and thus perfect mixing is likely to be impossible. The aim in a pharmaceutical mixture is generally to produce random arrangements of powders. In the case of a chess board, this would imply that each square is equally likely to be either black or white. There is then a possibility that two, three, or even more adjacent squares may be all of the same color. The probability that any given sample composition will occur can be estimated, and the variation can be calculated.

Random Mixing. By definition, random mixing is a process in which a bed of particles is repeatedly split and recombined until there is an equal chance of any individual particle being at any given point in the mix at any one time.[11] In most powder mixing cases, the maximum randomization achievable is when the probability of sampling a given type of particle is proportional to the number of such particles in the total mixture.[9] In other words, the mixing operation produces a mixture such that, when a sample is removed from the system, the relative proportions of the components of that sample are the same as the mixture as a whole.

Unlike molecules in a solution, which will mix spontaneously by diffusion, powder particles do not mix, but remain in their relative positions. Therefore, energy must be put into the system in order to start mixing. The powder bed expands and the particles separate from one another, leading to relative motion among them. One might intuitively expect that the randomization of a mixture progressively increases with time. However, one should determine at what point in time a particular mixture has been mixed long enough to produce an acceptable randomization of particles without using excessive time and energy. On the other hand, under certain conditions an optimum mixing time occurs, beyond which the mixture shows a tendency to separate back into its components (i.e., "demixing" or segregation). Interactions between particles include both gravitational and surface electrical forces in a random mix, although the gravitational force dominates the interaction of the particles.[12] Thus, particle size, shape, and density may have a significant impact on the homogeneity obtained during a random mixing process.

To determine the degree of mixing obtained in the blend unit operation, it is necessary to take samples of the mixture and determine the variation within the mixture. Carefully consider the following factors during the assessment of the mixture:

- sample size (i.e., amount of a sample);
- number of samples to take;

- device to take a sample;
- analytical test procedure;
- the statistical method used to analyze the particle size data.

Without doubt, the method of sampling is more important than the statistical method used to draw a conclusion. The samples taken from the mixture must accurately represent the system. A large number of statistical analyses have been applied to the mixing of powders.[9,13] Determination of blend homogeneity and sampling methodology will be further discussed later in this chapter.

Ordered Mixing. Hersey[14] first introduced the concept of ordered mixing to explain the behavior of interacting particles in a powder mixture. If a powder mixture contains fine particles of drug substance (less than 10 μm) and larger particles of excipients (carriers), the fine powder may adhere to or coat other larger particles to form so-called ordered units. When an ordered mix is complete, there is an even coating of fine particles (usually drug substance) surrounding the coarse (usually excipients) particles. In an ordered mix, the gravitational force is usually weak.[12] Potential adhesive or cohesive forces responsible for the formation of ordered units may include London–van der Waals and other dipole forces,[15] surface electrical (electrostatic) force,[16] forces due to the presence of water (such as surface tension forces), and capillary suction potential forces.[17] Ordered mixes are better than the best random mixes in terms of mixing homogeneity.[18] However, in a direct compression formulation containing wide particle size distributions, randomization and ordering are both present in a state of equilibrium. This is a "total" mix.[12] The size of carrier particles controls the size of the single ordered unit and, therefore, the level of segregation and the homogeneity of the mixture. A homogenous carrier particle size avoids potential segregation,[19] and macroporous or rough-surfaced carriers have better interparticulate interactions with fine particles.[18] More excipients as carriers in the mixture may adversely affect it by removing fine drug particles, but as each new excipient is added into the mixture, the mix behaves differently.[11]

Powders can acquire an electrostatic charge during processing, the extent of which is related to the aggressiveness of the process. By giving two dissimilar particles opposite charges through the making and breaking of surface contacts (i.e., triboelectrification), the ordered mix may be stabilized. The extent of the electrostatic charge accumulation will increase as the surfaces collide and contact (e.g., by increasing the agitation time and intensity of a powder in a mixer). The net results will therefore increase the spot charge over the particle surfaces and the adhesive characteristics. Since the drug is usually charged negatively and the excipients positively, this can be used to maintain the homogeneity of a mix through processing conditions.[20,21] In the mixing unit operation, powder mixing is rarely a purely random event, however. Certain interactions between particles will occur, leading to a partially random and partially ordered mix. Ordered mixing is an important factor that prevents segregation of powder mixes, especially for a low-dose drug product.

7.3.3 Segregation of Mixed Powders

In a powder mix system containing particles with similar physical properties, mixing for a sufficient time should achieve random mixing. However, in many pharmaceutical cases, formulations require multiple excipients with different properties. Similar particles tend to congregate within the powder mixture to cause segregation. Segregation, also known as demixing, is the separation of coarse and fine material during the flow of a powder or the vibration of a bed of powders. Segregation can occur during transport and storage of mixed powders. Movement of the powder mixture from hoppers and bins during processing can promote segregation sampling. The main factors at a particulate level are differences in particle size, shape, and density, as well as resilience of the constituent particles. However, difference in particle size is by far the most important factor. Four primary mechanisms are responsible for most particle segregation problems:

1. *Sifting segregation*: This is the most common mechanism by which particles segregate. The movement of smaller particles through a mixture of larger particles causes sifting. Since a powder mixture has a size distribution, smaller particles can move into the void spaces between larger particles during the disturbance. Therefore, there is a tendency for small particles to migrate downward in the direction of gravity in a storage hopper or upon pouring a powder into a pile. A very small size difference is sometimes sufficient to cause measurable segregation.
2. *Trajectory segregation*: When a powder cloud is in flight, fine particles can travel farther than single large particles. For coarse particles, larger particles tend to travel the farthest.
3. *Fluidization (elutriation segregation)*: Because fine particle beds generally have a lower permeability than coarse particle arrangements, they tend to retain air longer in their void spaces. Pouring a powder mixture into the top of a hopper or discharging it from a hopper displaces a large volume of air. The air velocity may exceed the terminal velocity of the smaller particles, which can cause the fine particles to suspend while the coarse particles settle out. The fine particles eventually settle on top of the suspension and form a layer on top of the powder.
4. *Rise of coarse particles upon vibration*: Particles often differ in their resilience, inertia, and other dynamic characteristics. These differences can cause them to segregate, particularly when they are forming a pile (such as when charged into a bin or discharged from a chute). Vibration can cause a single larger particle to rise through a container of fine particles that are percolating down by the sifting mechanism.

For a low-dose formulation, low concentration of micronized drug substance is mixed with larger particles of excipients to achieve an ordered mix. Although the ordered mix is more homogeneous and stable than a random mix, segregation may still occur in multiple ways:[13]

- Ordered unit segregation occurs when there is a size difference between the carrier/excipient particles; this leads to drug-rich areas (hot spots) in the mix.

- Displacement segregation involves another component in a formulation competing for the available binding sites on the carriers, thus displacing some adhering drug particles.
- Saturation segregation involves any excess fine particles with no available binding sites on carrier particles. Formulations with excessive drug loading act this way in certain circumstances.

Avoiding segregation may not be possible in all cases, but it can be minimized. The first and most important strategy for low-dose drug product development is design and optimization of formulation compositions. Changes in particulate characteristics of drug and excipients may decrease the differences in particle size and size distribution, or improve adhesion between a coarse diluent and fine drug particles. Secondly, selecting an appropriate mixer or blender may improve the quality of a mix, which can decrease the possibility of segregation. Lastly, avoid pouring mixed powders to form a sloping surface during manufacture.

7.3.4 Lubricity

Lubrication is an important unit operation in manufacturing solid oral dosage forms, particularly when using a direct compression platform. Pharmaceutical lubricants can have a significant impact on product performance (e.g., disintegration and dissolution) as well as manufacturability. Lubrication is one of the most critical aspects of a tablet formulation. A lubricant is intended to reduce the friction between the tablet surface and die wall during and after compaction to enable easy ejection of the tablet. In low-dose drug product development, three issues are associated with lubricating a direct compression formulation:

1. The type and amount of lubricant needed for adequate lubrication has to be determined.
2. Fine lubricant particles competing with the drug substance for the available adhesion sites on the carrier particles in an ordered mix increase the potential for segregation.
3. Lubricant interfering with interparticulate bonding during compression results in production of tablets with unacceptable strength.

Since the mean particle size of a direct compression powder mix is typically smaller than the granules from wet or dry granulation, direct compression often requires a relatively higher concentration of lubricant. Metallic stearates such as magnesium stearate are the most widely used lubricants. The activity of stearates may be due to polar molecular portions on their surfaces adhering to the surfaces of one particle species, while nonpolar surface components adhere to the other species' surfaces. The lubricant activity of metallic stearates relates to its readiness to form films on the die wall surface. It also displays the same film-forming propensity on the surface of drug and excipient particles, leading to reduced tablet hardness upon compression. This effect is more significant in direct compression formulations that use fillers that deform plastically. When plastic-deforming fillers are compressed, the film of metallic stearates around the particles remains relatively intact. This causes the interparticulate bonds to be primarily between lubricant particles that are inherently weak.

Besides the lubricant level, blending time for lubrication is also important. Standard blending time for granulations may or may not lead to coverage of all primary surfaces in a direct compression mixture. Thus, length of blending becomes much more critical in direct compression than in lubrication of coarse granules. Shah et al.[22] found that ejection force, hardness, disintegration, and dissolution of directly compressed tablets of lactose and microcrystalline cellulose were all significantly affected by blending time. Therefore, if using direct compression, evaluate the impact of lubrication on tablet properties as early as possible.

7.4 FORMULATION DEVELOPMENT FOR LOW-DOSE DRUG PRODUCTS USING DIRECT COMPRESSION

A formulation is the composition of a drug product that contains a drug substance (i.e., active pharmaceutical ingredient and other inactive ingredients). Science-based formulation design is key to a stable and bioavailable drug product and robust manufacturing processes. Successful development of low-dose tablet formulations using direct compression platform technology depends on careful consideration of several factors:

- drug substance properties;
- excipient properties;
- optimization of the compressibility of the powder blend;
- optimization of the flowability of the powder blend;
- optimization of the lubricity of the powder blend.

The following sections outline general considerations and formulation design/optimization for low-dose direct compression drug products.

7.4.1 A Good Understanding of Drug Substance

A better understanding of the physical, chemical, and biopharmaceutical properties of a drug substance is very important for formulation design. Table 7.2 lists the properties of a drug substance that should be characterized. As discussed earlier, for a low-dose formulation, the particle size of a drug substance is the first attribute to evaluate for impact on blending and content uniformity. It can be necessary to mill or micronize the drug substance to reduce its particle size. As part of the selection of the milling operation, examine the physical and chemical stability during and after milling. Since aggregation is a common issue for micronized powders, make efforts to control the aggregates of a fine drug substance. This can reduce difficulties

TABLE 7.2 Characterization of Drug Substance

Properties	Attributes
Physical	Particle size and size distribution
	True density
	Bulk and tapped densities
	Surface area
	Electric charge of surface
	Stability of solid state
	Porosity
	Hygroscopicity
	Compactibility
	Intrinsic dissolution
Chemical	Solubility at different pHs
	Stability in different pHs
	Oxidation
	Compatibility with excipients
Biopharmaceutical	Solubility in physiological fluids
	Permeability

during material handling and product manufacture. In some cases, it may be important to assess the surface area of the drug substance in addition to particle size. The combination of particle size and surface area of the drug substance may provide better control for final uniformity of the dose unit and long-term product stability.

To assess the impact of drug substance particle size and size distribution on a formulation, prepare two to three batches of drug substance with different mean particle sizes for formulation and process evaluation. This helps establish a specification to control particle size and size distribution of the drug substance.

Chemical properties are important when designing a formulation for direct compression. If a drug has tendency to oxidize, mixing an antioxidant with the drug substance may not be an effective way to place the antioxidant in close proximity to the drug substance to prevent the oxidation reaction. Similarly, direct compression cannot offer an optimum way to incorporate a wetting agent into a formulation. Thus, it may be necessary to revisit the formulation strategy for such a compound.

7.4.2 Selection of Critical Excipients—Fillers

Generally, when developing a direct compression formulation, efforts to match particle size distribution and density of drug substance to the major excipients help minimize segregation. Meanwhile, the particle size distribution should be relatively narrow (100 μm range) to ensure a satisfactory flow for the blend. The commonly used excipients for preparing direct compression blends can be categorized by the function performed in a formulation. Excipients are grouped into six functionalities in direct compression blends:

- fillers-binders (so-called carriers, diluent, and bulking agent);
- disintegrants;
- flow aids or glidants;
- adsorbents;
- stabilizers (pH modifiers and antioxidants);
- lubricants.

However, some excipients have multiple functions. For example, microcrystalline cellulose can function as a filler, a binder, and a disintegrant. As seen in Table 7.3, a typical low-dose formulation could include more than 85% filler—binders. Thus, physical and chemical properties for these specialty excipients are extremely important in a low-dose formulation for manufacturability, product performance, and long-term stability. Because the poor physicomechanical properties of components are not altered during manufacture as they are in the wet or dry granulation process, critical material properties and their impact on product quality attributes should be well characterized and understood.[23] Discussion in this section will focus on fillers–binders. For those requiring more information on excipients, several excellent books and review articles are available in the literature.[24–27]

There are many commercially available direct compression filler–binders. The most commonly used filler–binders include spray-dried lactose, mannitol, microcrystalline cellulose, pregelatinized starch, and dibasic calcium phosphate. Many factors affect the selection of a filler–binder for a direct compression tablet formulation. The most important requirements for a directly compressible filler–binder used in a low-dose formulation are listed below:

- high compactibility and compressibility to ensure that the powder mixture can be compressed efficiently and the compacted tablet will remain bonded after the release of the compaction pressure;
- good flowability as a result of appropriate particle density, size, and size distribution to ensure that the powder blend flows homogenously and rapidly during tableting;

TABLE 7.3 Typical Low-Dose Drug Formulation Composition for Direct Compression

Ingredient	Amount (% w/w)
API	<2
Filler–binders	>85
Disintegrant	4–8
Stabilizer (pH modifier, antioxidant)	<1
Glidant	<1
Lubricant	1–3

- low lubrication sensitivity to reduce potential over-lubrication;
- nonhygroscopicity;
- good compatibility with drug substance to ensure long-term product stability;
- good physical and chemical stability to ensure product quality attributes are unchanged during storage;
- good batch-to-batch reproducibility of physical and mechanical properties to ensure constant quality materials;
- good commercial availability and regulatory acceptability throughout the world.

Certainly, not a single excipient meets all the optimum requirements. Therefore, it is common to use a combination of two filler–binders in order to obtain a formulation with excellent tableting properties.

Lactose. Lactose, an animal-origin excipient, is the oldest and still one of most widely used direct compression filler–binders. Lactose is commercially available in various grades that differ in properties such as shape, particle size distribution, and flow characteristics. This permits the selection of the most suitable material for a particular application. Direct compression grades of lactose are available in three forms:

1. a primarily β-lactose anhydrous form or a mixture of β-lactose and α-lactose;
2. granulated/agglomerated α-lactose monohydrate containing small amounts of anhydrous lactose;
3. spray-dried α-lactose monohydrate containing some amorphous lactose (10–20%).

Table 7.4 lists the physical characteristics of directly compressible lactose.

Spray-dried lactose is a good excipient for use in low-dose formulations. It has excellent flow characteristics due to its spherical particle shape and narrow particle size distribution. In addition, the particles consist of an optimal mix of very small crystals of α-lactose monohydrate and amorphous lactose, which improves compactibility. The porous surface structure of spray-dried lactose provides sufficient adsorption sites for fine particles, ensures excellent mixing characteristics, and prevents segregation. Spray-dried lactose is available from a number of commercial sources in a number of grades (Table 7.4).[28–30] Because the processing conditions used by different manufacturers may vary, all spray-dried lactose products do not necessarily have the same physical properties, particularly degree of agglomeration, which affects both flowability and compactibility. As with all direct compression filler–binders, investigate and validate alternative sources of supply.

The presence of amorphous lactose in the excipient may have a negative effect on compactibility and product stability. Direct compression grades of lactose monohydrate are available as granulated/agglomerated particles from multiple vendors. These physical properties are listed in Table 7.4.[28,29,31] Commercial products combine the good flowability of coarse lactose crystals and the good compressibility

TABLE 7.4 Typical Physical Properties of Selected Lactose as Directly Compressible Filler–Binders

Chemical	Trade Name	Manufacturer	Bulk Density	Particle Size	Comments
Lactose anhydrous	Pharmatose DCL 21	DMV International	0.68 g/mL	15% <45 μm, 50% <150 μm, 85% <250 μm	Good for moisture-sensitive drug
	Pharmatose DCL 22	DMV International	0.67 g/mL	15% <45 μm, 35% <150 μm, 75% <250 μm	Good for low and high drug dose
	Lactose anhydrous NF DT	Kerry Bio-Sciences		35–50% >180 μm	Good compactibility, low friability, good dissolution, improved moisture stability
	Lactose anhydrous NF DT High Velocity	Kerry Bio-Sciences		40–60% >180 μm, 15–35% >250 μm	Faster flow and improved tablet uniformity
Lactose monohydrate	Pharmatose DCL15	DMV International	0.50 g/mL	25% <45 μm, 60% <150 μm, 97% <355 μm	Granulated for direct compression
	Tablettose 70	Meggle	0.51 g/mL	6% <63 μm, 70% <200 μm, 98% <500 μm	Agglomerated for direct compression
	Tablettose 80	Meggle	0.57 g/mL	75% <180 μm, 85% <400 μm, 97% <630 μm	Agglomerated for direct compression
	Lactose monohydrate NF 180 MS HV	Kerry Bio-Sciences		42–55% >106 μm, 25–35% >150 μm	
Lactose, spray-dried	Pharmatose DCL 14	DMV International	0.61 g/mL	10% <45 μm, 40% <100 μm, 100% <250 μm	Good for low-dose drug
	NF Lactose-316 Fast Flo	Foremost Farms	0.58 g/mL	60–80% <75 μm, 30–55% <140 μm, 0.5% <250 μm	Good flowability
	FlowLac 100	Meggle	0.62 g/mL	10% <32 μm, 20–45% <100 μm, 80% <200 μm	Good for low-dose drug

of a fine milled lactose. Angle of repose values are 33° for Pharmatose DCL15 and 32° for Tablettose 70 and Tablettose 80, respectively.[32] In addition, these materials are insensitive to lubrication level and to moisture uptake.

Anhydrous lactose is a free-flowing crystalline β-lactose without water of hydration, first described in the literature in 1966.[33] It is available in a white crystalline powder that has good flowability and high compactibility. Anhydrous lactose can be reworked or milled, resulting in a smaller loss of compactibility than with other forms of lactose (due to its high fragmentation propensity). Table 7.4 lists the physical properties of the product. The product is very suitable for moisture-sensitive drug formulations.

Pharmatose® DCL22 is a new anhydrous lactose grade with a unique particle surface structure. Its excellent mixing properties are suitable for direct compression with both low- and high-dose formulations.[28] However, at high relative humidity levels, anhydrous lactose will pick up moisture, forming the hydrated form. This often results in an increase in the volume of the tablets if the excipient is a large percentage of the total tablet.

Several incompatibility issues are associated with lactose. Chemically, lactose is a reducing sugar and may react with drugs containing a primary amine or amino acids by the Maillard reaction. Control the amount of amorphous lactose in the product when using it in a low-dose formulation containing a moisture-sensitive drug. The amorphous form of lactose may absorb moisture and change the microenvironment in the formulation, facilitating a chemical reaction or degradation of drug substance. In addition, lactose may contain trace amounts of peroxides that lead to chemical incompatibility with drug substances sensitive to oxidation.[34]

Mannitol. Recently there has been an increased interest in direct compression mannitol. Mannitol is a hexahydric alcohol related to mannose and is isomeric with sorbitol. Mannitol exists as a white, odorless, and crystalline powder with polymorphic forms.[35] Mannitol is vegetable-derived and has no regulatory concerns of transmissible spongiform encephalopathy, bovine spongiform encephalopathy, and genetically modified organism. For oral solid dosage forms, it is primarily used as a filler–binder in tablet formulations, where it is of particular value since it is not hygroscopic and may thus be used with moisture-sensitive active ingredients.[36] Granular or spray-dried mannitol grades are commercially available for direct compression tablet applications.

Table 7.5 lists typical physical properties of selected commercially available grades of direct compression mannitol. These products are free flowing and have good compactibility with low friability. Angle of repose estimates are 38° for Pearlitol® 200SD and 39° for Pearlitol® 100SD, respectively. Spray-dried mannitol such as Pearlitol® 200SD has nearly spherical particle shape with a porous surface that provides strong adsorption sites for fine particles in low-dose drug products. Thus, when the content uniformity and the mix homogeneity are of utmost importance, use specialty mannitol as a filler–binder for low-dose formulations.

TABLE 7.5 Typical Physical Properties of Selected Mannitol as Directly Compressible Filler–Binders

Chemical	Trade Name	Manufacturer	Bulk Density (g/mL)	Particle Size (μm)
Mannitol, spray-dried	Pearlitol 100SD	Roqette	0.48	
	Pearlitol 200SD	Roqette	0.45	
	Mannogem-EZ	SPI Pharma	0.46	Mean at 142, 60% at 75–150
Mannitol, granular	Pearlitol 300DC	Roqette	0.62	
	Pearlitol 400DC	Roqette	0.68	
	Pearlitol 500DC	Roqette	0.64	
	Mannitol Granular	SPI Pharma	0.66	60% at 75–1190
	Mannitol Granular 2080	SPI Pharma	0.64	Mean at 447
	Parteck M200	Merck KgaA	0.51	Mean at 150
	Parteck M200	Merck KgaA	0.49	Mean at 250

Microcrystalline Cellulose. Microcrystalline cellulose is a purified, partially depolymerized cellulose that occurs as a white, odorless, tasteless, crystalline powder composed of porous particles. It is widely used in pharmaceutical dosage forms, primarily as a filler–binder in oral tablets and capsules with both wet granulation and direct compression processes. Microcrystalline cellulose was marketed first in 1964 by the FMC Corporation under name Avicel® PH in four different particle size grades, each with different properties.[37] Addition of Avicel® into a spray-dried lactose-based formulation overcame compressibility problems. At the same time, the lactose enhanced the flowability of the Avicel products available at that time. The direct compression tableting process became a reality, rather than a concept, partially because of the availability of Avicel. As of 2007, Avicel® PH is commercially available in 10 types with different particle size, density, and moisture grades that have different properties and applications (Table 7.6).[38] Other brands of microcrystalline cellulose are also available on the pharmaceutical market, including Pharmacel® 101 and 102 from DMV International and Emcocel® 50 M and 90 M from JRS Pharma.

Microcrystalline cellulose is one of the most commonly used filler–binders in direct compression formulations because it provides good binding properties as a dry binder, excellent compactibility, and a high dilution potential. It also contributes good disintegration and lubrication characteristics to direct compression formulas. When compressed, microcrystalline cellulose undergoes plastic deformation. The acid hydrolysis portion of the production process introduces slip planes and dislocations into the material. Slip planes, dislocations, and the small size of the individual crystals aid in the plastic flow that takes place. The spray-dried particle itself, which has a higher porosity compared with the absolute porosity of cellulose, also deforms

TABLE 7.6 Different Grades of Avicel PH Microcrystalline Cellulose

Grade of Avicel	Nominal Mean Particle Size (μm)	Bulk Density (g/mL)	Moisture Content (%)	Characteristics
PH 101	50	0.26–0.31	≤5.0	Wet granulation
PH 102	100	0.28–0.33	≤5.0	Direct compression
PH 105	20	0.20–0.30	≤5.0	Superior compactibility
102-SCG	150	0.28–0.34	≤5.0	Superior flow
PH 200	180	0.29–0.36	≤5.0	Superior flow
PH 103	50	0.26–0.31	≤3.0	Low moisture
PH 113	50	0.27–0.34	≤2	Low moisture
PH 112	100	0.28–0.34	≤1.5	Low moisture
PH 301	50	0.34–0.45	≤5.0	High density
PH 302	100	0.35–0.46	≤5.0	High density

under compaction pressure. The strength of microcrystalline cellulose tablets results from hydrogen bonding between the plastically deformed, large surface area particles.[39–41]

Microcrystalline cellulose is the most compressible of any direct compression excipient. Producing a tablet of a given hardness requires less compression force for other materials. Therefore, it is usually mixed with another filler to achieve ideal compactibility and flowability of a direct compression formulation. Large particle size grades of microcrystalline cellulose are made by spray-dried processes to form dry and porous particle surfaces. The porous surfaces provide adsorption sites needed for fine drug particles in low-dose formulations. However, microcrystalline cellulose contains trace amounts of peroxides that may lead to chemical incompatibility with oxidatively sensitive drug substances.[34]

Pregelatinized Starch. Starches and their derivatives are among the most widely used excipients for oral solid dosage forms. Starch in its natural state does not possess two critical properties necessary for making good tablets: compactibility and flowability. There have been many attempts to modify starch to improve its compaction and flow characteristics. The only modification of starch that has received widespread acceptance in direct compression is pregelatinized starch. Pregelatinized starch such as Lycatab C is starch that is chemically and/or mechanically processed to rupture all or part of the starch granules. This renders the starch flowable and directly compressible. Typically, pregelatinized starch contains 5% free amylose, 15% free amylopectin, and 80% unmodified starch. In a tablet formulation, it can be used as a binder, filler, and disintegrant.[42] It has extremely high moisture content (>7%), but there is little indication that this moisture is readily available to accelerate the decomposition of moisture-sensitive drugs.[43] As a binder, it compresses well, predominately deforming plastically.

Analytical results on Lycatab C are 0.64 g/mL bulk density, 35° angle of repose, and mean particle size of 100 μm.[44] Another similar product, Starch 1500, supplied by Colorcon, can be used with other excipients such as microcrystalline cellulose, lactose, and dicalcium phosphate. This combination produces tablets with excellent hardness and low friability at compacting forces typically used in tableting operations.[45] Ahmed et al.[46] reported that Starch 1500, when premixed with an API as a carrier (filler–binder), yielded excellent content uniformity on a production scale of 4 million tablets. The average assay of the tablets was reported at 99% of the label claim (RSD of 2%), even though the API in the tablet formulation was only 0.07% (w/w). In another study, Starch 1500, in a low-dose indomethacin formulation (0.5% API), consistently yielded blends with significantly better homogeneity and minimal API agglomeration when compared with lactose (Fast Flo) and dibasic calcium phosphate dihydrate (Emcompress).[47]

The ability of Starch 1500 to achieve good homogeneity of the API may be ascribed to a uniform distribution of fine particles of API "nestling" into crevices of Starch 1500 substrate. The moisture contained within Starch 1500 may mediate strong adsorption of the API within the crevices via a hydrogen bonding mechanism. Thus, pregelatinized starch may be used as a carrier in low-dose formulations for good blending homogeneity and content uniformity. However, because of its plastic behavior under pressure, Starch 1500 is extremely sensitive to mixing with lubricant. Generally, avoid using alkaline stearates (or keep below 0.25%) when using Starch 1500 as a filler–binder in formulations. Alternatively, stearic acid and hydrogenated vegetable oil are acceptable to replace magnesium stearate.[44]

Dibasic Calcium Phosphate. The most widely used inorganic direct compression filler is unmilled dibasic calcium phosphate dihydrate, which consists of free-flowing aggregates of small microcrystals that shatter upon compression. It is a white, nonhygroscopic, odorless, and tasteless powder. Although this hydrate is stable at room temperature, it can lose water of crystallization when exposed to temperatures of 40–60°C.[48] This loss is more likely to occur in a humid environment. When combined with a highly hygroscopic filler like microcrystalline cellulose, the loss of moisture may be sufficient to cause a softening of the tablet matrix due to weakening of the interparticulate bonds. The ability of the hygroscopic filler to extract the water of crystallization may also accelerate decomposition of moisture-sensitive drugs.

In addition to the hydrate form, anhydrous dibasic calcium phosphate is also a directly compressible filler–binder. This form is also nonhygroscopic and stable at room temperature.

Both calcium phosphates have good flowability. The predominant deformation mechanism for both forms under compression is brittle fracture, which reduces the strain-rate sensitivity of the materials.[49] However, unlike the hydrate form, anhydrous dicalcium phosphate, when compacted under high-pressure, can exhibit lamination and capping.

Fujicalin is an anhydrous dibasic calcium phosphate designed as a direct compression excipient. It has improved flowability and compaction characteristics compared with the conventional product, and maintains the ability to rapidly disintegrate.[50] Fujicalin's patented manufacturing process yields porous spheres with a

TABLE 7.7 Physical Properties of Fujicalin and Conventional Dicalcium Phosphates

Property	Fujicalin SG (Dibasic Calcium Phosphate, Dehydrate)	Dibasic Calcium Phosphate, Dehydrate	Dibasic Calcium Phosphate, Anhydrous
Bulk density (g/mL)	0.42	0.83	0.76
Tapped density (g/mL)	0.45	0.91	1.11
BET specific surface area (m^2/g)	40	0.57	1.95
Mean particle size (μm)	112	127	43
Angle of repose (deg)	32	38	36

Source: Fuji Chemical Industry Co.

high specific surface area.[51] Table 7.7 gives physical properties of Fujicalin and conventional dicalcium phosphates. Particularly, the unique surface characteristics of Fujicalin may provide an advantage for low-dose formulations because it produces a filler–binder that has sufficient adsorption sites available for fine drug substances.

Co-Processed Excipients. Material science plays an important role in modifying the physicomechanical properties of a material, especially with regard to its compression and flow behavior. Coprocessing excipients provides an interesting method of altering the physicomechanical characteristics of materials. Materials are classified as elastic, plastic, or brittle based on their behavior under compression; however, a filler–binder usually exhibits all three types of behavior, with one type being the predominant response. Coprocessing is generally conducted with one excipient that is plastic and another that is brittle, because a combination of plastic and brittle materials is necessary for optimum tableting performance.[52]

Cellactose is a co-processed filler–binder containing 75% lactose (brittle material) and 25% cellulose (plastic material).[53] This particular combination prevents the storage of too much elastic energy during compression, which results in a small amount of stress relaxation and a reduced tendency of capping and lamination. Coprocessing two kinds of materials produces a synergistic effect, in terms of compressibility, by selectively overcoming the disadvantages of a single ingredient. Such combinations can help improve functionalities such as compaction performance, flow properties, strain-rate sensitivity, lubricant sensitivity or sensitivity to moisture, or reduced hornification.[52] Coprocessed filler–binder excipients for direct compression include:

- Starlac™—a spray-dried compound consisting of 85% alpha-lactose monohydrate and 15% maize starch;
- Cellactose® 80—a spray-dried compound consisting of 75% alpha-lactose monohydrate and 25% cellulose powder;

- MicroceLac® 100—a spray-dried compound consisting of 75% alpha-lactose monohydrate and 25% microcrystalline cellulose;
- Ludipress®—an excipient consisting of 93% alpha-lactose monohydrate, 3.5% povidone, and 3.5% crospovidone;
- Ludipress® LCE—an excipient consisting of 96.5% alpha-lactose monohydrate and 3.5% povidone;
- Cel-O-Cal—an excipient consisting of microcrystalline cellulose and calcium sulfate;
- Prosolv SMCC®—silicified microcrystalline cellulose consisting of microcrystalline cellulose and colloidal silicon dioxide.

Coprocessed excipients can be generally regarded as safe (GRAS) if the parent excipients are also GRAS-certified by the regulatory agencies due to the absence of chemical changes to the parent excipients during the manufacture process.[54] Therefore, these excipients do not require additional toxicological studies.

7.4.3 Formulation Design and Optimization

Formulation design is based on the physical, chemical, and biopharmaceutical properties of a drug substance. A formulation for direct compression is composed of active pharmaceutical ingredients and other inactive ingredients such as fillers, binders, disintegrants, flow aids, and lubricants. Simplicity is the basis of good formulation design. Minimally, a direct compression tablet formulation must meet requirements for manufacturability, uniformity of dose, physical and chemical stability, appropriate drug release profiles, and bioavailability. In addition, the formulation must meet many quality standards and special requirements to ensure the efficacy and safety of the product.

Prototype Formulation. Before selecting a formulation composition, perform a drug-excipient compatibility study and stress testing under conditions of different temperature, pH, light, and oxidizing agents. The results will determine selection of physically and chemically compatible excipients and the need for stabilizers such as pH modifiers and antioxidants. As listed in Table 7.3, a formulation scientist may need to select one excipient out of many in each functional category. Design of experiments and statistical analysis can be useful tools in prototype formulation screening. Usually, factorial designs (full or fractional) can be used in the preliminary screen stage. The goal of this study is to determine the optimal choice in each excipient category. The common formulation factors may include:

- filler–binder—lactose, mannitol, microcrystalline cellulose (MCC), or starch;
- disintegrant—crospovidone, sodium starch glycolate, or sodium croscarmellose;
- flow aid—talc or colloidal silicon dioxide;
- lubricant—magnesium stearate, stearic acid, or sodium stearyl fumarate.

For a two-level factorial design, only two excipients can be selected for each factor. However, for the filler–binder, a combination of brittle and plastic materials is preferred for optimum compaction properties. Therefore, different combinations such as lactose with MCC or mannitol with starch can count as a single factor. Experimental responses can be powder blend flowability, compactibility, blend uniformity, uniformity of dose unit, dissolution, disintegration, and stability under stressed storage conditions. The major advantage of using a DOE to screen prototype formulations is that it allows evaluation of all potential factors simultaneously, systematically, and efficiently. It helps the scientist understand the effect of each formulation factor on each response, as well as potential interaction between factors. It also helps the scientist identify the critical factors based on statistical analysis. DOE results can define a prototype formulation that will meet the predefined requirements for product performance stability and manufacturing.

After selecting a prototype, evaluate requirements of particle size and size distribution of drug substance. Prepare two to three batches of drug substance with different particle sizes and supply them to the formulation scientists to establish a specification on the particle size of the drug substance. It is important to understand the effect of particle size of the drug substance associated with drug load on blending homogeneity and product content uniformity as early as possible.

Be aware that the DOE study is a time-consuming and labor-intensive activity. The study may generate a significant amount of data. However, without a good understanding of the objective of the study and the factors-responses to be investigated, the DOE study may not provide any value to defining a formulation composition, but instead may waste development time and resources.

Compactibility, Flowability, and Segregation Studies. Designing and selecting a prototype formulation requires three studies related to manufacturability: compactibility, flowability, and segregation potential of the powder blends.

The first step is to design a direct compression formulation for optimizing tablet hardness with appropriate compression force, while at the same time assuring rapid tablet disintegration and drug dissolution. In other words, the formulation blend should have excellent compactibility. Next, the powder mixture must first flow through a stationary orifice (the outlet of a hopper), followed by flow into moving orifices (the tablet dies). Thus, the formulation blend should have good flowability to reduce tablet weight variation and improve product content uniformity. For low-dose formulations in which the drug makes up a relatively minor proportion of the tablet, flowability is usually not a problem because of the many innovative excipients with excellent flow properties available on the market today. Finally, carefully consider and select the particle size, shape, and density for the different components in a formulation to minimize the segregation potential during manufacture. A formulation scientist can design and optimize an acceptable direct compression formulation with excellent compactibility and flowability using a combination of excipients that have different physicomechanical characteristics.

A direct compression formulation should form a strong compact that can withstand coating, storage, and transportation requirements. An optimum formulation can be compacted into tablets with the desired strength without applying excessive compression force. For a low-dose formulation in which the drug substance makes up a relatively minor proportion of the tablet, compaction is usually not a problem since most directly compressible filler–binders are highly compactable. However, a mixture of different grades of Pearlitol SD and Avicel® PH may have significantly different compression profiles and some formulation blends can only generate relatively soft tablets (Fig. 7.2). Pearlitol 100SD has better compactibility than Pearlitol 200SD, while Avicel PH® 200 shows better compactibility than Avicel® PH102. A combination of Pearlitol 100SD and Avicel® PH102 at a ratio of 1 : 3 possesses an excellent compression profile. Generally, direct compression formulations are less compactable than wet granulation formulations. However, this clearly depends largely on the choice of materials, as selecting appropriate compositions of excipients can achieve desired compactibility.

It is essential to characterize formulation flow properties—and the factors which impact on it (Table 7.8)—at the beginning of the formulation design and optimization stages. Several different methods are available for determining the flow properties of powder mixtures that can serve as tools for prototype formulation screening:[55]

- flow rate through an orifice;
- Carr index;

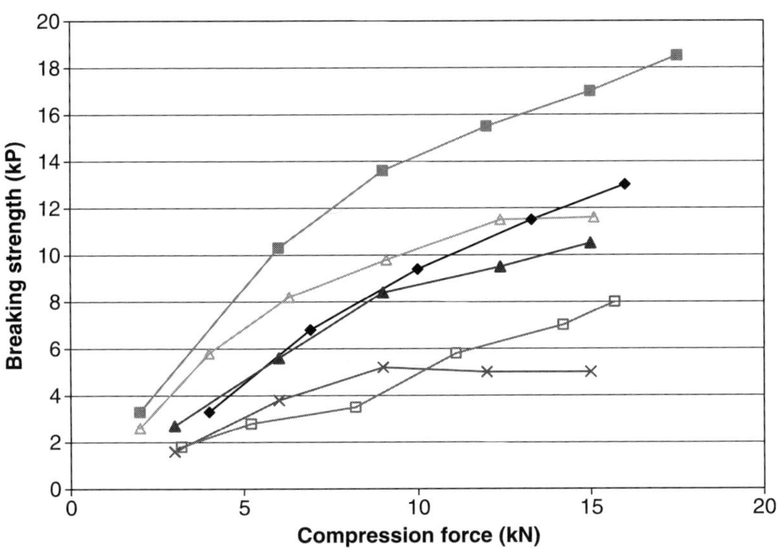

Figure 7.2 Compressibility of directly compressed mannitol–Avicel PH-based formulations containing 6% sodium croscarmellose and 1.4% magnesium stearate (◆, Pearlitol 100SD-Avicel PH102, 3 : 1; ■, Pearlitol 100SD-Avicel PH102®, 1 : 3; ▲, Pearlitol 100SD-Avicel® PH200, 3 : 1; ×, Pearlitol 200SD-Avicel PH102®, 3 : 1; □, Pearlitol 200SD-Avicel® PH200, 3 : 1; △, Pearlitol 200SD-Avicel PH200®, 1 : 3; 7 mm round shape with 150 mg tablet weight).

TABLE 7.8 Factors Impacting on Powder Flowability

Powder/Formulation Attributes	External Factors
Particle size	Flow rate
Particle size distribution	Degree of compaction
Density (bulk and tapped)	Vibration
Particle shape	Environmental humidity
Particle morphology (surface texture)	Environmental temperature
Cohesivity	Electro-static charge
Interaction between particles	Aeration
Attrition	Surface of liners in the container
Moisture content	Container shape
Hardness	Container size
Elasticity	Storage duration
Particle packing properties	
Thermal properties	

- angle of repose;
- shear cell method.

Flow rate through an orifice is used only for materials that have some capacity to flow. It is not useful for cohesive materials. The flow rate through an orifice is generally measured as the mass per time flowing from any of a number of types of containers (cylinders, funnels, hoppers). Measurement of the flow rate can be either in discrete increments or continuous. The orifice diameter and shape are critical factors in determining powder flow rate.[56] Because flow rate through an orifice is not an intrinsic property of the powder, it is used (in combination with other measurements such as angle of repose and Carr index) to screen prototype formulations with good flow and to distinguish good-flowing powders from poorer-flowing formulations.

The bulk density (ρ_b) of a powder mixture is its mass divided by the bulk volume it occupies. The tapped density (ρ_t) is the density of a powder mixture that has been compacted by tapping or vibration following a specified procedure. Carr[57] reported that the more a material is compacted in a compaction or bulk/tapped density test, the poorer its flow properties. Carr index (i.e., compressibility), is defined as:

$$\text{Carr index (\%)} = 100\,(\rho_t - \rho_b)/\rho_t \tag{7.2}$$

A Carr index less than 21 for a powder mixture indicates good flow, while one between 21 and 25 suggests a marginal flow property. A more commonly used term is the Hausner ratio, which is simply ρ_t/ρ_b, or the tapped density divided by bulk density. This ratio was introduced by Hausner in 1967 to characterize metal powders,[58] but is commonly used today for pharmaceutical powders. The higher the Hausner ratio, the poorer the flow. The Hausner ratio varies from about 1.2 for a free-flowing powder to 1.6 for cohesive powder.

When a powder pours from a funnel onto a flat surface, it forms a pile or mound of powder. A formulation mixture that is not cohesive and flows well spreads out and forms a lower mound. Mixtures that are more cohesive form higher mounds that are less spread out. The angle of repose is the angle of the free surface of a pile of powder mixture to the horizontal plane. This method is simple in concept, but not particularly discerning. The measurements obtained are highly dependent on the device used. As a rough guide, angles less than 35° are usually indicative of good flow, while powders with angles greater than 45° are likely to be poor flow materials.[59]

Heistand[60] related the repose angle to the intrinsic cohesion and frictional coefficient of powders. Angular tests may be more applicable to relatively free-flowing powders containing particles larger than 100 μm. It is not possible to investigate such powders in scientifically more satisfactory methods such as shear cell and tensile strength test due to their low cohesion and tensile strength. Thus, the angular test, usually in combination with other tests, provides a simple and sometimes useful method for screening the flow properties of prototype formulations. Table 7.9 gives the generally accepted scale of flowability for the Carr index, the Hausner ratio, and the angle of repose.

The weaknesses associated with the flow through an orifice and angle of repose measurements limit their application for powder flow studies and hopper designs. Consequently, several powder shear testers and methods that permit a more thorough and precisely defined assessment of powder flow characteristics were developed. Shear testers that measure the frictional characteristics of a powder bed under load yield valuable information with regard to powder flow in high-speed tablet equipment. A number of types of shear cell testers are available, but the most common types used in the pharmaceutical industry are the Jenike shear cell and the Schulze ring shear tester.[61,62]

The Jenike shear cell tester is classified as a direct shear tester that is capable of providing information on a solids' "cohesive strength" as well as its "wall friction" properties. The tester allows us to measure the strength of a powder blend as a function of pressure applied to it. These are two main considerations when design a bin or hopper to ensure reliable material flow. The tester consists of a base, a moveable shear ring resting on top of the base, and a top cover lid (Fig. 7.3).[61] The base is fixed while the lid rotates at a constant low rate. Powder blend is placed in the ring and base and a

TABLE 7.9 Scale of Flowability Determined with Different Methods

Flow Property	Angle of Repose (deg)	Carr Index (%)	Hausner Ratio
Excellent	25–30	1–10	1.00–1.11
Good	31–35	11–15	1.12–1.18
Fair (aid not needed)	36–40	16–20	1.19–1.25
Passable (may hang up)	41–45	21–25	1.26–1.34
Poor (must agitate, vibrate)	46–55	26–31	1.35–1.45
Very poor	56–65	32–37	1.46–1.59
Very, very poor	>66	>38	>1.60

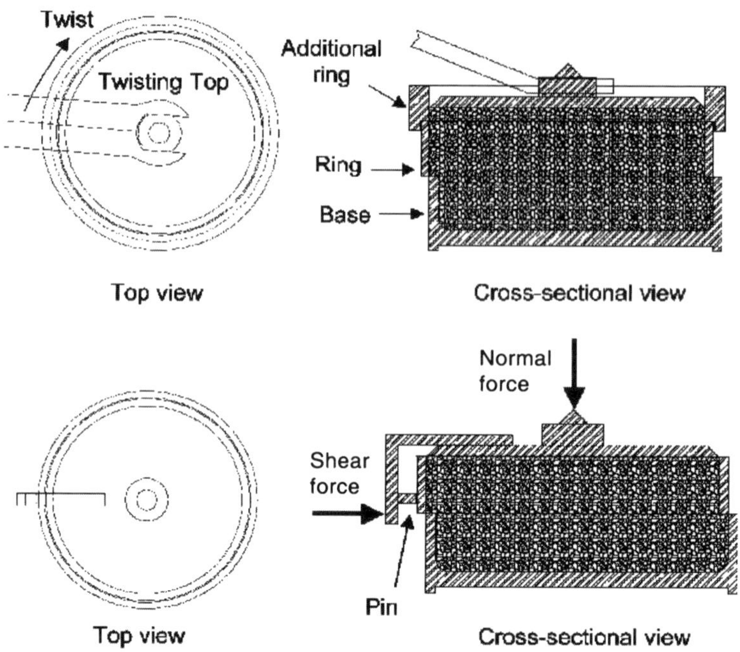

Figure 7.3 Schematic of the Jenike cell showing the twisting (top) and shearing (bottom) stages. (Adapted from Bilgili et al.[61])

special twisting top applied. As the total shear in the Jenike cell is limited, the standard testing procedure suggests preconsolidating (compacting) the blend within the cell by applying a weight onto the top of the cell and rotating the twisting top to produce a stress state in the test cell that is close to desired critical state. Then, the mold ring and twisting top are removed, and the shearing top and consolidation weight are placed on the blend in the specimen. The blend is sheared to achieve a constant shear force (steady-state). The consolidation load placed on the specimen is then reduced, and the specimen is sheared again to measure the maximum shear force required to fail the specimen in the tester. Repeat the process with the same consolidating load but with lower shearing loads until the yield locus is obtained. If developing a series of yield loci, use a series of consolidating forces. Base a flow-factor plot on at least three consolidation pressures. This method is extremely time-consuming and tedious, and the testing result is operator-dependent.

The Schulze ring shear tester is a modified version of the Jenike shear tester. In the Schulze ring shear tester, the powder sample is contained in an annular trough (Fig. 7.4). An angular lid attached to a crossbeam lies on top of the sample. Small bars attached to the bottom side of the lid and the bottom of the cell prevent the powder from sliding against the lid or bottom. Crossbeams attached to a fixed beam prevent the lid from rotating while the shear cell rotates. The movement of the cell with respect to the fixed lid causes the power bed to shear, which is measured with load cells attached to tie rods. Weights hung from a crossbeam apply force on the

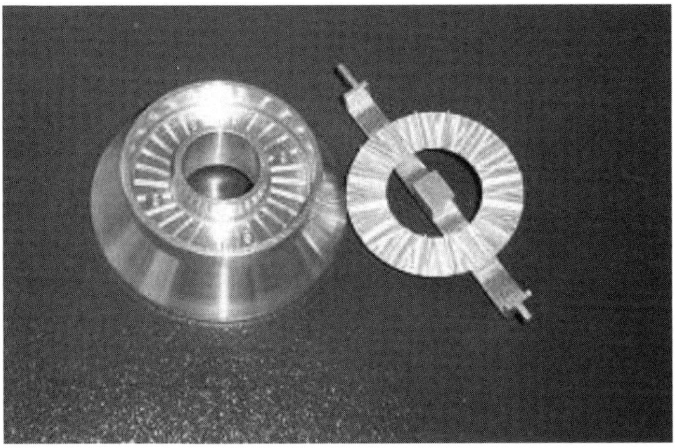

Figure 7.4 Schulze ring shear tester annular trough.

sample. This can be done during the shearing and conditioning of the power sample. The scientist can also remove the cell and conduct time consolidation by placing weights on the sample outside of the test device, in a similar manner to that with the Jenike shear tester.

The Schulze ring shear tester has several important advantages over the Jenike cell tester. It offers a constant area of shear, to make handling easier and consolidation and shear faster. After consolidating the bed, it is possible to generate a full locus without reconsolidating after each load. The consolidation step becomes more automated and uniform, eliminating much of the operator's variability during the testing process. Table 7.10 lists classification of powder flow properties using the Schulze ring shear tester.

Understanding the segregation potential of low-dose drug formulations is an important aspect of drug product development. This assessment should occur during design of the prototype formulations and initial process development stages. Further processing of a segregated, heterogeneous mixture can result in final product quality issues such as poor content uniformity for individual dosage units and nonuniform appearance for tablet dosage forms. Segregation can also affect manufacturing process robustness through erratic or unstable powder flow. This can cause unequal filling of the die cavities, resulting in variations in tablet hardness, friability,

TABLE 7.10 Classification of Powder Flow Properties Using the Schulze Ring Shear Tester

FFC Value	Nature of the Powders	Example
$FFC < 1$	Non-flowing	Caked sugar
$1 < FFC < 2$	Poor flowing	Moist clay
$2 < FFC < 4$	Cohesive	Flour
$4 < FFC < 10$	Good flowing	Fine moist sand
$10 < FFC$	Free flowing	Fine dry sand

weight uniformity, and thickness. The extent of segregation that will occur is a function of not only the formulation composition and its tendency to segregate, but also the equipment (e.g., blender design), process (e.g., transfer rate), and environment (e.g., temperature and moisture content).

Besides theoretical prediction tools,[63] commonly used devices include fluidization segregation testers and sifting segregation testers. The Jenike and Johanson fluidization tester is standardized through ASTM International.[64] The tester fluidizes a powder sample (80 mL) in a column of air and allows the particles to settle in the column. The tester has a mechanism to retrieve top, middle, and bottom samples of the settled powder. The sample is then analyzed to determine if there is a property gradient within the column. However, the tester can be improved by making it material-sparing, more efficient, and more reproducible.

Hedden et al.[65] reported that a modified fluidization tester offers several improvements over the current ASTM standardized method. This modified tester requires less than 20 mL of powder to characterize the fluidization segregation potential of a sample. In addition, the tester includes unique features for powder containment of potent compounds, in-process monitoring of the fluidization conditions, and sample retrieval without the need for sub-sampling or riffling for typical analyses.

The sifting segregation tester consists of an upper hopper, a low hopper, a guide cylinder connected to the low hopper, and a material collecting cup. Load a representative, one-liter sample of formulation powders carefully into the upper hopper and allow it to fall into the lower hopper. Then, open the lower hopper slide gate and the powders fill in the guide cylinder in a funnel flow pattern. Collect the powders in the guide cylinder into the 55 mL collecting cup. For one liter of powder, a total of 19 samples can be collected. Using proper subdivision techniques such as a rotary riffler, the size of the sample should be suitable for potency and particle size analysis. The trend from the beginning to the end of discharge is an indication of segregation potential. Usually, sifting segregation favors the initial discharge of fine particles with increasing quantities of coarse particles at the end of discharge. Other methods used to measure segregation tendency of a formulation can also be found in the literature,[66,67] including the free-fall method, the die filling method, the vibratory drum method, rotating horizontal method, and inclined rotating drum method.

Formulation Optimization. Formula optimization follows the selection of a formulation composition from the preliminary screening work. Formulation optimization focuses on determining the optimal level of each excipient to enable definition of a design space for each individual excipient. A proper DOE study is an effective and efficient way of defining the excipient levels and aiding in the selection of the optimal formulation. Factors in an optimization DOE study may include:

- drug substance load—0.5% and 1%;
- Fast Flo lactose—Avicel® PH200: 3 : 1 and 1 : 3;
- sodium starch glycolate—4% and 8%;
- magnesium stearate—0.75% and 1.5%.

Using a full factorial design, a DOE study could require a total of 2^4 (i.e., 16) trials. The batch size could be 2–5 kg. The responses may include blend uniformity, powder flowability, compactibility (compression profiles), tablet ejection force, uniformity of dose units (UDU), dissolution, disintegration, and stability. If a middle level is relevant for each of the factors, replicate independent trials are often performed with each of the factors set at their mid level. These trials help assess whether there is evidence that at least one of the factors may have curvature associated with it. This is calculated by comparing the average responses of the center point trials to the average responses of the factorial trials. Curvature is assumed if the center point responses cannot be predicted from a linear relationship between the factorial trial responses. Other DOE approaches applied in formulation optimization include fractional factorial design, central composite design, mixture design, D-optimal design, and Box–Behnken design.

7.5 MANUFACTURING PROCESS DEVELOPMENT FOR LOW-DOSE DRUG PRODUCTS

A good formulation must not only be stable and bioavailable after administration, but must also have a robust manufacturing process capable of consistently producing high-quality product. Exploration of preliminary process conditions occurred during formulation screening and optimization. After defining the unit formula for the commercial drug product, the scientist should perform additional studies to optimize the manufacturing process. Figure 7.5 illustrates a flow diagram for tablet manufacture using direct compression.

A blending operation mixes the drug substance, filler–binder, and a disintegrant. If necessary, first preblend the drug substance with a portion of filler–binders. Either pass the blend through a sieve or mill by a cone mill to break down agglomerates of drug substance. Then, mix the resultant blend with the remaining filler–binder(s) and a disintegrant. Incorporate a glidant, if necessary, and a lubricant by subsequent blending operations. Finally, discharge the lubricated blend into an IBC, and compress into tablets. Each processing step involves multiple process parameters. Table 7.11 lists the process variables and quality and performance attributes for each unit operation.

For a given formulation, it is important to evaluate thoroughly all processing steps in order to develop a robust manufacturing process. The scale could be a few kg to 1/10th scale for the commercial batch size, thus necessitating a significant quantity of bulk drug substance. The following sections further discuss the critical steps in direct compression for tablet manufacture.

7.5.1 API Deagglomeration

Micronizing a drug substance increases the surface area and surface energy, resulting in cohesiveness between the particles. This cohesiveness may promote aggregation and agglomeration of the drug substance, causing poor homogeneity of the final mix. Compression of this final mix may lead to poor tablet UDU. In developing a

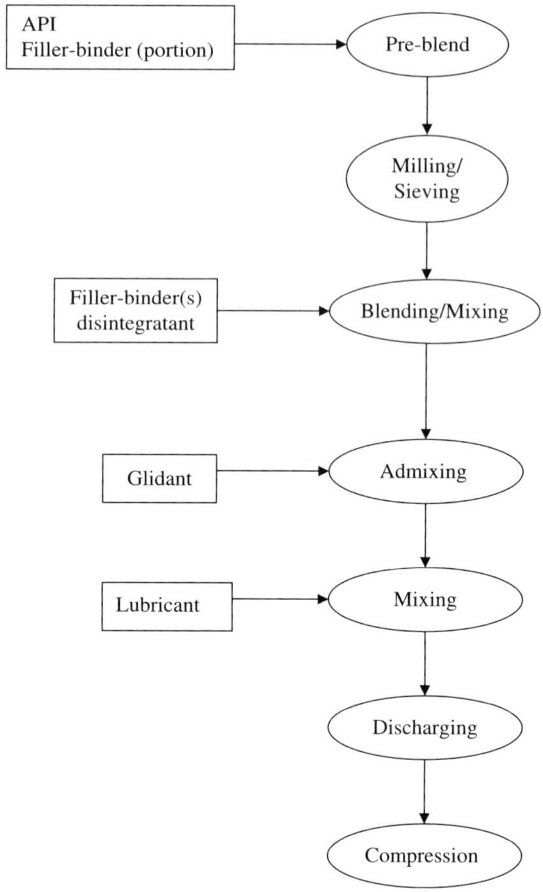

Figure 7.5 Manufacturing flow diagram using direct compression platform.

low-dose formulation, a deagglomeration operation is important step in evenly distributing the cohesive drug substance throughout the powder blend. This unit operation is highly recommended for low-dose formulations in order to achieve the required UDU and, consequently, a consistent and safe drug product. With very low drug concentrations, geometric dilutions or trituration become less effective for deagglomeration. Several methods are used in the pharmaceutical industry for effectively dispensing agglomerates, namely:

- sieving a preblend mixture of micronized drug and filler–binder;
- milling a preblend mixture of micronized drug and filler–binder;
- using high-shear equipment.

It is important to understand the nature of the agglomerates to be dispersed. If the agglomerates are only held together by cohesive surface forces, the techniques

TABLE 7.11 Process Variables and Quality Attributes Using Direct Compression for Tablet Manufacture

Unit Operation	Variables	Product Quality Attributes
Pre-blending	Load level Rotation speed Mixing time	Content uniformity
Milling	Screen size Feed rate Speed	Content uniformity
Mixing	Load level Rotation speed Mixing time	Blend homogeneity Content uniformity
Blending with lubricant	Load level Rotation speed Mixing time	Blending homogeneity Compression characteristics Dissolution Disintegration
Discharge	Container size Discharge rate	Content uniformity
Compression	Press speed Force feeder speed Compression force	Content uniformity Tablet hardness Friability Dissolution profile Disintegration time

have a good chance to work. If the agglomerates are bound together tightly, a more aggressive milling approach may be needed.

Sieving drug–filler premixes is a simple unit operation and, in many cases, is an adequate approach to limiting the agglomerates to a subcritical level. Egermann[68] observed a content variation of 29.1% for 1 mg medazepam tablets prepared without sieving step after 30 min of mixing time. If the drug alone was passed through a 0.5 mm sieve before mixing, sufficient deagglomeration could not be achieved because agglomeration took place again after passage through the sieve. In fact, 0.9% of the drug was found as lumps in the powder mixture, with the largest agglomerate weighing 1.2 mg. Sieving a 10% drug-filler blend through a 0.5 mm sieve effectively prevented agglomeration and resulted in the absence of lumps in the powder mixture and a UDU result of approximately 1%.

The appropriate mesh size for sieving a preblend is also important. Choice of size depends substantially on the drug dose strength and the required degree of homogeneity, and can be quantified only by approximation.[69] It is estimated that reducing the maximum agglomerate weight to 5% of the labeled drug content is adequate based on the requirements of the USP content uniformity test. According to this estimate, sieving of the preblend is practical even at extremely small dose levels; for a 10 μg dose, the mesh size is still larger than 100 μm.[68]

An alternative approach to sieving for deagglomeration is to mill the drug–filler preblend using a cone mill. This approach could easily work at commercial scale. A 1% blend of red iron oxide [nominal size of 2 μm in spray-dried lactose (Pharmatose DCL11) with a mean size of approximately 100 μm] required two passes through the cone mill using the smallest screen at 1400 rpm to effectively deagglomerate the pigment.[70]

Another example focuses on blending a cohesive drug using rotating bins of different sizes, followed by passing the blend through a conical cone mill after discharge from the rotating bin. The conical mill provides shear and ensures that the blend will be entirely and uniformly exposed to shear.

Conical mills improve the distribution of the drug substance and minimize drug agglomerates.[71] However, do not regard use of mills following discharge as a universal solution. If the blend is highly heterogeneous, the stream traversing the mill will exhibit differences in composition as a function of time. Lacking back-mixing capacity, a mill cannot eliminate such insufficiencies in homogenization. This should not be a concern, however, for low-dose formulation development, since an additional mixing unit operation with the remaining filler–binders (90%) occurs after this unit operation. Usually, deagglomeration by sieving or milling the drug-filler blend is suitable for a low-dose formulation with drug load of 0.5% and above.

When drug load in a formulation is lower than 0.5%, use a blender equipped with a high-speed intensifier bar. The intensifier bar is also suggested when a toxic drug substance requires a contained deagglomeration operation. Figures 7.6 and 7.7 show an intensifier bar situated within a tumbling blender. This configuration gives added versatility to these blenders due to the high shear attainable by the intensifier bar when operated at a speed of 1200–3450 rpm. This allows for effective deagglomeration and intimate mixing of a small amount of drug substance using a wide range of shearing force. Serial dilution, if necessary, is easy to achieve when incorporating low-dose active ingredients into the mixture. However, it is essential to control the blending time when using the intensifier bar. Using an intensifier bar for more than 5 min is not recommended. Longer mixing times may, in fact, adversely affect batch homogeneity and cause attrition of large, more friable particles in a mixture.

In conclusion, when blending small quantities of a micronized drug substance, the key process risk is the survival of particle agglomerates that can cause poor UDU results. Using deagglomeration steps can significantly help alleviate this issue, provided that the agglomerates do not re-form during subsequent mixing steps.

7.5.2 Powder Mixing

Powder blending or mixing after deagglomeration is the most important unit operation in direct compression, as it has a direct impact on content uniformity. Among the available equipment for powder mixing, tumbling blenders remain the most prevalent in the pharmaceutical industry. Tumbling blenders are hollow containers attached to a rotating shaft. The container is loaded with the powders and rotated

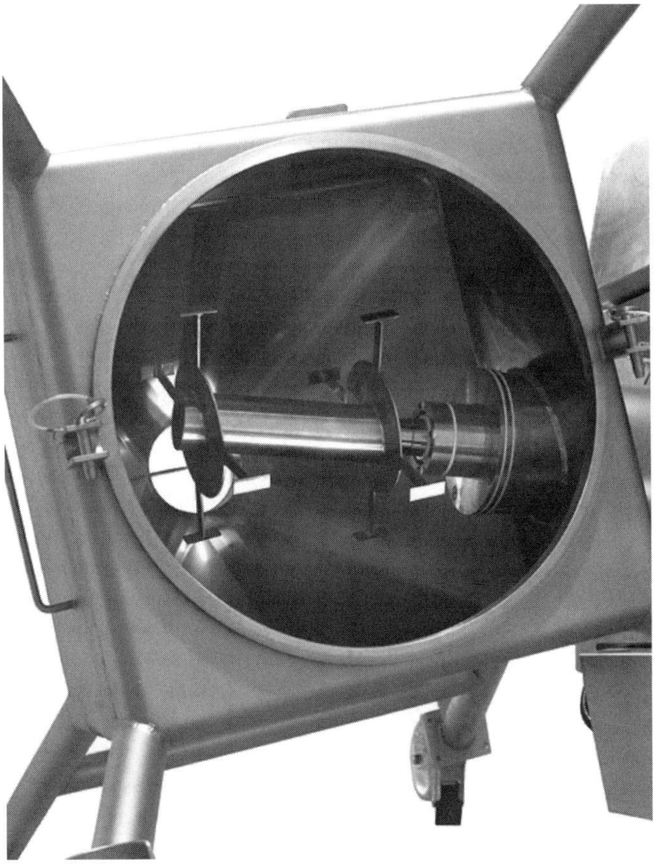

Figure 7.6 Tumbling bin blender with an intensifier bar. (Courtesy of Patterson–Kelley Co., Pennsylvania.)

for a fixed number of revolutions. The major advantages of tumbling blenders are large capacities, low-shear stresses, and ease of cleaning.

A number of different geometries are available from blender manufacturers, including V-blenders (e.g., the twin-shell blender), double cones, rotating cylinders,

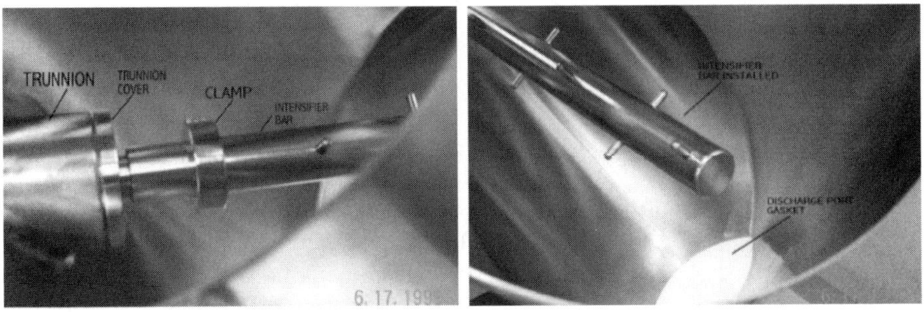

Figure 7.7 Pin intensifier bar installed in V-shaped blender. (Courtesy of GlobePharma, New Jersey.)

cube blenders, and bin blenders. It is possible to remove the bin blender from the rotating shaft after the blending operation(s) and transport it to the next process of operation (e.g., compression) without discharging its blend into a secondary vessel (i.e., hopper, barrel). This added functionality eliminates the need for additional transport containers, avoids tying up the production line, and minimizes operator contact with a potent drug. Additionally, avoiding a bin-to-bin transfer reduces the potential for segregation. Many experimental investigations regarding the performance of tumbling blenders can be found in the literature.[72–75]

Using V-shaped and bin blenders to mix fine, cohesive drug particles with free-flowing excipients can achieve adequate uniformity in a low-dose formulation.[13] However, the mixing mechanism in the V-shaped or bin blenders is mediated by diffusive mixing; therefore, strong agglomerates cannot be broken down during mixing. Hence, a deagglomeration operation, as discussed in the previous section, is necessary prior to the blending step to facilitate good content uniformity for the powder blend.

Fill level or blender load affects mixing efficiency in tumbling blenders. A reduced amount of materials in the blender should result in faster, or more efficient, mixing. However, very low fill levels (<25%) may interfere with the natural mixing mechanism and hinder mixing rate. Filling the blender to more than 80% of its capacity may result in dead zones in the middle of the mixture that do not interact with the rest of the materials.[72,76] In general, a fill level at approximately 60–80% is recommended, although the fill level in a blender may be related to type of blender.

Rotation speed of tumbling blenders can be another factor affecting blending efficiency. When mixing small amounts of micronized drug substance with free-flowing fillers, shear becomes the dominant factor for blend homogeneity. In addition, rotation speed may play a decisive role in determining mixing rates.[77] Conduct experimental studies at a scale of at least 1/10th commercial batch size to understand effects of fill level, rotation speed, and blending time on blend homogeneity. It is necessary to establish the relationship between blending time and blending homogeneity in order to meet the requirements of U.S. 21 CFR211.110 for demonstrating the adequacy of mixing to ensure uniformity of in-process powder blends and finished dosage units.

Quantitatively evaluate blend uniformity or homogeneity to determine optimum mixing time. Typically, a measure based on total mixture homogeneity is used as the means to track the evolution of mixture quality in blenders. There are three key factors to consider:

- sampling and sampling method;
- sample analysis;
- acceptance criteria.

Sampling is an important part of estimates of blending quality. In most cases, scientists do not have mixing problems, but actually have sampling problems.[8] Ideally, a powder for testing should be sampled when it is in motion and the whole of the stream of powder should be taken for many short increments of time instead of part of the stream being taken for a longer time.[78,79] However, it is usually not possible to take the powder mixture from a moving stream in blenders because of the equipment design and batch size.

The most commonly used devices for sample retrieval in blending homogeneity testing are thief probes. Several different sampling thieves have been developed and used for many years in the pharmaceutical industry.[72] A major problem with most thieves is that the retrieved sample is not representative of the true concentration at the location from which the sample is supposed to be obtained. Contamination with powders from other locations in the mixture during probe insertion causes these sampling errors. Also, nonuniform flow of different components into the sampling cavity can skew the sample concentration.

Some studies show that two samplers—the groove sampler and the core sampler—are more effective, accurate, and reliable than typical side-sampling or end-sampling thieves.[80–82] The groove thief consists of a hollow sleeve surrounding a solid inner steel rod with a groove bored along most of the length of the rod. The inner rod has a sampling cavity that is approximately 0.5 inch deep and wide along the middle 80% of the rod. Rotating the inner rod relative to the outer sleeve opens and closes the sampler. Insert the sampler into the powder bed while closed. Open the sampler to allow powder to flow into the sampling cavity, then close the sampler to trap the material within the sampler. After removing the sampler from the powder bin, place it horizontally on a stand while open. Rotate the entire device to discharge the collected material into a series of small trays.

Sample size can vary depending on the size of the sampler or the width of the container into which the material is discharged. Avoiding contamination during sample collection is vital, but determining the location and number of samples to extract from the mixture is equally important. Often, samples are taken from throughout the powder bed to ensure complete coverage of the entire mixture. Although this approach guarantees thoroughness, it can lead to wasted time, effort, and material if more efficient means are available. Carefully identify 10–15 sampling locations with three replicates in the blender to represent potential areas of poor blending.[83,84] In tumbling blenders such as V-shaped blenders, double cones, or drum mixers, select samples from at least two depths along the axis of the blender. The minimum number of sampling locations suggested is based on current scientific knowledge of blenders. For convective blenders (such as a ribbon blender), make a special effort to implement uniform volumetric sampling to include the corners and discharge area. Sample at least 20 locations to adequately validate the mixing.

Define effects of sample size on analytical results while developing a technique capable of measuring the true uniformity of the blend. Usually, 1–3 times the dosage unit weight is preferred, and sample quantities larger than three times (e.g., 4–10×) can be used with adequate scientific justification.[84] Quantitatively test one sample per location without sub-sampling for drug substance content using a validated analytical method. All individual results within 90.0–110.0% (absolute) of the mean of the results and a relative standard deviation of all individual results of $\leq$5% demonstrates adequacy of mixing and thus allows determination of optimum mixing time. On the other hand, significant within-location variance in the blend data can be an indication of one factor or a combination of factors such as inadequacy of blend mix, sampling error, or agglomeration. Significant between-location variance in the blend data can indicate that the blending operation is inadequate.

In the literature, the various mixing indices, over 30 in all, have been proposed to measure and compare homogeneity or degree of mixedness. The indices are derived or empirically modified from binary systems which contain monosized particles having the same density.[8] Those indices could be important tools to investigate the mechanism of mixing and to develop some basic mixing theory. However, the indices may not be practical for real-world mixing processes in the pharmaceutical industry.

7.5.3 Mixing with Lubricant

As discussed earlier, lubrication of direct compression formulations is one of the more complex and difficult problems faced by a pharmaceutical scientist. The ideal lubrication operation provides the mildest mixing conditions that guarantee sufficient homogeneity of the lubricant. Magnesium stearate, provided as a finely divided powder, is one of the most widely used lubricants in the pharmaceutical industry. Many formulations are sensitive to the lubrication process when the formulation uses magnesium stearate powder.

The shear applied during the mixing process is a critical variable. If the mixing process is inadequate, the lubricant might be poorly distributed, resulting in variability in tablet mechanical strength and tablet dissolution. If applying excessive shear, however, the magnesium stearate can adversely affect the flow of the final mix or suppress the dissolution of the tablets across the batch.[73] Evaluate processing parameters of the blender load, rotation rate, and blending time for their impact on tablet hardness, ejection force, and dissolution once the optimum lubricant level in a formulation has been established. A factorial DOE study containing three variables (load level, rotation speed, and blending time) at two levels can be applied effectively to optimize the lubrication process. As a rule of thumb, the mixing time for the lubricant should be set as the minimum time required to produce the desired lubricating effect.

7.5.4 Discharging from a Blender

At the end of final blending and lubrication, the mixture has to be discharged from the blender into a conveyer or a tablet press. In some cases, discharging into a secondary container has a mixing effect and thus leads to mixing quality changes. For a formulation with strong segregation tendencies, discharging may cause segregation of the blend. Therefore, evaluate the homogeneity of the final powder mixture after it is discharged into an intermediate bulk container. The sampling method and acceptance criteria are similar to that described in the blending homogeneity analysis. Developing robust blending and transfer processes that will minimize postblending segregation of the mixture, and that result in a product with acceptable content uniformity and performance.

7.5.5 Compression

The pharmaceutical industry produces tablets almost exclusively on rotary tablet presses from pilot plant to commercial manufacture. The output from different tablet presses may range from a few thousand tablets per hour to more than 1 million tablets per hour. By design, the compression event occurs using three parts: a die, lower punch, and upper punch. The dies and punches are mounted on a rotating turret. The shape of the die controls the shape of the tablets, while the distance between the lower and upper punch tips at the maximum compression force determines the thickness of the tablets. The tablet compression process is divided into three steps: powder filling into the die, compression, and tablet ejection from the die.[85]

First, the die is filled when it passes beneath a stationary feed frame and the lower punch is in the filling position. Tablet weight variation is dependent on uniform powder filling into the die cavity. Since the residence time of the die under the feed frame is very short, the formulation blend must flow easily and reproducibly.

Second, movement of both punches between the compression rollers compresses powders in the die. The distance between the punch tips decreases under compression force and progressively reduces the porosity of the powder bed in the die. Once the particles are close enough together, interparticulate forces lead to bond formation and the individual particles aggregate, forming a tablet.

Some tablet presses are equipped with two sets of rollers: a smaller roller located between the feed frame, and the main compression roller which allows a small degree of compression (e.g., precompression) to take place. Precompression can remove air from the powder bed in order to minimize tablet capping and lamination. Good compactibility of the powder blend is essential to tablet formation under the influence of compression forces and ensures that tablets will remain intact compact when the compression force is removed.

Third, after the tablet is compressed, the upper punch is withdrawn from the die and lower punch moves upwards to eject the tablet. Successful ejection of tablets without chipping or sticking requires sufficient lubrication of the powder blend so there is minimum adhesion between the tablet and the die wall. Lower ejection forces are preferred during tablet production to avoid unnecessary mechanical wear on the tablet press.

A small rotary press is most likely used when the initial formulation and process is developed at small scale. However, a large rotary press, used in a production area, may have significant differences in the number of stations, dwell time, and compression speed compared with smaller compression machines. Thus, early formulation design should consider the performance requirements of commercial production. Compaction simulators provide a useful tool able to reproduce the punch speeds of production machines and require only small quantities of powder blends for testing.[86] The simulators can play an important role in formulation and process development and can also facilitate the technical transfer from development to commercialization.

Systematic optimization of the compression process for a given formulation is necessary, and a DOE approach can be applied to understand the critical parameters and control space. Process variables may include tablet press speed, precompression force, compression force, and force feeder speed. Typical response variables include ejection force, compression profile, weight/hardness/thickness variations, friability, disintegration time, dissolution, and UDU. A robust manufacturing process and good process understanding gained through a meaningful experimental design and statistical analysis will, in turn, contribute to the successful scale-up and validation of the process.

7.6 SCALE-UP FOR BLENDING OPERATION

To ensure that specifications established for critical product quality attributes are met in a large-scale operation, the formulation and manufacturing process developed in the laboratory must be transferred to production and validated. It is necessary to start with a small scale in pharmaceutical research and development. Unfortunately, small-scale mixers necessary during the early development phase will not necessarily have the same characteristics as a commercial-scale mixer. Currently no mathematical techniques exist to predict the blending behavior of multicomponent solid mixtures; therefore, experimental work to ensure the proper scale-up and transfer to the production facility is required. Consider the following process parameters for a tumbling blender during scale-up trials:

- differences between blender geometry;
- filling level of powders;
- rotation rate;
- blending time.

When performing small-scale experimental work, the equipment should be as similar as possible to the intended large-scale blender, thereby minimizing differences in powder flow patterns. Keep the fill level constant with changes in scale to maintain similar velocity of flow and quantity of powder per unit volume within the mixer, given a geometrically similar blender and the same mixture composition. Maintaining a rotation speed within the recommended operating range does not have significant effects on the mixing quality for free-flowing powders when using small-scale twin shell and double cones mixers.[87,88] Thus, the number of revolutions is the most important parameter governing the mixing. Unlike free-flowing powders, mixing cohesive powders depends on shear and, consequently, rotation rates are very important.[73] Mixing of cohesive powders is common during the preblending operation of micronized bulk drug substances.

In the literature, the Froude number ($Fr = \Omega^2 R/g$; where Ω is the rotation rate, R is the vessel radius, and g is the acceleration from gravity) is often suggested for tumbling blender scale-up.[89] This relationship balances gravitational and inertial forces and can be derived from the general equations of motion for a general fluid. However, there have been no experimental data to support the validity of this approach. Attempts have been made to develop nondimensional scaling criteria according to particle surface velocities in the blender.[90] Unfortunately, the lack of scale-up models necessitates a significant number of commercial-scale trials to ensure robustness of the blending process.

7.7 FORMULATION EXAMPLES FOR DIRECT COMPRESSION

As discussed above, the development of low-dose formulations for direct compression is both an art and a science. In order to achieve good quality of drug products, a formulation scientist should carefully evaluate multiple factors related to the formulation composition and manufacturing process, including properties of drug substance and excipients, their sources of supply, unit formula and unit operations. Once the formulation and process is defined and optimized, any change, including material sources of supply, specifications of API and excipients and unit operations, should not be made without additional validation work done. A few low-dose formulations for direct compression are given below to illustrate key points discussed in this chapter.

7.7.1 Example 1: 0.5 mg Tablets

The drug substance was micronized and the particle size was controlled per specification of $X_{50} < 15\ \mu m$ and $X_{90} < 50\ \mu m$ determined using a laser diffraction method. The unit formula of example 1 is listed in Table 7.12. Early experiments revealed the appearance of what appeared to be agglomerates of API. For this reason, preblend and milling steps were introduced to eliminate the presence of API agglomerates. The preblend was produced by blending the entire quantity of API with a portion of the lactose (30–50%) using a V-shape blender mixer for 10 min. The preblend was then passed through a conical screen cone mill (round screen, 0.024 inch opening) and operated at approximately 2000 rpm. The preblend was mixed with the remaining lactose, microcrystalline cellulose (Avicel® PH102), and croscarmellose sodium for approximately 15 min using a bin blender. The colloidal silicon dioxide was then passed through a #30 mesh screen into the bin blender and mixed for approximately 5 min. Finally the magnesium stearate was passed through a #30 mesh screen into the bin blender and mixed for approximately 5 min. The final blend was compressed to

TABLE 7.12 Unit Formula of Example 1–0.5 mg Tablets

Ingredient	Composition (%)	Quantity per Tablet (mg)	Function
API	0.46	0.69	Active
Spray-dried lactose	69.59	104.39	Filler
Avicel® PH102	23.20	34.8	Filler–binder
Croscarmellose sodium	5.0	7.5	Disintegrant
Colloidal silicon dioxide	0.75	1.13	Glidant
Magnesium stearate	1.0	1.5	Lubricant
	100.0	150.0	

tablets with a rotary press and the tablet weight was 150 mg using 7 mm standard round concave tooling.

Spray-dried lactose in the formulation may be replaced by spray-dried mannitol such as Pearlitol® SD100. Also, the ratio of the lactose to Avicel® PH102 should be optimized for required product quality attributes including blending uniformity, content uniformity, potency, drug release, and breaking strength.

7.7.2 Example 2: 1 mg Tablets

In this case, the API was a poorly water soluble compound. To improve the bioavailability, the API was micronized to reduce its particle size and also sodium lauryl sulfate (surfactant) was added into the formulation as a wetting agent. The particle size of the API was controlled per specification of $X_{50} < 20\ \mu m$ and $X_{90} < 45\ \mu m$ determined using a laser diffraction method. The unit formula of example 2 for 1 mg tablets is listed in Table 7.13. The tablets were manufactured by a direct compression process with multiple blend steps. All ingredients were passed through a security screen prior to mixing. The API was mixed with Starch 1500 in a bin mixer and the resultant mixture was then blended with lactose, hypromellose, sodium lauryl sulfate, and Avicel® PH101 in an appropriate bin mixer. The blend was dischared, passed through a conical cone mill, and mixed with colloidal silicon dioxide and magnesium stearate. The final blend was compressed into 200 mg tablets using a rotary press.

7.7.3 Example 3: 0.2 mg Tablets

The unit formula of example 3 is listed in Table 7.14. The batch size manufactured was 10 kg. The API was preblended with Avicel® PH101 using a Patterson–Kelly tumble bin blender equipped with an intensifier bar (0.5 ft^3, Fig. 7.6) at 15 rpm with the intensifier bar speed of 2000 rpm for 15 min. The preblend was mixed with lactose, sodium starch glycolate and colloidal silicon dioxide in a 1 ft^3 tumble

TABLE 7.13 Unit Formula of Example 2–1 mg Tablets

Ingredient	Composition (%)	Quantity per Tablet (mg)	Function
API	0.5	1.0	Active
Lactose, anhydrous	60.0	120.0	Filler
Starch 1500, pregelatinized	20.0	40.0	Filler
Hypromellose	2.5	5.0	Binder
Sodium lauryl sulfate	0.5	1.0	Wetting agent
Avicel® PH101	15.0	30.0	Disintegrant
Colloidal silicon dioxide	0.5	1.0	Glidant
Magnesium stearate	1.0	2.0	Lubricant
	100.0	200.0	

TABLE 7.14 Unit Formula of Example 3–0.2 mg Tablets

Ingredient	Composition (%)	Quantity per Tablet (mg)	Function
API	0.20	0.20	Active
Spray-dried lactose	68.3	68.3	Filler
Avicel® PH101	25.0	25.0	Filler–binder
Sodium starch glycolate	5.0	5.0	Disintegrant
Colloidal silicon dioxide	0.5	0.5	Glidant
Magnesium stearate	1.0	1.0	Lubricant
	100.0	10.0	

bin blender at 12 rpm with the intensifier bar speed of 2000 rpm for 15 min. Finally, the blend was mixed with magnesium stearate in the blender for 3 min at 12 rpm. The final blend was compressed to 100 mg tablets on a rotary press using 6 mm round tooling. To achieve acceptable content uniformity, the particle size of the API was micronized to $D_{90} < 15$ μm determined by a laser diffraction method. It was noticed that larger variation in assay values could be obtained when the D_{90} of the API was greater than 90 μm.

7.8 CONCLUSIONS

The simplicity of the direct compression process for tablet manufacture presents an economic advantage over other manufacturing platforms because it requires fewer unit operations and, consequently, less capital expense for facilities and equipment. In addition, because it is a dry process, direct compression is a process of choice for thermolabile and moisture-sensitive drugs. The challenges facing the pharmaceutical scientists for low-dose drug products by direct compression are related to achieving and maintaining a homogeneous blend. The small particle size of a drug substance obtained from a micronization process may lead to cohesion, agglomeration, and nonhomogeneity. Deaggregation methods such as sieving and milling, or use of mixers equipped with an intensifier bar minimize the risk of a nonuniform blend. Alterations in the particulate characteristics of the drug and/or excipients can favor the formation of ordered mixes and thereby promote the creation of homogenous blends that tend not to segregate. Give careful consideration to development of the entire formulation design and manufacturing process to ensure a successful drug product by direct compression.

ACKNOWLEDGMENTS

The author wish to thank Dr David Moeckly at Eli Lilly and Company for review of the manuscript. Special thanks are expressed to Ms Karen Boleyn for help with preparation of the manuscript.

REFERENCES

1. Shangraw RF, Demarest DA Jr. 1993. A survey of current industrial practices in the formulation and manufacture of tablets and capsules. Pharm. Technol. 17(1): 32–44.
2. Johnson MCR. 1972. Particle size distribution of the active ingredient for solid dosage forms of low dosage. Pharm. Acta Helv. 47: 546–559.
3. Rohrs BR, Amidon GE, Meury RH, Secreast PJ, King HM, Skoug CJ. 2006. Particle size limits to meet USP content uniformity criteria for tablets and capsules. J. Pharm. Sci. 98: 1049–1059.
4. Johnson MCR. 1975. The effect of particle size upon mixture homogeneity. Pharm. Acta Helv. 50: 60–63.
5. Egermann H, Kemptner I, Pichler E. 1985. Effects of interparticulate interactions on mixing homogeneity. Drug. Dev. Ind. Pharm. 11: 663–676.
6. Yalkowsky SH, Bolton S. 1990. Particle size and content uniformity. Pharm. Res. 7(9): 962–966.
7. Zhang Y, Johnson KC. 1997. Effect of particle size on content uniformity of low-dose solid form. Int. J. Pharm. 154: 179–183.
8. Lantz RJ Jr, Schwartz JB. 1990. Mixing. In: Lieberman HL, Lachman L, Schwarts JB, editors. Pharmaceutical dosage forms: Tablets vol. 2, 2nd ed. New York: Marcel Dekker; 1–71.
9. Williams JC. 1968/1969. The mixing of dry powders. Powder Technol. 2: 13–20.
10. Train D. 1960. Pharmaceutical aspects of mixing solids. Pharm. J. 185: 129–134.
11. Staniforth JN. 1982. Advances in powder mixing and segregation in relation to pharmaceutical processing. Int. J. Pharm. Tech. Prod. Manuf. 3(suppl.): 1–12.
12. Staniforth JN. 1981. Total mixing. Int. J. Pharm. Tech. Prod. Manuf. 2(1): 7–12.
13. Venables HJ, Wells JI. 2001. Powder mixing. Drug Dev. Ind. Pharm. 27(7): 599–612.
14. Hersey JA. 1975. Ordered mixing: a new concept in powder mixing practice. Powder Technol. 11: 41–44.
15. Staniforth JN, Rees JE, Lai FK, Hersey JA. 1981. Determination of interparticulate force in ordered powder mixes. J. Pharm. Pharmac. 1981; 33: 485–490.
16. Staniforth JN, Rees JE. 1982. Electrostatic charge interactions in ordered powder mixes. J. Pharm. Pharmac. 34: 69–76.
17. Stephenson PL, Thiel WJ. 1980. The effect of humidity on the production of ordered mixtures. Powder Technol. 25: 115–119.
18. Staniforth JN. 1987. Order out of chaos. J. Pharm. Pharmac. 39: 329–334.
19. Hersey JA. 1977. Preparation and properties of ordered mixtures. Aust. J. Pharm. Sci. 6: 29–31.
20. Staniforth JN, Rees JE. 1981. Short communication. Powder mixing by triboelectrification. Powder Technol. 30(2): 255–256.
21. Kulvanich P, Stewart PJ. 1987. The effect of particle size and concentration on the adhesive characteristics of a model drug-carrier interactive system. J. Pharm. Pharmac. 39: 673–678.
22. Shah AC, Mlodozeniec AR. 1977. Mechanism of surface lubrication: influence of duration of lubricant–excipient mixing on processing characteristics of powders and properties of compressed tablets. J. Pharm. Sci. 66(10): 1377–1382.

23. Hlinak TJ, Kuriyan K, Morris KR, Reklaitis, GV, Basu PK. 2006. Understanding critical material properties for solid dosage form design. J. Pharm. Innov. 1(1): 12–17.
24. McCarty JA. 2004. Direct powder blends for encapsulation and tablet compression Part II: Materials. Am. Pharm. Rev. 7(1): 94–100.
25. Chang D, Chang RK. 2007. Review of current issues in pharmaceutical excipients. Pharm. Technol. 31(5): 56–66.
26. Bolhuis GK, Chowhan ZT. 1996. Materials for direct compaction. In: Alderborn D, Nystrom C, editors. Pharmaceutical powder compaction. New York: Marcel Dekker; 419–500.
27. Shangraw RF. 1989. Compressed tablets by direct compression. In: Loeberman HA, Lachman L, Schwartz JB, editors. Pharmaceutical dosage forms: Tablets, vol. 2. New York: Marcel Dekker, 1989; 195–245.
28. DMV International. 2006. Technical Literature: Pharmatose.
29. Kerry Bio-Sciences (Sheffield Products). 2006. Technical Literature: Lactose monohydrate NF 180 MS HV, lactose anhydrous NF DT, lactose anhydrous NF DT high velocity.
30. Foremost Forms U.S.A. 2006. Technical Literature: Lactose.
31. Meggle GmbH. 2006. Technical Literature: Lactose excipients (http://www.meggle-pharma.de/). Accessed 11 November 2007.
32. Rowe RC, Sheskey PJ, Owen SC. 2006. Handbook of pharmaceutical excipients, 5th ed. London: Pharmaceutical Press and American Pharmaceutical Association; 385–398.
33. Butujios NA. 1966. Anhydrous lactose in direct tablet compression. J. Pharm. Sci. 55: 727–730.
34. Wasylaschuk WR, Harmon PA, Wagner G, Harman AB, Templeton AC, Xu H, Reed RA. 2007. Evaluation of hydroperoxides in common pharmaceutical excipients. J. Pharm. Sci. 96(1): 106–116.
35. Bauer H, Herkert T, Bartels M. 2000. Investigations on polymorphism of mannitol/sorbitol mixtures after spray drying using different scanning calorimetry, X-ray diffraction and near infrared spectroscopy. Pharm. Ind. 62(3): 231–235.
36. Allen LV. 2000. Featured excipients: capsule and tablet diluent. Int. J. Pharm. Compound 4(4): 306–325.
37. Marshall K, Sixsmith D. 1974/1975. Some physical characteristics of microcrystalline cellulose (1) powders for pharmaceutical use. Drug Dev. Commun. 1: 51–71.
38. FMC Corporation. 2007. Technical Literature: Avicel PH (http://www.fmcbiopolymer.com). Accessed 12 October 2007.
39. Reier GE, Shangraw RF. 1966. Microcrystalline cellulose in tableting. J. Pharm. Sci. 55: 510–514.
40. Huttenrauch R. 1971. Pharmazie 66: 645–655.
41. David ST, Augsburger LL. 1977. Plastic flow during compression of directly compressible fillers and its effect on tablet strength. J. Pharm. Sci. 66(2): 155–159.
42. Kibbe AH. 2006. Starch, pregelatinized. In: Rowe RC, Sheskey PJ, Owen SC, editors. Handbook of pharmaceutical excipients, 5th ed. London: Pharmaceutical Press and American Pharmaceutical Association; 385–398.
43. Manudhane KS, Contractor AM, Kim HY, Shangraw RF. 1969. Tableting properties of a directly compressible starch. J. Pharm. Sci. 58: 616–620.

44. Roquette. 2000. Technical Literature: Lycatab C for capsule filling, direct compression and wet granulation.
45. Colorcon. 1997. Technical Literature: Starch 1500.
46. Ahmed H, Shah N. 2000. Formulation of low dose medicines—theory and practice. Am. Pharm. Rev. 3(3): 9–14.
47. Kausar N, Cornelius V, Snowden MJ, Mitchell J, Mwesigwa E, Do N, Farrell T. 2006. Assessment of low-dose content uniformity of indomethacin in excipient blends using FT-Raman mapping spectroscopy. AAPS Annual Meeting and Exposition, San Antonio, TX.
48. Landin M, Rowe RC, York P. 1994. Structural changes during the dehydration of dicalcium phosphate dehydrate. Eur. J. Pharm. Sci. 2: 245–252.
49. Rowe RC, Sheskey PJ, Owen SC. 2006. Handbook of pharmaceutical excipients, 5th ed. London: Pharmaceutical Press and American Pharmaceutical Association; 93–99.
50. Fuji Chemical Industry Co. Technical Literature: Bulk Pharmaceuticals Fujicalin. (http://www.fujichemical.co.jp/). Accessed 12 October 2007.
51. Fuji Chemical Industry Co. 1996. Calcium hydrogen phosphate, a method for preparing it and an excipient utilizing it. U.S. patent no. 5,486,365.
52. Nachaegari SK, Bansal AK. 2004. Coprocessed excipients for solid dosage forms. Pharm. Technol. 28(1): 52–64.
53. Maarschalk KVDV, Bolhius GK. 1999. Improving properties of material for direct compression. Pharm. Technol. 23(5): 34–46.
54. Moreton RC. 1996. Tablet excipients to the year 2001: a look into the crystal ball. Drug Dev. Ind. Pharm. 22(1): 11–23.
55. Rios M. 2006. Developments in powder flow testing. Pharm. Technol. 30(2): 38–49.
56. European Pharmacopoeia, 5th ed. 2006. Chapter 2.9.36. Powder flow.
57. Carr RL Jr. 1965. Classifying flow properties of solids. Chem. Engng 7: 163–167.
58. Hausner HH. 1967. Friction conditions in a mass of metal powder. Int. J. Powder Metal. 3(4): 7–13.
59. Pilpel N. 1971. Cohesive pharmaceutical powders. In: Bean HS, Beckett AH, Charles JE, editors. Advances in pharmaceutical sciences, vol. 3. Academic Press: London; 179–219.
60. Hiestand EN. 1966. Powders: particle–particle interactions. J. Pharm. Sci. 35: 1325–1344.
61. Bilgili E, Yepes J, Stephenson L, Johanson K, Scarlett B. 2004. Stress inhomogeneity in powder specimens tested in the Jenike shear cell: Myth or fact? Part. Part. System Charact. 21(4): 293–302.
62. Standard shear test method for bulk solids using the Schulze ring tester. ASTM International, Designation D6773-02, 2006.
63. Abatzoglou N. 2005. Prediction of segregation tendency occurrence in dry particulate pharmaceutical mixtures: development of a mathematical tool adapted for granular system application. Pharm. Dev. Technol. 1: 59–70.
64. Standard practice for measuring segregation tendencies of powders. ASTM Standard D6941-03, 2006. American Society for Testing and Materials International.
65. Dedden DB, Brone DL, Clement S, McCall M, Olsofsky A, Patel PJ, Prescott J, Hancock BC. 2006. Development of an improved fluidization segregation tester for use with pharmaceutical powders. Pharm. Technol. 30(12): 54–64.

66. Williams JC. 1976. The segregation of particulate materials: a review. Powder Technol. 15: 245–251.
67. Chowhan ZT. 1995. Segregation of particulate solids, Part II. Pharm Technol. 19: 81–94.
68. Egermann H. 1982. Problems on assessing actual content uniformity by spot sample assays. Int. J. Pharm. Tech. Manuf. 3(2): 59–66.
69. Egermann H. 1979. Mixing: agglomeration during sieving. Sci. Pharm. 47: 25–31.
70. Martino A. 2004. Robust tablet design: developing low-dose products with increased probability of meeting PAT criteria – prevalidation approaches. Land O'Lakes Pharmaceutical Annual Meeting, University of Wisconsin at Madison, WI.
71. Poska RP, Hill TR, van Schaik JW. 1993. The use of statistical indices to gauge the mixing efficiency of a conical screening mill. Pharm. Res. 10(8): 1248–1251.
72. Alexander A, Arratia P, Goodridge C, Sudah O, Brone D, Muzzio F. 2004. Characterization of performance of bin blenders. Part 1 of 3: Methodology. Pharm. Technol. 28(5): 70–86.
73. Alexander A, Arratia P, Goodridge C, Sudah O, Brone D, Muzzio F. 2004. Characterization of performance of bin blenders. Part 3 of 3: Cohesive powders. Pharm. Technol. 28(9): 54–74.
74. Carstensen JT, Patel MR. 1977. Blending of irregularly shaped particles. Powder Technol. 17: 273–282.
75. Samyn JC, Murthy KS. 1974. Experiments in powder blending and unblending. J. Pharm. Sci. 63(3): 370–373.
76. Sudah OS, Coffin-Beach D, Muzzio FJ. 2002. Effects of blender rotational speed and discharge on the homogeneity of cohesive and free-flowing mixtures. Int. J. Pharm. 247: 57–68.
77. Prescott JK, Garcia TP. 2001. A solid dosage and blend content uniformity troubleshooting diagram. Pharm. Technol. 25(3): 68–88.
78. Allen T. 1975. Particle size measurement, 2nd ed. London: Chapman and Hall.
79. Muzzio FJ, Robinson P, Wightman C, Brone D. 1997. Sampling practice in powder blending. Int. J. Pharm. 155: 153–178.
80. Muzzio FJ, et al. 1997. Sampling practice in powder blending. Int. J. Pharm. 155: 153–178.
81. Muzzio FJ, et al. 2003. Sampling and characterization of pharmaceutical powder and granular blends. Int. J. Pharm. 250(1): 51–64.
82. Muzzio FJ, et al. 1999. An improved powder sampling tool. Pharm. Technol. 23(4): 92–110.
83. U.S. FDA Center for Drug Evaluation and Research. 2003. Guidance for Industry: powder blends and finished dosage units – stratified in-process dosage unit sampling and assessment. Draft guidance. http://www.fda.gov/cder/guidance/index.htm. Accessed 25 October 2007.
84. Boehm G, Clark J, Dietrick J, Foust L, Garcia T, Gavini M, Gelber L, Geoffroy J, Hoblizell J, Jimenez P, Mergen G, Muzzio F, Planchard J, Prescott J, Timmermans J, Takiar N. 2003. The use of stratified sampling of blend and dosage units to demonstrate adequacy of mix for powder blends. PDA J. Pharm. Sci. Technol. 57(2): 64–74.
85. Davies P. 2004. Oral solid dosage form. In: Gibson M, editor. Pharmaceutical preformulation and formulation. Interpharm/CRC: New York; 379–456.

86. Wang, JJ, Guillot MA, Bateman SD, Morris KR. 2004. Modeling of adhesion in tablet compression. II. Compaction studies using a compaction simulator and an instrumented tablet press. J. Pharm. Sci. 93(2): 407–417.
87. Brone D, Alexander A, Muzzio FJ. 1998. Quantitative characterization of mixing of dry powders in V-blenders. AIChE J. 44(2): 271–278.
88. Brone D, Muzzio FJ. 2000. Enhanced mixing in double-cone blenders. Powder Technol. 110(3): 179–189.
89. Wang RH, Fan LT. 1974. Methods for scaling-up tumbling mixers. Chem. Engng 81(11): 88–94.
90. Alexander AW, Muzzio FJ. 2006. Batch size increase in dry blending and mixing. In: Levin M, editor. Pharmaceutical process scale-up. 2nd ed. New York: Taylor & Francis.

CHAPTER 8

REDUCTION OF PARTICLE SIZE OF DRUG SUBSTANCE FOR LOW-DOSE DRUG PRODUCTS

CHRISTOPHER L. BURCHAM, PAUL C. COLLINS, DANIEL J. JARMER, and KEVIN D. SEIBERT
Chemical Product R&D, Lilly Research Laboratories, Eli Lilly and Company, Indianapolis, IN 40285

8.1 INTRODUCTION

Particle size control of the API is often an important development strategy to consider, particularly when considering the impact of particle size on the quality attributes of the final drug product or the drug product manufacturing process. The physical properties of the API can affect the drug product quality in several ways:

1. They can affect the dissolution rate of a poorly soluble compound in gastric fluids.
2. They can affect blending and content uniformity, especially in the case of low-dose compound manufacture.
3. They can affect the flowability of powder blends.
4. Any combination of one or more of the above can occur.

In the case of compounds that exhibit low solubility in gastric fluids, the rate of dissolution may limit the availability of the compound *in vivo*. The dissolution rate can be improved by increasing the surface area of the compound. In this case, the API physical property (either surface area or particle size distribution) will likely be a critical quality attribute, as it could directly impact the safety, identity, strength, purity and quality (SISPQ) of the drug product.[1,2]

The *Biopharmaceutics Classification System* (BCS)[3] defines four classes of compounds based upon solubility and permeability. Particle size and size distribution

Formulation and Analytical Development for Low-Dose Oral Drug Products. Edited by Jack Zheng

affect the dissolution rate of the API and therefore are most relevant when dealing with Class II and Class IV compounds.

In the case of low-dose drug products, content uniformity of the dosage form can be negatively affected if the particle size of the API is either too large or the size distribution is too broad. This could result in the need to deliver API below a certain size to ensure content uniformity. Recently, Rohr et al.[4] expanded upon previous work to develop a statistical model predicting the volume mean diameter of API necessary to meet USP stage 1 criteria on content uniformity for tablets with a 99% confidence level [Eq. (8.1)]:

$$d_{50} = \sqrt[3]{\left(\frac{6D}{\pi\rho}\right) \exp\left(-4.5 \ln^2 \sigma_g \left(\frac{CV}{100}\right)^2\right) 10^3} \qquad (8.1)$$

where CV is the coefficient of variation (%), D is the dose (mg), ρ is the density of the solid particles (g/cm^3) and σ_g is the log–normal standard deviation of the distribution.

Lastly, manufacturability of a drug product can be affected by the physical properties of the drug substance. Manufacturability refers to the ability to execute a process efficiently, without excessive operator intervention, and without the need for specialized equipment designed solely to overcome specific product properties. In the case of drug product manufacturing, this typically includes the ability to transfer powder blends through each drug product unit operation. The physical properties of the API such as particle size and shape can affect the flowability of the intermediate and final powder blends.

If the drug loading is greater than 5–10%, then the API physical properties can have a significant impact on mixing and/or filling operations of the drug product, especially for direct compression and roller compaction processing. Powder flowability and tablet/capsule filling performance are a function of the size, shape, and solids density of the powder particles. Pharmaceutical excipients are typically manufactured in a way to optimize powder flowability. As the drug loading increases, the physical properties of the API begin to have an impact on the flowability and subsequent manufacturability of the drug product.

As a particle becomes more needle-like, or the aspect ratio (defined as the length of the particle to the breadth of the particle) increases, so too does the resistance to flow.[5] Poor flowability has been demonstrated to result in poor capsule filling performance.[6] Danjo et al.[7] report a rapid decrease in flowability when the particle shape index* drops below the 0.5–0.3 range. This translates to a particle aspect target ratio range between 3 : 1 and 5 : 1 for rod-like particles and is in agreement with a generally recognized rule-of-thumb that, for free-flowing materials, the aspect ratio should be less than 5 : 1. Particle size also has an affect on flowability. Tan and Newton[6] report that flowability generally decreases with decreasing particle size. As a result

*Particle shape index is defined as the projected area of the particle divided by the area of a circle having a diameter equivalent to the maximum projected length of the particle.

it is important to design the API physical properties to meet the requirements of the downstream drug product manufacturing process, provided that bioavailability and content uniformity are not impacted.

While smaller particle size distributions (PSD) may translate into an advantage for content uniformity and bio-availability, this smaller size range is often disadvantageous for powder flow operations. These competing drivers need to be considered when designing a drug product manufacturing process; the actual PSD of the API may need to reside in an intermediate range. When considering API physical properties for usage in low-dose or poorly soluble drug products, requirements are typically restricted to a small PSD range for the purpose of achieving content uniformity or improving dissolution rate, as discussed in the previous chapter. When referring to the restricted size material needed, the term "micronization" is often employed. In fact, micronization is not strictly defined, although most definitions tend to imply a reduction in size to a diameter of a few microns.[8–11] For the purpose of this chapter, in discussing the various methods of achieving micronization, the target PSD will be $d_{90} < 10\,\mu\text{m}$, where d_{90} is defined as the size in the overall PSD where 90% of the distribution (by volume) is less than that size.

Micronization can be achieved by a variety of technologies. The technologies can be divided roughly into two categories: (1) mechanical breakage techniques (milling); and (2) particle formation techniques (crystallization and precipitation). Both of these categories will be discussed in more detail, but limited to applications achieving the definition of micronization as defined above. Reviews covering a broader spectrum of particle sizes and their control techniques are available.[12]

8.2 REDUCTION OF PARTICLE SIZE OF DRUG SUBSTANCE BY MILLING TECHNOLOGIES

Milling can be classified a number of ways. Classification by the media in which the particles are milled, that is, wet or dry, is a common way to classify milling techniques. Fracture mechanism (compression or impaction) is an alternative means of classification. The milling approach selected for the specific API requires knowledge of both the input and desired output PSD. Additionally, the intrinsic properties of the solid particle define the degree of fracture that a particle will undergo given a specific milling type.

Various types of dry milling equipment have been developed for reduction of particle size distributions (Table 8.1). The selection of milling equipment appropriate for a target particle size distribution may vary depending upon the initial particle size distribution, the breadth of the distribution, the friability of the crystal, and other system operating parameters. While this is may be used as guidance, there are numerous situations when mill types may be used to afford particle size distributions outside of the predicted range of operation. The majority of our discussion will be limited to those mills that have higher probability of achieving micronization for variety of APIs.

TABLE 8.1 Approximate Particle Size Obtainable by Various Milling Techniques

	Size (μm)	Hammer Mill	Universal and Pin Mill	Jet Mill	Jet Mills with Internal Classifier	Media Mills	Toothed Rotor–Stator	Colloid Mill
Type	—	Dry	Dry	Dry	Dry	Wet	Wet	Wet
Very fine	50–150	Yes	Yes	No	Yes	No	Yes	No
Super fine	10–50	Yes	Yes	Yes	Yes	Yes	Yes	Yes
Ultra fine	<10	No	Yes	Yes	Yes	Yes	No	Yes
Colloidal	<1	No	No	No	Yes	Yes	No	Yes

8.2.1 Dry Milling

Dry milling is a commonly employed approach to particle size reduction. As with all milling, the unit operation is associated with the control strategy for upstream API processing. For instance, isolation of API is most often performed through a solids isolation strategy (e.g., crystallization) followed by filtration of the solids and a terminal drying step. Based upon the thermodynamic and kinetic properties of the system, the physical properties of the solids of interest and the dynamics of the environment within the crystallizer, several outcomes are possible. Crystallizations that end in final isolated particles at the desired PSD specification require no further processing to be carried into the downstream processing train, and are often the result of targeted particle engineering efforts.[13–15] Particles below the target PSD can either be tested for processability in the drug product manufacturing, or the size increased through modified crystallization strategies to yield larger particles of the desired PSD.[16] Most often, and generally by design, the isolated crystals are larger than the target PSD as established through formulation development or bioavailability testing. In these situations the resulting dried material must be milled to reduce the PSD to the target.

Deliberately growing particles larger than the target PSD may offer processing advantages in the form of cycle-time savings from reduced processing time during isolation. For the isolation of solids from a slurry, the pressure drop per unit length for a given liquid flow across a packed bed of particles is well represented by the Carman–Kozeny relation, which has been shown to be applicable for filtration.

$$-\frac{\Delta p}{L} = \frac{k\mu\nu(1-\varepsilon)^2 S^2}{\varepsilon^3} \tag{8.2}$$

where μ is the viscosity of the filtrate, ν is the linear velocity of the fluid passing through the bed, ε is the void fraction of the cake and S is the specific surface area of the crystals defined as surface area per volume of solid particle; k is a constant for various particle shapes and sizes, and is equal to 4.17 for random packed particles. Equation (8.2) illustrates that, for situations of constant pressure, the time to filter is proportional to the pressure drop per unit length, and therefore to the specific surface area of the particles. Additionally, filtration time is inversely proportional to the cube of the void fraction. As a result, larger particles are inherently easier to filter. Alternatively, unimodal particle size distributions generally result in smaller specific cake resistances as the void fraction approaches that for randomly packed spheres. For broad PSDs, smaller particles tend to fill voids left by larger particles, therefore reducing the void fraction, and increasing the overall filtration time.

While the filtration time can be reduced through increased pressure, equipment limitations and nonlinearity associated with compressible solids may result in diminishing returns. As a result, it is often advantageous to attempt to grow larger particles through various crystallization strategies and isolate larger particles in the final wet processing steps of an API synthesis. In situations with solution instability this may be the only suitable processing option. Therefore, in considering the overall manufacturing efficiency associated with making API, the purposeful generation of large particles, which are later reduced in size, is a viable option to consider. In such a scenario dry milling is the preferred technology for micronization.

Dry milling is the process of reducing particle size in the absence of any liquids. This may be accomplished by grinding or high force collisions of particles with a moving pin or hammer of a mill. Alternatively, it may be accomplished by high energy particle–particle as is the case with jet mills. Solids are conveyed by either gravitational flow through the milling apparatus, screw conveyance, or by conveyance with a carrier gas such as nitrogen. For reduction of PSDs to sub-micron, typically dry milling strategies are not adequate to reduce to the colloidal range, and therefore wet-milling strategies are typically employed.

Hammer Mill. While not typically utilized for the reduction of particle sizes to below 10 μm, hammer mills are occasionally capable of significantly reducing particle size. Hammer mills involve introduction of solids to a hopper or delivery device, then through a series of spinning hammers. Attrition of particles is accomplished through the impact of the particulates with hammers and the mill internals. A sieve screen is generally held in place to limit the size of the milled primary particle that can be removed from the system. To obtain sub-10 μm solids, other higher energy milling strategies are more often utilized for micronization of API material.

Universal/Pin Mill. The term "universal" mill usually refers to a mill configuration whereby multiple milling heads can be utilized. These mills often can be fitted with pin, turbo-rotor, and hammer-type heads. Of these, pin mills are most likely to provide material in the micronized regime. Pin mills work by similar action to hammer mills, but with typically faster tip speeds and lower tolerances between rotating and stationary pins. Solids are fed from a hopper to a milling chamber. The milling chamber typically contains a high-speed rotor/stator configuration of intermeshing pins which impact the particles as solids are directed through the intermeshing pins (Fig. 8.1). Control parameters to adjust and vary the output PSD include pin gap or pin spacing, the rotational speed of the rotor, solids feed rate, size of the mill, and velocity of the carrier gas used to convey the solids out of the milling chamber. In

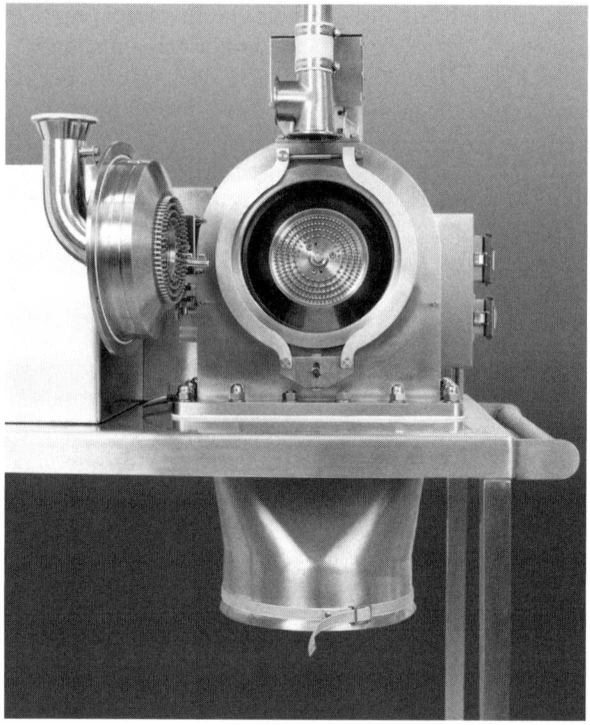

Figure 8.1 Pin mill internals. (Photo courtesy of Hosokawa Micron Powder Systems.)

addition to the control parameters, typically the outlet PSD is also strongly affected by the input PSD of the material to be milled.

Jet Mill. Jet mills are an alternative to hammer or pin milling, where the primary mode of action is the mechanical impact with the particle. With jet milling, micronization is accomplished through the action of fluid energy, resulting in particle–particle collisions and the subsequent reduction in size. Spiral jet mills, loop jet mills and fluidized bed jet mills are examples of fluid energy mills.

All of the types of jet mills work using the same general principle. Through the introduction of high pressure air or other carrier gas (i.e., nitrogen) into specially designed nozzles, the potential energy of the compressed gas is converted into a grinding stream at sonic or supersonic velocities. Differences in the various mills are predominantly in the geometry of the grinding chamber itself.

Spiral mills create a high velocity helix of gas that rotates around the center of the jet mill. Solids are introduced via a venturi feed injector (Fig. 8.2) and become entrained in the turbulent helical flow. The resulting high energy collisions between particles as well as with the particles and the mill internals fracture particles to micron and submicron size.

For loop jet mills, air or carrier gas is also injected into a grinding loop or "race track" through specially designed nozzles. Solid particle are injected into this

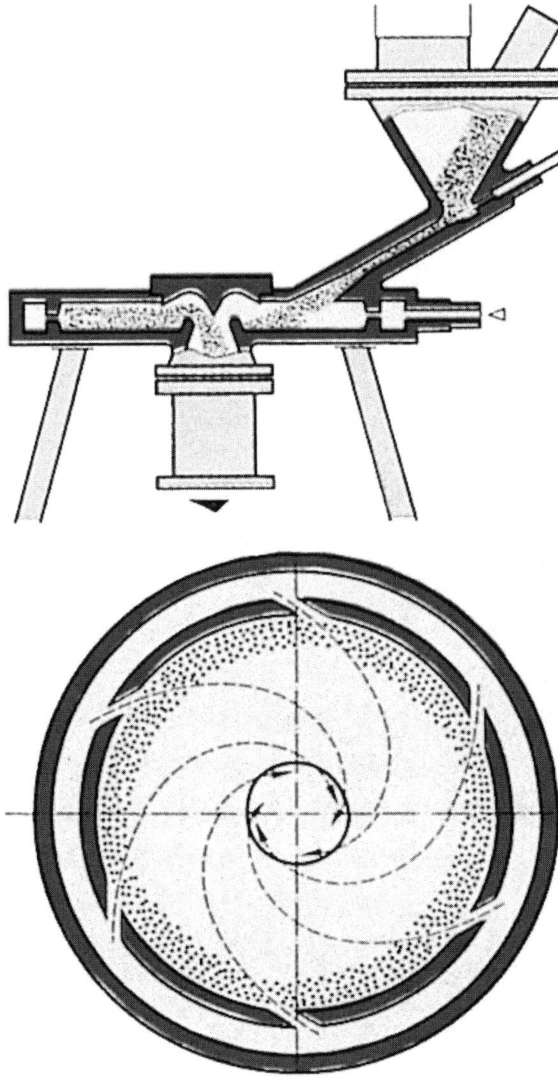

Figure 8.2 Spiral jet or "pancake" mill. (Photo courtesy of Hosokawa Micron Powder Systems.)

stream, resulting in high-velocity particle–particle collisions. In both designs, particles will stratify based on their relative inertia toward the outlet of the mill, resulting in larger particles being returned to the grinding chamber while smaller particles are carried out of the mill to the collection cyclone or chamber.

Fluidized bed jet mills work in similar fashion, with the grinding chamber oriented as a fluidized bed. Specially designed nozzles introduce the grinding gas at the bottom of the fluidized bed, creating high-intensity collisions between particles

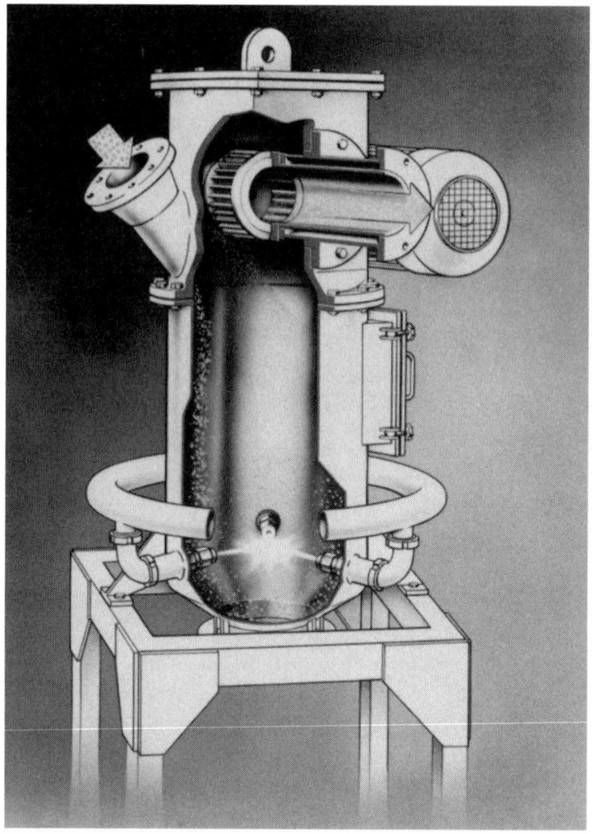

Figure 8.3 Fluidized bed jet mill with classification. (Photo courtesy of Hosokawa Micron Powder Systems.)

(Fig. 8.3). Vertical gas flow is in turn used to fluidized the milled material out of the grinding chamber. Typically fluidized bed jet mills are fitted with a classification wheel. Based on the rotational speed of the classifier wheel, particles of too large a size have a radial momentum imparted upon them returning these particles back to the grinding zone of the fluidized bed. This type of arrangement will typically lead to much narrower particle size distributions than other types of jet milling equipment.

In most size reduction milling equipment, residence time in the milling apparatus is the predominant parameter in determining outlet particle size. As a result, the feed rate becomes a significant part of the control strategy and must be carefully considered when determining scale-up parameters for milling equipment.

8.2.2 Wet Milling

Milling a solid suspended in liquid is referred to as either wet or slurry milling. The utilization of a wet mill offers many advantages to dry milling, though there are some limitations. One significant advantage with wet milling is the ability to eliminate a separate unit operation of dry milling. Wet milling can be carried out as part of the final crystallization–isolation sequence. This approach eliminates the cycle time and cost associated with an extra unit operation, which can be particularly significant if special containment is necessary (see next section). An additional process design benefit is potentially realized with this milling option, as it allows for greater flexibility in terms of how a crystallization process is developed. As an example, as a crystallization progresses the size of the crystal suspension can be simultaneously reduced by milling during the crystallization process. This is time-sparing, and also presents crystallization benefits by continually exposing new surface area for use in the ongoing crystallization. Wet mills are also preferred if the material being milled exhibits undesirable physical properties or phase changes at higher temperatures as the increased heat capacity of the liquid carrier media allows for lower temperature fluctuations during milling. This can be especially important for materials that have either a low melting point, or are susceptible to form conversion at lower temperature. Additionally, dry milling imparts large amounts of energy, and has been observed to cause chemical instability.[17] While milling-induced disorder likely occurs during a wet milling process, contact of the crystal with a liquid media facilities surface annealing.

Slurry milling also affords better containment than dry milling by lowering the amount of dry powder handling. While advances have been made in containment technologies, exposure or opportunity for exposure is increased as dry product has a propensity to migrate and become airborne more so than product in a suspension.

Wet mills can be operated in multiple ways. Operation as single-pass mode involves passing all the product through the mill once with no recycle. Alternatively, the wet mill offers the versatility to operate in recycle mode, in which product is passed through the mill, back to a well-mixed holding tank, and back through the mill again. In this case, multiple reactor residence times are necessary to ensure that all the material has passed through the mill at least once. As with dry mills, multiple types of wet mills are available. The three most commonly used in pharmaceutical manufacturing are toothed rotor-stator mills, colloid mills and media mills.

Toothed Rotor Stator Mills. Rotor-stator mills (Fig. 8.4a) consist of a rotating shaft (rotor), with by an axially fixed concentric stator. Toothed rotor–stator mills have one or more rows of intermeshing teeth on both the rotor and the stator with a small gap between the rotor and stator. Variations in the number of teeth, teeth spacing, angle of incidence, etc., all impact the milling efficiency of toothed rotor-stator mills.

The differential speed between the rotor and the stator imparts extremely high shear and turbulent energy in the gap between the rotor and stator. In this configuration, particle size is reduced by both the high-shear created in the annular region between the teeth and by the collisions of particles on the leading edge of the teeth (Fig. 8.4b). Size is affected by selecting rotor-stator pairs with different gap thickness, or by operating at different rotational rates (or tip speeds) of the rotor. Tip speed is a very important factor when considering the amount of shear input

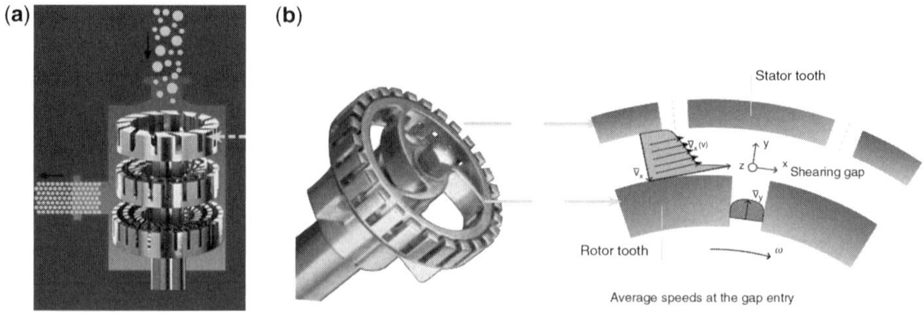

Figure 8.4 Wet mill internals (a) and rotor–stator working principle (b). (IKA.)

into the product. Tip speed is determined according to the following equation:

$$v_{ts} = \pi D \omega \tag{8.3}$$

where D is the rotor diameter and ω is the rotation rate (rpm).

The shear created between the rotor and stator is a function of the tip speed and the gap thickness. The shear rate is given by:

$$\dot{\gamma} = \frac{v_{ts}}{\mathrm{h}} \tag{8.4}$$

where h is the gap distance.

Another important factor is the number of occurrences that rotor and stator openings mesh. This is known as the shear frequency given by:

$$f_s = N_r N_s \omega \tag{8.5}$$

The shear number is given by:

$$N_{sk} = f_s \dot{\gamma} \tag{8.6}$$

Depending upon the rotor–stator design, the number of rows should be accounted for when calculating the shear number.

Colloid Mills. Colloid mills are another form of rotor stator mill. A colloid mill is composed of a conical rotor rotating in a conical stator (Fig. 8.5). The surface of the rotor and stator can be smooth, rough, or slotted. The spacing between the rotor and stator is adjustable by varying the axial location of the rotor to the stator. The gap can be as little as a few hundred microns to a couple of millimeters.[18] Varying the gap varies not only the shear imparted to the particles but also the mill residence time and the power density applied. Particle size is affected by adjusting the gap and the rotation rate. It is possible to produce particles in the 1–10 μm size range.

Media Mills. Media mills, also referred to as pearl or bead mills, are much different in operation than a rotor–stator mill. The mill is composed of a milling chamber, milling shaft and product recirculation chamber. The milling shaft extends the

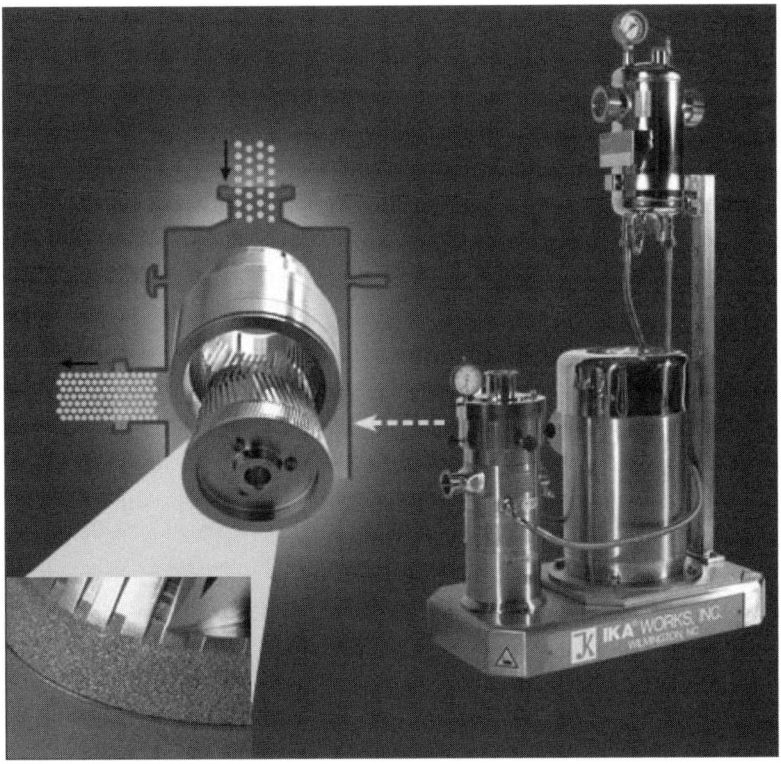

Figure 8.5 Colloid mill. (IKA.)

length of the chamber. A shaft can have either radial protrusions or fingers extending into the milling chamber, a series of disks located along the length of the chamber, or a relatively thin annular gap between the shaft and mill chamber. The chamber is filled with spherical milling media less than 2 mm in diameter and typically 1 mm in diameter or less. Media is retained in the mill by a mesh screen located at the exit of the mill. The rotation of the shaft causes the protrusions to move the milling media, creating high shear forces.[19] Scale-up of media mills is accomplished by maintaining the same residence time, keeping the milling media size constant and holding energy input constant.

The high energy and shear that result from the movement of the milling media is imparted to the particles as the material is circulated through the milling chamber. The result is the ability to create submicron particles. Thermally labile material is easily handled as the milling chamber is jacketed. By utilizing smaller media (less than 100 μm) nano-sized (20 nm) particles are achievable.

At the small size scales achievable by media milling, particle–particle interactions caused by van der Waals forces can begin to dominate.[20] By inclusion of certain additives to the dispersion fluid, the possible agglomeration and resulting reduced efficiency and reduced effectiveness of the mill can be mitigated. Surfactants can inhibit agglomeration by both electrostatic and steric stabilization. Similarly, polymeric stabilizers can also be used to retard agglomeration. The smaller the particle produced, the greater the amount of surfactant needed since the specific surface area of the particle increase with decreasing with one over the radius of the particles.

Milling media is available as several materials: glass, metals, ceramics such as zirconium oxide, and polymeric such as a highly cross-linked polystyrene resin. The proper selection of the milling media is an important criterion in the milling process. Materials such as glass and metals are typically not used for APIs since some abrasion of the milling media can occur, leading to concerns about extraneous material. As a result, either polymeric or ceramic media are typically used.[19]

Wet Milling Limitations. The largest impediment to utilizing wet mills for produce micronized API is around isolation of neat API. Filtration of micronized or submicron material can result in extremely long filtration times (see above). This impediment can be overcome if the micronized slurry can be used directly in the drug product, for examples as the feed for a wet granulation process or a spray coating process. If the product is filtered and dried, it should be delumped as it exits the dryer to ensure that the particles are not agglomerated.

8.3 REDUCTION OF PARTICLE SIZE OF DRUG SUBSTANCE USING CRYSTALLIZATION TECHNOLOGIES

8.3.1 Direct Crystallization

Scenarios exist whereby milling is undesirable for micronization. Depending on the milling technique employed, controlling the size distribution and crystal morphology can be difficult, especially for micronized material. In addition, high-energy milling can induce changes in the surface properties of the API, such as a loss of crystallinity, which can directly impact physical stability.[21] Some APIs will melt or undergo polymorphic form conversion while milling to achieve micronization. Isolated material is often electrostatically charged and cohesive following a milling operation. Milling can be labor-intensive and introduce environmental exposure concerns, which may require installation and maintenance of expensive engineering and containment controls.[12] To address the shortcomings of traditional milling methods, it is often desirable to produce particles with a defined particle size directly from solution, and circumvent the need for a terminal milling step. Crystallization strategies that can be employed to achieve this goal include antisolvent and reactive crystallization with an in-line mixing device, as well as crystallization with supercritical fluids.

8.3.2 Antisolvent and Reactive Crystallization with In-Line Mixing

Crystallization, triggered by the addition of a miscible nonsolvent (antisolvent) to a solute-containing solvent system, can be used to produce microscale particles with narrow particle size distributions. The process is complex as it involves the coupling of thermodynamics, hydrodynamics, mass transfer, and crystallization kinetics. A goal in most crystallizer designs is to manipulate fluid mechanics within the crystallizer to allow rapid, homogeneous mixing between the solute containing solution and the antisolvent. This provides a homogeneous, supersaturated environment before the onset of crystallization. In order to minimize the effect of imperfect mixing on the crystallization kinetics, the characteristic times for mixing (i.e., macromixing, mesomixing, and micromixing) must be less than the characteristic times for particle nucleation and growth.[22,23] Under these conditions, crystallization becomes kinetically limited and is controlled by the particle nucleation and growth rate. This requirement is currently being met by design and development of in-line mixers that are capable of rapidly mixing two fluid streams. These in-line devices often require confined injection geometries in which turbulence is intense, energy dissipation rates are large, and contact times between fluid streams are short.[24–26] Various mixer geometries have been investigated, but impinging jets, confined impinging jets, and vortex mixer designs can achieve this high degree of mixing quality at scale and in an economical manner.

With an impinging jet in-line mixer, two streams at high velocity impinge upon one another resulting in a rapid, intense micromixing of the streams.[24,25] In confined impinging jets, the chamber size affects the mixing quality.[27] In either geometry, if the mixer is designed properly, the scale of mixedness can be achieved and the molar-flow ratios are preserved during the rapid mixing process. As a result of the rapid mixing, a high degree of supersaturation is generated which fosters a nucleation-dominant crystallization producing fine particles. Industrial operation of an impinging jet crystallizer is discussed by Midler et al.,[28] with variations of this design by Linrud et al.[29] Scale-up criteria for impinging jets are discussed by Mahajan et al.[26] Johnson and Prud'homme[27] examined the performance and scaling criteria for a confined impinging jets mixer.

When supersaturation is generated by a chemical reaction, and the product crystallizes from solution, the operation is often termed "reactive crystallization." The reaction may either be between two organic compounds or a neutralization by an acid or base to form an organic salt.[30] Reaction rates are often fast relative to both mixing and crystallization. This can lead to high local levels of supersaturation and extensive nucleation, resulting in small particles. Similar to antisolvent crystallization, in-line mixers are applicable to reactive crystallization where the goal is to homogeneously mix two fluid streams prior to the onset of crystallization. An example of industrial operation of an impinging jet crystallizer with focus on reactive crystallization is given by am Ende et al.[31]

8.3.3 Supercritical Fluid Crystallization

Supercritical fluid crystallization (SFC) is a technique for precipitating or crystallizing solutes dissolved in liquid solvents by injecting or mixing the solvent system with a compressed or supercritical fluid antisolvent. SFC is unique in that it uses a compressed gas to trigger the crystallization. Two benefits often associated with SFC include single-step processing of particulate pharmaceuticals with controlled characteristics[32,33] and the efficient separation (by decompression) of the antisolvent from both the solvent and solid products. Jarmer et al.[34] have described appropriate use of and scale-up criteria for such systems.

8.4 SCALE-UP CONSIDERATIONS

Each of the mentioned milling technologies is capable of micronizing a compound depending on permissive physical properties of the premilled material. In choosing one of the techniques for long-term use, other factors may be important beyond the capability of the equipment to reach the desired PSD specification. Worker exposure, explosivity of the milled compound, and ability of the milling operation to scale/translate across development and manufacturing facilities should all be considered in choosing a platform for micronization.

The minimum ignition energy (MIE) of a compound refers to the minimum energy necessary to ignite a sample of the material dispersed in air. The MIE is related to particle size[35–38] such that smaller size material has lower ignition energy. For micronization, a large percentage of the technologies being considered must take into account these explosivity concerns. The risks associated with explosivity are primarily associated with dry milling techniques; however, all dry handling carried out after micronization requires the proper engineering safeguards to be put in place.

Worker exposure to generated dust will vary along with the type of mill being utilized. In combination with the exposure control limit of the compound, which is typically molecule-specific, certain mill technologies carry much greater risk of overexposure. Wet milling and direct crystallization methods of controlling PSD are inherently safer from an exposure perspective as the primary particle size is controlled in the slurry. While dry handling occurs downstream of these operations, the amount of dust generated in these operations, such as delumping and packaging, is generally much less than that observed with dry milling equipment and the associated dust containment. Dry milling containment can be designed such that operator exposure is minimized; however, this comes at a cost—often much greater than that associated with the milling equipment itself.

Wet milling has potential limitations with regards to micronization, as mentioned in a previous section of this chapter. In the situation where the solids in question can be micronized by wet mill technologies, these technologies are favorable for low exposure and can be readily scaled. Scaling and transferability across manufacturing sites are important as campaigning of products in multiuse equipment is common in the pharmaceutical industry. As such, different sites and equipment configurations may be employed from one product campaign to the next and milling processes that are not scaled appropriately across equipment may not yield equivalent performance. Several correlations have been developed for scaling wet mills.[39–41] Most correlations involve the tip speed of the rotor, geometric descriptions of the system such as rotor-stator gap, number of rotor and stator teeth, and number of passes through the milling system.

Dry milling techniques are more difficult to scale across sets. While the output PSD is largely a function of mill energy input (tip speed for pin mill and gas pressures for jet mills) and residence time in the mill, it is the residence time that may be a problematic control parameter. The residence time is typically derived through a combination of the mass feed rate and gas flow through the system. Loss-in-mass feeders do exist but are typically not utilized in the pharmaceutical industry. Volumetric-based systems rely on an inferred solids bulk density allowing calculation of mass feed rate. Bulk density of the material at the point of solids introduction to the mill can vary, however, as a function of the height of material in the feed hopper, as well as hopper discharge mechanics. As a result, volumetric feed mechanisms are subject to potential dynamic changes resulting in fluctuations in mass feed rate. Careful consideration needs to be given to the design and operation of the solid feed and conveyance to a mill.

8.5 EMERGING TECHNOLOGIES AND FUTURE DIRECTIONS

While process analytical technologies (PAT) are commonly employed in commodity chemical industries for feedback control of solids processing,[42–46] they have not been widely adopted in the pharmaceutical industry. Likewise, while mathematical modeling of inorganic materials has been attempted for the purpose of predicting breakage properties, modeling is not widely utilized in pharmaceuticals. Both PAT and modeling represent an opportunity to combine emerging technologies with predictive control. Current control of milling operations for APIs typically involve determination of the milling parameters applicable to the mill type in use. Holding milling parameters constant, given potential differences in input PSD from upstream processing variability, can lead to potential output variability. Other opportunities for improvement include feed-forward modeling utilizing existing off-line particle size measurements,[47] or feedback control utilizing on-line particle size analysis. Both feed-forward and feedback control schemes, while different in implementation, exploit the concept of controlling final API PSD to a constant number which is independent of differences to the input PSD.

ACKNOWLEDGMENTS

We gratefully acknowledge Pavan Akkisetty of Purdue University for his help in building a database of milling references.

REFERENCES

1. Amidon GL, Lennernas H, Shah VP, Crison JR. 1995. A theoretical basis for a biopharmaceutic drug classification: the correlation of in vitro drug product dissolution and in vivo bioavailability. Pharm. Res. 12: 413–420.
2. Oh DM, Curl R, Amidon G. 1993. Estimating the fraction dose absorbed from suspensions of poorly soluble compounds in humans: A mathematical model. Pharm. Res. 10: 264–270.

3. Waiver of in vivo bioavailability and bioequivalence studies for immediate-release solid oral dosage forms based on a biopharmaceutics classification system. U.S. Department of Health and Human Services Food and Drug Administration Center for Drug Evaluation and Research (CDER), August 2000.
4. Rohrs BR, Amidon GE, Meury RH, Secreast PJ, King HM, Skoug CJ. 1996. Particle size limits to meet USP content uniformity criteria for tablets and capsules. J. Pharm. Sci. 95(5): 1049–1059.
5. Popov KI, Krstic SB, Obradovic MC, Pavlovic MG, Irvanovic ER. 2003. The effect of the particle shape and structure on the flowability of electrolytic copper powder. I. Modeling of a representative powder particle. J. Seb. Chem. Soc. 68(10): 771–777.
6. Tan SB, Newton JM. 1990. Powder flowability as an indication of capsule filling performance. Int. J. Pharm. 61: 145–155.
7. Danjo K, Kinoshita K, Kitagawa K, Iida K, Sunada H, Otsuka A. 1989. Effect of particle shape on the compaction and flow properties of powders. Chem. Pharm. Bull. 37(11): 3070–3073.
8. Zeng XM, Martin GP, Tee SK, Ghoush AA, Marriott C. 1999. Effects of particle size and adding sequence of fine lactose on the deposition of salbutamol sulfate from a dry powder. Int. J. Pharm. 182(2): 133–144.
9. Shoyele SA, Cawthorne S. 2006. Particle engineering techniques for inhaled biopharmaceuticals. Adv. Drug Deliv. Rev. 58(9–10): 1009–1029.
10. Gonda I. 1992. Targeting by deposition. In: Hickey AJ, editor. Pharmaceutical inhalation aerosol technology. New York: Marcel Dekker; 61–82.
11. Hinds WC. 1982. Aerosol technology. New York: John Wiley and Sons.
12. Fisher E. 2006. Milling of active pharmaceutical ingredients. In: Encyclopedia of pharmaceutical technology, 3rd ed. Informa Healthcare; 2339–2351.
13. Liotta V, Sabesan V. 2004. Monitoring and feedback control of supersaturation using ATR-FTIR to produce and active pharmaceutical ingredient of a desired crystal size. OPR&D 8: 488–494.
14. Dennehy RD. 2003. Particle engineering using power ultrasound. OPR&D 7: 1002–1006.
15. Kim S, Lotz B, Lindrud M, Girard K, Moore T, Nagarajan K, Alvarez M, Lee T, Nikfar F, Davidovich M, Srivastava S, Kiang S. 2005. Control of particle properties of a drug substance by crystallization engineering and the effect on drug product formulation. OPR&D 9: 894–901.
16. Paul EL, Tung HH, Midler M. 2005. Organic crystallization processes. Powder Technol. 150(2): 133–143.
17. Price R, Young PM. 2005. On the physical transformations of processed pharmaceutical solids. Micron 36: 519–524.
18. Urban K, Wagner G, Schaffner D, Röglin D, Ulrich J. 2006. Rotor–stator and disc systems for emulsification processes. Chem. Engng Technol. 29(1): 24–31.
19. Kwade A, Schwedes J. 2007. Wet grinding in stirred media mills. In: Handbook of powder technology; 229–249.
20. Russell WB, Saville DA, Schowalter WR. 1991. Colloidal dispersions. New York: Cambridge University Press.
21. Beach S, Latham D, Sidgwick C, Hanna M, York P. 1999. Control of the physical form of salmeterol xinafoate. Org. Process Res. Dev. 3: 370–376.

22. Baldyga J, Bourne JR. Turbulent mixing and chemical reactions. New York: John Wiley & Sons.
23. Shekunov BY, Baldyga J, York P. 2001. Particle formation by mixing with supercritical antisolvent at high Reynolds numbers. Chem. Engng Sci. 56: 2421–2433.
24. Demyanovich RJ, Bourne JR. 1989. Rapid micromixing by the impingement of thin liquid sheets. 2. Mixing study. Ind. Engng Chem. Res. 28: 825–830.
25. Demyanovich RJ, Bourne JR. 1989. Rapid micromixing by the photographic study of the impingement of thin liquid sheets. 1. A flow pattern. Ind. Engng Chem. Res. 28: 830–839.
26. Mahajan AJ, Kirwan DJ. 1996. Micromixing effects in a two-impinging-jets precipitator. AIChE J. 42: 1801–1814.
27. Johnson BK, Prud'homme RK. 2003. Chemical processing and micromixing in confined impinging jets. AIChE J. 49: 2264–2282.
28. Midler M, Paul EL, Whittington E, Futran M, Liu P, Hsu J, Pan S. 1994. Crystallization method to improve crystal structure and size. U.S. patent 5,314,506.
29. Linrud MD, Kim S, Wei C. 2001. Sonic impinging jet crystallization apparatus and process. U.S. patent 6,302,958.
30. Paul EL, Tung HH, Midler M. 2005. Organic crystallization processes. Powder Technol. 150: 133–143.
31. Am Ende D, Crawford TC, Weston NP. 2003. Reactive crystallization method to improve particle size. U.S. patent 5,471,001.
32. Palakodaty S, York P. 1999. Phase behavior effects on particle formation processes using supercritical fluids. Pharm. Res. 16(7): 976–985.
33. Kordikowski A, Shekunov T, York P. 2001. Polymorph control of sulfathiazole in supercritical CO_2. Pharm. Res. 18(5): 682–688.
34. Jarmer DJ, Lengsfeld CS, Randolph TW. 2006. Scale-up criteria for an injector with a confined mixing chamber during precipitation with a compressed fluid antisolvent. J. Supercritical Fluids 37: 242–253.
35. Cashdollar K. 1996. Coal dust explosivity. J. Loss Prev. Process Ind. 9(1): 65–76.
36. Nifuku M, Koyanaka S, Ohya H, Barre C, Hatori M, Fujiwara S, Horiguchi S, Sochet I. 2007. Ignitability characteristics of aluminium and magnesium dusts that are generated during the shredding of post-consumer wastes. J. Loss Prev. Process Ind. 20: 322–329.
37. Kalker N, Schecker H. 1979. Theoretische uberlegungen zum einfluss der teilchengrosse auf die mindestzundenergie von stauben. Chem. Ing. Technol. 51: 1248–1249.
38. Eckhoff RK. 2003. Dust explosions in the process industries, 3rd ed. Gulf Professional Publishing.
39. Shelley S. 2007. High-shear mixers: still widely misunderstood. Chem. Engng Prog. 103(11): 7–12.
40. Lee I, Variankaval N, Lindemann C, Starbuck C. 2004. Rotor–stator milling of APIs—emperical scale up parameters and theoretical relationships between the morphology and breakage of crystals. Am. Pharm. Rev. 7(5): 120–123.
41. Atiemo-Obeng V, Calabrese R. 2003. Rotor stator mixing devices. In: Paul EL, Atiemo-Obeng V, Kresta S, editors. Handbook of industrial mixing, 1st ed. New York: John Wiley & Sons.
42. Galan O, Barton GW, Romagnoli JA. 2002. Robust control of a SAG mill. Powder Technol. 124: 264–271.

43. Holve DJ, Harvill TL. 1996. Particle size distribution measurements for in-process monitoring and control. Adv. Powder Metal. Part. Mat. 1(4): 81–93.
44. Collin A. 1997. Online control of particle size distribution. Spectra Anal. 26(196): 31–33.
45. Terray M. 2001. Process improvements for leading manufacturer of glass beads. Rec. Prog. Gen. Procedes 15: 557–560.
46. Harvill TL, Hoog JH, Holve DJ. 1995. In-process particle size distribution measurements and control. Part. Syst. Charact. 12(6): 309–313.
47. Collins PC, Roginski RT. 2006. Feed-forward modeling approach to particle size control in milling operations. AIChE Annual Meeting, San Francisco, CA, November.

CHAPTER 9

FUNCTION, QUALITY, AND REGULATIONS OF PHARMACEUTICAL EXCIPIENTS FOR ORAL SOLID DOSAGE FORMS

JACK Y. ZHENG
Pharmaceutical Sciences R&D, Lilly Research Laboratories, Eli Lilly and Company, Indianapolis, IN 40285

9.1 INTRODUCTION

Drug products, regardless of their dosage form, formulation composition, manufacturing process, and route of administration, must meet the following basic requirements to assure the safety, identity, strength, purity, and quality of the product:

- good patient compliance;
- efficacy and safety (patient outcomes);
- product quality attributes maintained throughout the shelf-life;
- reproducible and cost-effective manufacturing process with good control strategy;
- continuous improvement on process for consistent quality over time.

Pharmaceutical excipients used in the formulation of various dosage forms help meet these requirements. A pharmaceutical excipient is any substance other than the active drug substance or prodrug that has been appropriately evaluated for safety and is included in the manufacturing process or is contained in a finished pharmaceutical dosage form.[1] Pharmaceutical excipients with a variety of physical and chemical properties can aid in the processing of the drug product during its manufacture; maintain or enhance the product stability, bioavailability, or patient acceptability; assist in product identification; or enhance any other attribute of the overall safety, effectiveness, or delivery of the drug during storage or use.

Formulation and Analytical Development for Low-Dose Oral Drug Products. Edited by Jack Zheng

For a low-dose solid dosage form, excipients are indispensable components of the drug product and comprise the greatest proportion of the single dosage unit. Clearly, the intended function of an excipient is a prerequisite to the successful design, development, and manufacture of optimal pharmaceutical dosage forms. Technical information about pharmaceutical excipients is readily available.[2,3] This chapter provides a general overview of topics regarding pharmaceutical excipients and their function, quality, and regulations. More detailed information on individual applications, performance, and associated problems can be found in the literature.

9.2 CLASSIFICATION OF PHARMACEUTICAL EXCIPIENTS IN SOLID DOSAGE FORMS

Pharmaceutical excipients are an essential component in the successful design, development, and manufacture of drug products. Especially in low-dose drug products, the amount of excipients used in the formulation is significantly higher than that of active pharmaceutical ingredient. A review of the literature shows approximately 1300 excipients currently used in the pharmaceutical industry. Excipients are classified by the functions in a pharmaceutical dosage form. Table 9.1 lists the most commonly used excipients in oral solid dosage forms and their major functions. Fillers (diluents), disintegrants, binders, glidants, lubricants, and coating materials are the most commonly used excipients in solid dosage forms. Antioxidants, wetting agents, solublizing agents, and absorption enhancers are added into formulations as needed. Special functions of excipients related to manufacturability are addressed in Chapters 4–7 on individual manufacturing platform technology for those interested in a more in-depth treatment of the topic.

In general, pharmaceutical excipients are considered GRAS materials, using a term from the food industry.[4] Traditionally, the excipients used in a drug product are

TABLE 9.1 The Most Common Pharmaceutical Excipients and Their Functions for Oral Solid Dosage Forms

Classification	Excipients
Fillers (diluents)	Lactose, mannitol, microcrystalline cellulose, starch, calcium phosphate dibasic
Binders	Povidone, hydroxypropyl cellulose, hypromellose
Disintegrants	Crospovidone, sodium starch glycolate, sodium croscarmellose
Glidants	Talc, silicon dioxide
Lubricants	Magnesium stearate, stearic acid, sodium stearyl fumarate
Film formers/coatings	Hypromellose, hydroxypropyl cellulose, methylcellolose
Antioxidant	Ethylenediamine tetraacetic acid, butylated hydroxytoluene
Wetting agents	Sodium lauryl sulfate, Polysorbate 80 (Tween 80)
Solubilizing agents	Cyclodextrins, ethyl alcohol, propylene glycol
Absorption enhancers	D-α-Tocopheryl polyethylene glycol 1000 succinate, oleic acid

required to be inert and pharmacologically/toxicologically inactive. However, excipients do not always meet these two basic requirements. Excipients, like any other chemicals, have their own internal thermodynamic energy, which results in a certain reactivity. Although this reactivity may be low, it may trigger reactions leading to degradation when influenced by physical and chemical factors in the microenvironment.[5–7] On the other hand, certain "active" excipients in oral formulations are reported to alter the rate and/or extent of drug absorption, thus affecting in vivo bioavailability or bioequivalence.[9] Hence, the basic requirements for a pharmaceutical excipient in a drug product may be defined as follows:

- no significant interaction with the drug substance and other excipients in the formulation to form impurities higher than toxicological limits;
- no significant impact on the desired pharmacokinetic profile upon administration;
- no significant changes in product quality attributes over shelf-life storage (such as appearance, potency, dissolution, and disintegration).

For a very long time, scientists generally underestimated the importance of excipients in pharmaceutical dosage forms. Excipients were cheap ingredients viewed solely as inert supports for medicaments. Today, with modern pharmaceutical excipients on the shelf, development of various novel drug delivery systems, and production with high-speed tablet/capsule machines, excipients are rather more than the sugar in the pill.[9,10]

9.3 PHYSICOCHEMICAL ATTRIBUTES OF PHARMACEUTICAL EXCIPIENTS

Chemically, excipients are of natural, semisynthetic, or synthetic origin. Pharmaceutical excipients encompass diverse chemical classes including celluloses, carbohydrates (such as sugars and starches), inorganic salts, fatty acids and derivatives, surfactants, and water-soluble and -insoluble polymers. The chemical composition and structure of excipients determines their key physicochemical properties and function in drug products. Chemical composition is usually used as an important control in specific monographs of pharmacopeias. For instance, changes in substitution of hydroxypropoxy and methoxy content of hypromellose can result in different hydration rates, and therefore different surface and interfacial activities for controlled-release solid dosage forms.[2] On the other hand, chemical reaction between excipients and drug substance is mainly dependent on functional groups in the molecules. The Maillard reaction between lactose and primary or secondary amines such as fluoxetine hydrochloride is a classic example of drug–excipient imcompatibility.[11]

However, for low-dose drug products, impurities from excipients can be more problematic for causing chemical stability issues with a drug product. Several commonly used excipients (including povidone, PEG400, polysorbate 80, and hydroxypropyl cellulose) contain substantial concentrations of a hydroperoxide impurity with significant lot-to-lot and manufacturer-to-manufacturer variation.[12] Chemical reaction of the hydroperoxides with nucleophilic groups (two-electron transfer) such as amines and thio-ethers can occur and lead to degradation of drug substance.[13,14] Also, the hydroperoxides can be catalytically decomposed by trace levels of transition metals (such as iron III), as well as by heat and light to form peroxy and alcoxyl radicals.[14–16] These radicals can initiate chain propagation of peroxy radicals, which subsequently react with and degrade oxidatively sensitive drug substances (single-electron transfer). Therefore, when formulating a compound prone to oxidation, test different types, batches, and sources of excipients for hydroperoxide levels. This may result in selection of excipients and manufacturing processes that minimize hydroperoxide concentration and improve the long-term product stability.

Physical characteristics of excipients that are closely linked to final product quality attributes (such as uniformity, dissolution, appearance, and mechanical strength) have been receiving more attention in recent years with the "quality-by-design" initiative in drug product development. The physical properties of excipients that should be considered important in formulation and manufacturing process development include bulk and tapped density, true density, crystallinity, polymorphic forms, compaction characteristics, hygroscopicity, flowability, melting point, moisture content, moisture-absorption isotherms, particle size distribution, particle morphology, specific surface area, static charges, and solubility.

Pharmaceutical excipients (such as lactose, mannitol, and magnesium stearate), like most organic compounds, exhibit polymorphism.[2] Different polymorphic forms of an excipient may differ in physical, chemical, electrical, material, and thermal properties. Nitrofurantoin has been found in four different crystal forms: anhydrous forms α and β, and monohydrous forms I and II.[17] The monohydrate forms are not stable under a low humidity environment and mechanical stress, and form undesired amorphous forms.[18] Also, anhydrous forms have better aqueous solubility than hydrates.[19] Thus, the anhydrous forms are preferred for development of stable drug product. Airaksinen et al.[20] found that excipient selection can significantly affect solid-state phase transformation of nitrofurantoin anhydrate during wet granulation. Amorphous excipients such as L-hydroxypropylcellulose and microcrystalline cellulose can inhibit hydrate formation of nitrofurantoin anhydrate at high water content during wet granulation. Crystalline excipients such as lactose are unable to control hydrate formation. Similarly, premixing with hypromellose in the presence of water or ethanol during wet granulation can inhibit solid-state phase transformation of ciprofloxacin anhydrate to the undesired hydrate form.[21]

Thermal behaviors of excipients include melting or sublimation, desolvation or dehydration, thermolability, and potential interaction with other components. Polyethylene glycols are often used to enhance the aqueous solubility or dissolution characteristics of poorly soluble compounds by making solid dispersions with an appropriate grade. The melting behavior of PEGs selected in the formulation could facilitate formation of a solid solution during a manufacturing process such as hot-melt extrusion or granulation.[22] Formation of hydrates such as lactose anhydrate during wet granulation processes and their subsequent partial dehydration during drying could lead to (1) an increase in lactose weight percentage and thus a decrease in potency of the final product, and (2) collapse of crystal structure and formation of the amorphous form that may promote chemical interaction with amines (such as the Maillard reaction).

Some excipients are prone to sublimation at relatively mild processing conditions, which affects final product quality. For instance, butylated hydroxytoluene, a commonly used anti-oxidant, sublimes at approximately 50°C.[23] When using such excipients, take care to avoid exposure to high temperatures during processing and storage, since loss of the functional excipient may have a negative impact on drug product stability. Furthermore, micrometritic characteristics such as particle size, shape, specific surface area, and porosity, are another important physical attribute of excipients.

Particle size of excipients, especially in direct compression and roller compaction, plays a key role in determining critical product and process attributes such as content uniformity, flowability of formulation blend, and lubricity. Poor flow behavior in direct compression formulation contributes to commonly encountered technical issues such as bridging, rat-holing, surging, and the uneven movement of particles into die cavities.[24] This can lead to tablet weight variation. Microcrystalline cellulose is available in several grades with different compactibility, particle size, shape, and bulk and tapped densities. One particular grade could be more suitable than another for meeting specific formulation and process requirements. Larger particle size granular grades such as Avicel® PH200 improve flowability of powder mixtures and are commonly selected for direct compression formulations. In addition, when mixing is critical in manufacturing processes, matching the particle size and densities of excipients with drug substance can help the drug substance distribute uniformly in the excipient matrix to avoid blend uniformity and powder segregation issues. Selection of excipients in formulations with a good understanding of their mechanical properties (such as compressibility and compactibility) helps in designing and developing robust formulation and manufacturing processes.

When granules or powder mixtures are compressed into tablets, the materials undergo several mechanical processes: consolidation, deformation, and fusion. Information on the plastic, elastic, and brittle properties of excipients used will guide the pharmaceutical scientist towards developing a robust formulation. Characterization of the consolidation behavior of powders using shear cell is gaining in popularity. This characterization allows better design of bins and hoppers and avoids flow issues such rat-holing, arching, and the flooding phenomenon of the powders during high-speed tablet manufacture.[25]

Solid dosage form design and process development, especially for low-dose drug products, depends greatly on the physical and chemical properties of excipients in the formulation. Over decades, formulation scientists have put more emphasis on chemical interaction between drug substance and excipients than on physical properties of excipients. Pharmaceutical scientists and processing engineers should make a greater effort to create standards, reliable knowledge bases, and predictive relationships of physical properties for common components to develop pharmaceutical products and manufacturing processes.

9.4 REGULATORY STATUS AND EXCIPIENT QUALITY

According to ICH Guideline Q8 Pharmaceutical Development, the marketing authorization application (MAA) should discuss the excipients chosen and their concentration. The MAA should show the characteristics that can influence the medical product performance and manufacturability relative to the respective function of each excipient. Additionally, the MAA should demonstrate the ability of excipients to provide their intended functionality throughout the intended period of validity of the formulation. Use the information on excipient performance as appropriate to justify the choice and quality attributes of the excipients.[26]

9.4.1 Regulations

Manufacture of excipients usually takes place on a large scale, which means that automated process controls and continuous stream processing are more likely. Production equipment and operations vary depending on the type of excipient, the scale of production, and the type of operation (e.g., batch vs continuous). Hence, batch-to-batch variation from the same manufacturer will not be a surprise, while an excipient from different sources might not have identical properties with respect to its use in a specific formulation. Federal Food, Drug, and Cosmetic Act Section 501 (a) (2) B requires that drugs, including excipients meeting the definition of a drug in Section 201 (g) of the Act, be manufactured in conformance with cGMP. Thus, according to the Act, manufacture of all excipients intended for use in a drug product must occur under cGMP regulations. However, FDA has not promulgated cGMP regulations for excipients. The cGMP requirements as published in the 21 CFR Part 210 and 211 strictly apply to finished pharmaceuticals, and the FDA only expects the pharmaceutical manufacturer to be compliant. To establish a suitable quality system for excipient manufactures, the GMP for bulk pharmaceutical excipients has recently been published as a general chapter <1078> in the *United States Pharmacopeia* (USP) 30/NF25.[27] Table 9.2 outlines the information used as the basis for a quality system in the manufacture of excipients.[27]

Generally speaking, procedures utilized in the manufacture and control of excipients should be written. Conformance to those procedures should be documented. A quality manual is a documented base intended to describe the quality policy and the commitment of the supplier to quality. The procedural system should have adequate formal controls related to procedure approval, revision, and distribution. These controls should provide assurance that the proper version of a procedure is used throughout the operation. On the other hand, cGMP requirements as regulated by the U.S. FDA expect pharmaceutical manufacturers to qualify their excipient suppliers, although the FDA does not have specific guidance for pharmaceutical companies on how to do that. As a result, the International Pharmaceutical Excipient Council (IPEC) has developed excellent guidelines on how to conduct an audit of a manufacturing operation that produces pharmaceutical excipients and how to audit their

TABLE 9.2 Excipient Quality Systems

General	Specific
1. Management and employee responsibility	• Quality policy • Organization • Personnel
2. Manufacturer and user responsibilities	• Contract review • Document and data control • Purchasing • Control of customer supplied products • Product identification and traceability
3. Process control	• Buildings and facilities • Equipment • Water systems and water quality • Aseptic and sterile manufacturing • Validation of process and control procedures • Stability • Expiration dating and re-evaluation • Process changes (change control) • Lot or batch production records • In-process blending or mixing • Solvent, mother liquors, and second crops
4. Inspection and testing	• Test status • Raw material testing • In-process testing • Finished product testing and release • Control of nonconforming product
5. Inspection, measuring and test equipment	
6. Handling, storage, preservation, packaging, and delivery	• Handling, storage, and preservation • Packaging system • Delivery
7. Quality record control	
8. Internal quality audits	
9. Training	

distribution and repackaging.[27,28] General auditing considerations should be given in the following areas:

- prevention of contamination;
- documentation;
- inspections;
- significant processing steps;
- documentation and record keeping;
- product lot or batch consistency and audit.

The Organization of International Standardization (ISO) 9000 series outlines a quality system standard of general application that can be applied to cover every aspect of manufacturing to the benefit of both the manufacturer and customer. It is internationally recognized as a general guideline for all manufacturing quality systems. Since there is no current regulatory requirement in Europe, Japan, or the United States for third-party certification, an excipient manufacturer may apply the standard with or without ISO certification. However, such certification has the benefit of providing assurance to pharmaceutical companies that conformance to this quality system has been independently confirmed. Pharmaceutical manufacturers worldwide increasingly regard compliance with ISO 9002 as an essential qualification for the excipient supplies. Incorporation of GMP requirements into the ISO 9000 quality system enhances not only the quality system, but also a company's operational procedures as well.

Excipient and vendor selections can greatly influence the new drug development timeline, product performance, and acceptance of final products. Compendial excipients have composition consistent with monographs published in compendia such as USP-NF; these are the better-characterized excipients. These excipients most likely possess desirable qualities and are preferred excipients for pharmaceutical formulations. Non-compendial excipients can also be used for drug products if they are supported by Type IV drug master files (DMFs) in regulatory dossiers. Overall, a good excipient supplier should:[29]

- maintain DMFs with FDA for noncompendial items;
- consistently conform to pharmacopeial monograph requirements;
- manufacture in ISO-9000-certified facilities;
- pass FDA inspection and auditing by either pharmaceutical companies or IPEA.

Although pharmaceutical excipients, unlike finished dosage forms, are not currently subject to regulatory control in terms of cGMP regulations, inattention to excipients, excipient suppliers, and regulations may lead to delay or failure to bring a new drug product to market. Thus, pharmaceutical scientists should become familiar with excipients selected for the drug product, their manufacturers, and regulations during commercial product development.

9.4.2 Control Strategies

Control of excipients is often built around the various pharmacopeial standards including the *British Pharmacopoeia* (BP), *European Pharmacopoeia* (PhEur), *Japanese Pharmacopeia* (JP) and the *United States Pharmacopeia/National Formulary* (USP/NF). The use of excipients that conform to a compendium ensures that the material meets the established specifications and acceptance criteria. This provides a handle on the batch-to-batch variability of the excipients used, as well as an option to select from multiple vendors for controlling the cost of goods. However, the pharmaceutical industry has long recognized that these standards are insufficient because they emphasize impurity, chemical stability, and assays, but have little to contribute at a similar level of rigor for the physical or mechanical properties of excipients. On the other hand, most of the standards in different pharmacopeias are not identical. As seen in Table 9.3, the standards of talc, a commonly used glidant, are very different in various pharmacopeias. Especially in JP, only identification, water-soluble substances, and iron tests are the same as those required in the PhEur and USP. Thus, one of the challenging issues today is establishing harmonized global quality standards for acceptance of excipients to eliminate redundant testing to save costs. The International Conference on Harmonization (ICH) has made significant progress towards harmonization of testing methods and specifications. Monographs for about 38 excipients have been harmonized so far.[30] Much progress has been made but we are still far from full harmonization.

Drug products might also utilize noncompendial excipients. Type IV DMFs in regulatory dossiers (i.e., new drug applications, abbreviated new drug applications, or investigational new drug applications) support the use of these noncompendial excipients. Excipient manufacturers should maintain these files with the regulatory agency. The files should support the safety of the excipient as well as the quality and consistency of excipient manufacturing.

Very few excipients are manufactured specifically for pharmaceutical use. Manufacturing plants are usually not devoted to the manufacture of a specific excipient. With continuous production cycles, the control and quality are often not at a

TABLE 9.3 Standards of Talc in Different Pharmacopeias

PhEur	JP	USP
Identification: (IR, or XRPD and formation of magnesium ammonium phosphate)	Identification	Identification (IR and formation of magnesium ammonium phosphate)
Microbial limit		Microbial limit
		Acidity and alkalinity
Loss on ignition		Loss on ignition
Water-soluble substances	Purity: acid, alkali, and water-soluble substances	Water-soluble substances
Limit of ion	Water-soluble iron	Limit of ion
Limit of lead		Limit of lead
Limit of calcium		Limit of calcium
Limit of aluminum		Limit of aluminum
		Absence of asbestos (IR, XRPD, optical microscopy)
Content of magnesium		Content of magnesium
	Purity: acid-soluble substances	
	Loss on drying	
	Arsenic	

pharmaceutical level. Thus, some excipient manufacturers do not label their products as compendial grade because of low demand from the pharmaceutical industry, increased GMP expectation, the prospect of FDA inspection, or the time and resources needed to perform required audits.[31] There is an increasing danger of excipient manufacturers not producing pharmaceutical-grade excipients that meet compendial criteria. This can create an enormous problem for the drug manufacturing industry. However, if the supplier stops designating the excipient as compendial grade for GMP reasons, do not use the material from such a supplier; instead, find a different acceptable supplier for that excipient.[32] From a regulatory perspective, removing the USP or NF labeling for an excipient does not obviate the requirements to meet applicable cGMP and official USP/NF standards if the excipient is used in a drug product.[32] Nevertheless, excipient manufacturers should have appropriate control processes in place, along with sufficient testing and measurement, to ensure that each finished lot of excipient meets all of its quality requirements.

9.4.3 Functionality Testing

With the FDA's recent quality-by-design initiative,[33] the quality of pharmaceutical excipients has emerged as a key attribute to building quality into a drug product. Physical and material properties of excipients play an important role in drug product performance, manufacturability, and reproducibility. Thus, a measure of the physical properties of excipients (e.g., functionality testing), has become a hot topic of debate for both pharmaceutical and excipient manufacturers for some years.[32,34,35] Functionality is a desirable property of a material that aids manufacturing and improves the manufacture, quality, or performance of the drug product. Clearly, each formulation or drug product will have its own unique requirements for functionality. Thus, functionality can only be properly tested by manufacturing and subsequently testing a batch of product. Pharmaceutical scientists should perform studies to identify the functionality that matters most in connection with their use of an excipient. Another approach is to identify a surrogate test (usually a physical test) that links to the required functionality of a formulation. PhEur defines such properties as "functionality-related characteristics," and includes this in General Text 5.15.[36] PhEur indicates that monographs on excipients may have a nonmandatory section entitled "Functionality-related characteristics" for the user. The USP/NF uses the term "Performance tests" for excipient functionality. USP/NF informational chapter <1059> "Excipient Performance" provides an overview of the key functional categories of excipients identified in USP/NF along with tests that relate to excipient performance. Careful consideration of the function of the excipient in the dosage form and the critical attributes that relate to the excipient's performance will determine the need for additional tests on the excipient. Table 9.4 shows an example of the different excipients typically used to achieve the desired functions in a formulation and the proposed functionality tests.

Of course, it is necessary to have reliable and reasonably objective methods to measure the physicochemical properties of the excipients. Table 9.5 summarizes analytical methods commonly used in excipient characterization. A better

TABLE 9.4 Typical Function of Some Excipients and Their Functionality Testing

Excipient	Function	Functionality Testing
Spray-dried lactose, starch, microcrystalline cellulose, spray-dried mannitol	Diluent or filler	Bulk density, tapped density, particle size and size distribution, flow
Sodium starch glycolate, crospovidone, croscarmellose sodium	Disintegrant	Hydration capacity, water uptake
Magnesium stearate, steatric acid, sodium stearyl fumarate	Lubricant	Particle size, surface area
Hypromellose, povidone	Binder	Viscosity

TABLE 9.5 Analytical Techniques Used to Characterize Physical and Material Properties of Excipients

Material Property	Characterization Techniques
Crystallinity and polymorphism	X-ray powder diffraction
	Differential scanning calorimetry (DSC)
	Infrared spectroscopy
	Solid state NMR
	Raman spectroscopy
	Thermogravimetric analysis (TGA)
Morphology/crystal habit	Microscopy/image analysis
	Scanning electron microscope
Particle size	Laser diffraction
	Coulter counter
	Photon correlation spectroscopy
	Microscopy
	Ro-Tap sieve analysis
Surface area	Nitrogen adsorption multipoint Brunauer–Emmett–Teller method
Wettability	Contact angle tensiometer
	Moisture sorption
	Dynamic moisture/vapor sorption analysis
Thermal property	DSC, TGA
	Isothermal microcalorimetry
	Hot stage microscopy
Flow	Angle of repose tester
	Shear cell tester
	Flow time
True density	Helium pycnometry
Bulk and tapped density	Density tester (graduated cylinder method)
Mechanical properties	Dynamic mechanical analyzer
	Texture analyzer
	Compaction simulator
	Instron material test system

understanding of critical physical and material properties for the specific dosage form is very important to conducting the functionality testing and controlling the quality of excipients. Control strategies concerning excipient functionality and/or performance-related tests should be based on the product quality requirements investigated during design and development of the formulation and manufacturing process, as well as the excipient manufacturer's process capabilities. The excipient user and excipient maker should work together to set the test parameters and control strategies for pharmaceutical excipients.

9.4.4 New Excipients

Pharmaceutical excipients available on the market seem sufficient to support typical oral solid dosage form development. In some cases, new drug candidates have physicochemical and biopharmaceutical properties that are less than ideal. These drugs present formulation challenges and may require either the discovery of new excipients or improvement of existing excipients. From a regulatory perspective, there is no answer for the question of registration of an excipient as a separate entity.

In Europe, any new excipient that has not been used in any drug product should be evaluated as new chemical entity.[37,38] Established excipients are included in MAAs for new drugs, with the assumption that their presence and characterization in pharmacopeias will not cause concern with European regulations. In Japan, the Pharmaceuticals and Medical Devices Evaluation Center (PMDE) conducts the assessment of new drug applications containing excipients with prior use in Japan. The Subcommittee on Pharmaceutical Excipients of the Central Pharmaceutical Affairs Council (CPAC) must evaluate new products that contain a new excipient. They do this concurrently with the approval process undertaken through the PMDE center.[39] Submit information to justify including the excipient, precedents of use, quality, stability, and safety for evaluation. In the United States, the FDA assesses and permits use of excipients as part of a new drug application (NDA). As in Europe, it is assumed that the use of an excipient in approved products will gain its acceptance in the new drug formulation. For a new excipient, submit appropriate safety evaluation data.[40] Conducting safety and toxicology evaluation of new excipients and generating DMF-required documents is expensive. Because of the economic hurdles, only a handful of new excipients with new chemical entities have been introduced into the market over the past 20 years.

The advancement of material science and technology has allowed excipient manufacturers to improve the performance of existing excipients that have already been used in approved products (Table 9.6). The modification of the traditional excipients is mainly focused on their physical properties, such as particle size, density, morphology, and the degree and form of crystallization. These modified excipients may improve compressibility and compactibility, increase dilution potential, decrease lubrication sensitivity, enhance flow properties and blending process, and improve product stability in formulation and process development. Such excipients will raise less regulatory concern during registration of the new drug product.

TABLE 9.6 Examples of Excipient Modification for Improved Performance

Modifications	Origin	Modified Excipient	Characteristics
Modification of particle size by milling, sieving, agglomerating, spray-drying	Starch Avicel PH101	Starch 1500 Avicel PH102, Avicel PH200	Better flowability Better compactibility
Modification of density	Dibasic calcium phosphate Avicel PH101	Fujicalin Avicel PH301, Avicel PH302	Better blending behavior
Modification of morphology	Lactose monohydrate Mannitol	FastFlo Lactose Pearlitol SD100, Pearlitol SD200	Better flowability Better compactibility
Coprocessing of excipients	Lactose + cellulose Lactose + starch Cellulose + colloidal silicon dioxide	Cellactose Starlac Prosolv SMCC	Better flowability Better compactibility Better blending behavior
Modification of moisture content	Avicel PH101	Avicel PH103, Avicel PH112	Compatible with moisture-sensitive drug

Therefore, functional improvement of existing excipients will be a continuing trend in new excipient development for pharmaceutical purposes.

9.5 SUMMARY

Design of pharmaceutical dosage form is as much science as it is art. It involves a good understanding of the formulation compositions and justifiable selection based on the best knowledge of the special characteristics of the compositions. In a drug product, both drug substance and excipients are essential to developing a robust formulation and manufacturing process. Especially for low-dose drug products, quality and functionality of excipients in a formulation can affect drug product critical characteristics, and thus pharmacological performance, after administration. Therefore, manufacture and control of pharmaceutical excipients is the first crucial step towards the success of a drug product.

ACKNOWLEDGMENTS

The author wish to thank Dr Paul Sirois at Eli Lilly and Company for review of the manuscript. Special thanks are expressed to Ms Karen Boleyn for help with preparation of the manuscript.

REFERENCES

1. International Pharmaceutical Excipients Council—Americas. What are pharmaceutical excipients?. Available at http://www.ipecamericas.org/public/faqs.html#question1. Accessed September 9, 2007.
2. Rowe RC, Sheskey PJ, Owen SC. 2006. Handbook of pharmaceutical excipients, 5th ed. Washington DC: Pharmaceutical Press.
3. Ash M, Ash I, editors. 2007. Handbook of pharmaceutical additives, 3rd ed. New York: Synapase Information Resources.
4. U.S. Food and Drug Administration. Inactive ingredient search for approved drug products, http://www.accessdata.fda.gov/scripts/cder/iig/index.cfm. Accessed September 12, 2007.
5. Akers MJ. 2002. Excipients–drug interactions in parenteral formulations. J. Pharm. Sci. 91(11): 2283–2300.
6. Sims JL, Carrieira JA, Carrier DJ, Crabtree SR, Easton L, Hancock SA, Simcox CE. 2003. A new approach to accelerated drug–excipient compatibility testing. Pharm. Dev. Technol. 8(2): 119–126.
7. Wyttenbach N, Birringer C, Alsenz J, Kuentz M. 2005. Drug–excipient compatibility testing using a high-throughput approach and statistical design. Pharm. Dev. Technol. 10: 499–505.
8. Chen ML, Straughn AB, Sadrieh N, Meyer M, Faustino PJ, Ciavarella AB, Meibohm B, Yates CR, Hussain AS. 2007. Pharm. Res. 24(1): 73–80.
9. Lesney MS. 2001. More than just the sugar in the pill. Today's Chemist at Work, January: 38–43.
10. Pifferi G, Restani P. 2003. The safety of pharmaceutical excipients. Il Farmaco 58: 541–550.
11. Wirth DD, Baertschi W, Johnson RA, Maple SR, Miller MS, Hallenbeck DK, Gregg SM. 1998. Maillard reaction of lactose and fluoxetine hydrochloride, a secondary amine. J. Pharm. Sci. 87: 31–39.
12. Wasylaschuk WR, Harmon PA, Wagner G, Harman AB, Templeton AC, Xu H, Reed RA. 2007. Evaluation of hydroperoxides in common pharmaceutical excipients. J. Pharm. Sci. 96: 106–116.
13. Hartauer KJ, Arbuthnot GN, Baertschi SW, Johnson RA, Luke WD, Person NG, Rickard EC, Tingle CA, Tsang PKS, Wiens RE. 2000. Influence of peroxide impurities in povidone and crospovidone on the stability of raloxifene hydrochloride in tablets: identification and control of an oxidative degradation product. Pharm. Dev. Technol. 5: 303–310.
14. Hovoroka SW, Schoneich C. 2001. Oxidative degradation of pharmaceuticals: theory, mechanism, and inhibition. J. Pharm. Sci. 90: 253–268.
15. Johnson DM, Gu LC. 1988. Autoxidation and antioxidants. In: Swarbrick J, Boylan JC, editors. Encyclopedia of pharmaceutical technology, vol. 1. New York: Wiley; 415–449.
16. Sheldon RA, Kochi JK. 1976. Metal-catalyzed oxidation of organic compounds in the liquid phase: A mechanistic approach. In: Ely DD, editor. Advances in catalysis. New York: Academic Press; 273–413.

17. Caira MR, Pienaar EW, Lotter AP. 1996. Polymorphism and pseudopolymorphism of the antibacterial nitrofurantoin. Mol. Cryst. Liq. Cryst. 279: 241–264.
18. Kishi A, Otsuka M, Matsuda Y. 2002. The effect of humidity on dehydration behavior of nitrofurantoin monohydrate studied by humidity controlled simultaneous instrument for X-ray diffractormetry and differential scanning calorimetry (XRD-DSC). Colloid. Surf. B: Biointerfaces 25: 281–291.
19. Khankari RK, Grant DJW. 1995. Pharmaceutical hydrates. Thermochim. Acta 248: 62–79.
20. Airaksinen S, Karjalainen M, Kivikero N, Westermarck S, Shevchenko A, Rantanen J, Yliruusi J. 2005. Excipient selection can significantly affect solid-state phase transformation in formulation during wet granulation. AAPS PharmSciTech. 6(2) article 41: E311–E322.
21. Li X, Zhi F, Hu Y. 2007. Investigation of excipient and processing on solid phase transformation and dissolution of ciprofloxacin. Int. J. Pharm. 328: 177–182.
22. Miralles MJ, McGinity JW, Martin A. 1982. Combined water-soluble carriers for coprecipitates of tolbutamide. J. Pharm. Sci. 71: 302–304.
23. Verhagen H. 1990. Toxicology of the food additives BHA and BHT. Pharm Weekly (Sci) 12: 164–166.
24. Prescott JK, Barnum RA. 2000. On powder flowability. Pharm. Technol. 24: 60–84.
25. Schwedes J, Schulze D. 1990. Measurement of flow properties of bulk solids. Powder Technol. 61: 59–68.
26. International Conferences of Harmonization. 2006. Guidance for industry: Q8 Pharmaceutical Development. http://www.fda.gov/cder/guidance/6746fnl.pdf. Accessed September 22, 2007.
27. <1078>Good Manufacturing Practices for Bulk Pharmaceutical Excipients. 2007. USP 30/NF25; 514.
28. Silerstein I. 2004. How IPEA's auditing program can help both producers and users. Am. Pharm. Rev. 7(3): 76–79.
29. Chang D, Chang RK. 2007. Review of current issues in pharmaceutical excipients. Pham. Technol. 31(5): 56–66.
30. Mohan G. 2005. Functionality testing of excipients and their impact on formulation development. Am. Pharm. Rev. 8(6): 64–67.
31. Larner G, Schoneker DR, Sheehan C, Uppoor R, Walsh P, Wiens R. 2006. PQRI survey of pharmaceutical excipient testing and control strategies used by excipient manufactures, excipient distributors, and drug-product manufactures. Pharm. Technol. 30(9): 90–98.
32. Carlin B, Carter D, Griffiths M, Larner G, Moore K, Rothman B, Schoneker D, Sheehan C, Uppoor R, Walsh P, Wiens R. 2007. Joint position paper on pharmaceutical excipient testing and control strategies. Pharm. Technol. 31(9): 84–104.
33. International Conference on Harmonization. 2006. Q8 Pharmaceutical Development. http://www.fda.gov/cder/guidance/index.htm. Accessed September 8, 2007.
34. Rios M. 2006. Debating excipient functionality. Pharm. Technol. 30(9): 50–60.
35. Moreton RC. 2006. Functionality and performance of excipients. Excipients performance. Pharm. Technol. suppl.: S4–S14.
36. European Pharmacopoeia. 2008. <5.15> Functionality-related characteristics of excipients, 6th ed.

37. Wotton PK, Khosla R. 1991. Acceptability of excipients in the European community and U.S.A. BIRA J. 10(7): 11–13.
38. Medical products for human use, presentation and contents of the dossier. 1998. The rules governing medicinal products in the European Union Notice to Applicants. Luxembourg: Office for Official Publications of the European Communities; 2B.
39. Uchiyama M. 1999. Regulatory status of excipients in Japan. Drug Inform. J. 33: 27–32.
40. The U.S. Food and Drug Administration. 2005. Guidance for industry: nonclinical studies for the safety evaluation of pharmaceutical excipients. http://www.fda.gov/cder/guidance/index.htm. Accessed August 18, 2007.

PART II

CHALLENGES IN ANALYTICAL METHOD DEVELOPMENT FOR ORAL LOW-DOSE DRUG PRODUCTS

CHAPTER 10

ANALYTICAL METHOD DEVELOPMENT: CHALLENGES AND SOLUTIONS FOR LOW-DOSE ORAL DOSAGE FORMS

BEVERLY NICKERSON, REENA M. JOSEPH, CHARLES PALMER, ALEX M. OPIO, and H. GEORGE BERESFORD

Pfizer Global Research & Development, Groton and New London Laboratories, Pfizer, Inc., Groton, CT 06340

10.1 INTRODUCTION

The analysis of high-potency, low-strength solid oral dosage forms poses a number of analytical challenges that can impact potency, purity and dissolution testing of the dosage form. The low quantity of active ingredient and corresponding degradants in these dosage forms results in sample solutions with extremely low analyte concentrations that pose difficulties for detection and quantitation. These low concentrations often necessitate the use of sample concentration techniques or the use of detectors with greater sensitivity than conventional UV detection (e.g., fluorescence, electrochemical). Low analyte concentrations may also make the use of conventional dissolution apparatus not viable. The high excipient to drug ratio in low-dose drug products poses additional challenges such as difficulties extracting all the active ingredient, leading to low potency or irreproducible assay results. Potency and purity results can also be impacted by interferences from the excipient or excipient-related impurities.

This chapter contains four case studies which illustrate some specific challenges of analyzing low-dose drug products. The first case study discusses the loss of an active ingredient due to adsorption of drug to sample vials, which impacts assay results. The second case study highlights several sources of extraneous or nondrug-related peaks, which can impact purity analysis. The third case study illustrates difficulties encountered while developing a single HPLC purity method for a fixed combination product where one active ingredient is present at a low dose and the

Formulation and Analytical Development for Low-Dose Oral Drug Products. Edited by Jack Zheng

other is at a much higher dose. And the last case study discusses how the challenge of low sample concentration for dissolution analysis was addressed using a nonconventional dissolution apparatus.

10.2 CASE STUDY 1: DRUG ADSORPTION TO SURFACES

Development of a robust analytical method with adequate recovery for assay and sensitivity for purity analysis of low-dose solid oral drug products is challenging. Development of the sample preparation step for the method has its own challenges, such as potential difficulties in extracting all the active ingredient from the excipient matrix or potential loss of the active ingredient through adsorption to surfaces. Loss of active ingredient, even in small quantities, will have a significant impact on the potency results when dealing with low-dose dosage forms.

Numerous examples of drug adsorption to surfaces such as glass (e.g., flasks and vials),[1–5] plastic (e.g., flasks, vials, tubes),[1,2,6–9] and filters[10,11] have been reported in the literature. While filter validation is typically performed to verify adequate recovery of drug, recovery studies are not typically conducted for HPLC sample vials or other component surfaces used during the analysis. Drug adsorption to sample vials posed an issue for Compound A, a low-dose compound under development. The structure of this compound contains an amine group as well as a hydrophobic region containing phenyl and naphthalene rings.

During development of Compound A, tablet strengths of 0.25 and 0.5 mg were investigated in clinical studies. The assay response for sample solutions was found to vary depending on the type of HPLC sample vials used as well as the sample diluent used. Sample vials and vial inserts are available in a number of different materials, including borosilicate glass, borosilicate amber glass, silanized or deactivated glass, and various types of plastics (e.g., polypropylene, polymethylpentene).[12–14] While type 1, class A borosilicate glass is commonly used, compounds such as Compound A that contain amine groups may have affinity for the polar silanol groups (Si–O–H) on the glass surface.[12] Amber glass vials are typically produced from type 1, class B borosilicate glass, which is more alkaline than type 1, class A borosilicate glass. A number of chemically "inert" glass vials are commercially available, where the silanol groups on the glass surface have been "silanized" or treated with an organosilane to produce a more hydrophobic surface ($Si–O–Si–R_3$) to minimize interactions of polar compounds with the glass surface. Plastic vials are another alternative for compounds that interact with glass. When using plastic vials, studies should be conducted to ensure that no leachable components from the plastic are extracted into the sample solution.

A study was conducted to investigate the variability in the assay results observed in the analysis of Compound A samples. One of the factors evaluated was the possibility of drug adsorption onto the sample vials. In this study, sample solutions were prepared in two different dissolving solvents. One set of samples was prepared in an aqueous acidic diluent (pH 2). The second set of samples was prepared in a dissolving solvent containing 85% of the same aqueous medium and 15% methanol.

As shown in Table 10.1, the solubility of the drug is higher in acidic aqueous media and in methanol compared to the other media listed. Several HPLC vial types were evaluated, including borosilicate glass, amber glass, silanized glass, and polypropylene HPLC vials. Sample solutions were prepared and aliquots were transferred to the vials for analysis. Six sample solutions in each diluent were analyzed per type of vial. Experiments were conducted such that the residence time for the sample solution in each vial type was approximately the same.

As shown in Fig. 10.1a, the drug, when prepared in the aqueous acidic diluent, has a higher area response for sample solutions in the borosilicate glass and amber glass vials than in the other vial types. The area response in the borosilicate and amber glass vials decreases slightly with time. This change in area response as a function of time could result in variable assay results during the course of an analysis. Compound A is a protonated amine under acidic conditions. A hydrophilic interaction between the protonated amine of the drug and the negatively charged silanol groups on the borosilicate glass and amber glass surface likely cause the drug to adsorb to the glass surface over time.

Figure 10.1a also shows that the area response of Compound A in the silanized glass vials is lower than the area response in the nondeactivated glass vials. And the area response in the polypropylene vials is even lower, approximately 7% lower than in the borosilicate glass vials. Besides the lower area response, the use of plastic vials results in the appearance of additional, noninterfering peaks in the HPLC chromatogram. The silanized vials and polypropylene vials have hydrophobic surfaces that appear to have an affinity for the hydrophobic phenyl and/or

TABLE 10.1 Solubility of Compound A in (a) Water and (b) Organic Solvents

	Solubility (mg/mL)
(a) Aqueous Solubility of Compound A	
pH	
1.4	36
2.1	4.1
3.1	1.5
4.1	0.6
5.4	0.1
7.0	<0.01
9.7	<0.01
11.4	<0.01
(b) Solubility of Compound A in Organic Solvents	
Solvent	
Acetonitrile	0.2
Methanol	6.6
Ethanol	0.8
Ethyl acetate	0.0

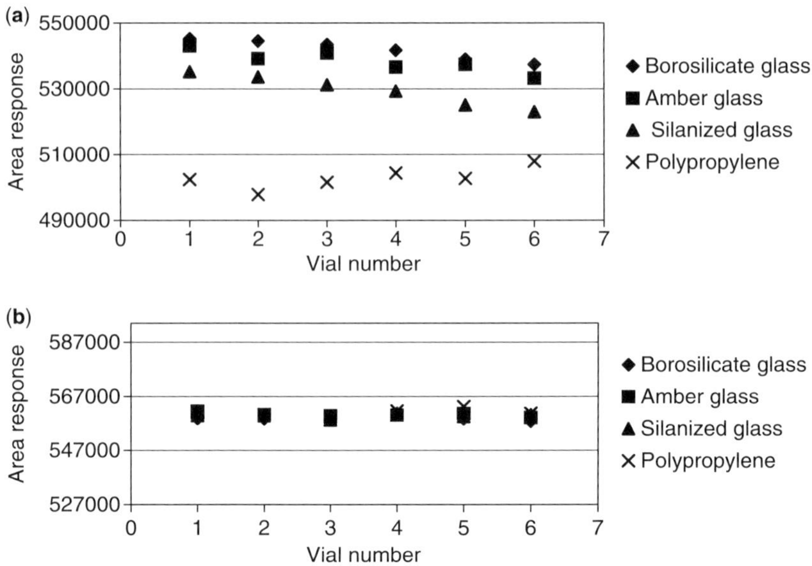

Figure 10.1 Area response for samples of Compound A in (a) aqueous acidic medium and (b) 85% aqueous acidic medium/15% methanol.

naphthalene rings of the drug. As shown in Fig. 10.1b, when 15% methanol is added to the aqueous diluent, the area response is consistent for all vial types and the response is also consistent over time. Addition of organic solvent to the diluent overcomes the weak interaction between the drug and the vial surface such that the analyte resides preferentially in the diluent. Hence, in this case addition of organic solvent to the sample diluent can be used to eliminate drug absorption to the vial surfaces and result in more accurate and reproducible assay results. Another potential resolution for this issue, which was not investigated in this case, might include the use of a higher ionic strength diluent or buffer. In this case the buffer ions might preferentially interact with the negatively charged silanol groups on the borosilicate glass and/or amber glass surfaces, thereby reducing the adsorption of drug to the surface. In addition, using a higher nominal concentration of drug in the sample solution would minimize the impact of the quantity of drug interacting with the vial surface.

In conclusion, for low-dose drug products, it is important to be aware of the possibility that adsorption of the drug from the sample solutions onto surfaces can lead to low or variable assay results. These surfaces include filters, volumetric flasks, and sample vials. Evaluation of the components that come in direct contact with the sample solutions for potential drug adsorption should be conducted as part of method development. This is especially true for compounds containing active sites such as amino groups, as described in this case study. While, most potency analyses involve the use of some organic solvents in the dissolving solvent, dissolution analyses could be problematic since the compendial media are aqueous buffers. For components such as HPLC vials, it is important to examine not only the type of vials, but also the vendor specific vials. Even the use of "deactivated" or silanized glass should be evaluated as some drugs may still interact with these surfaces.

10.3 CASE STUDY 2: CHALLENGES DUE TO NONDRUG-RELATED IMPURITIES

Purity analysis can be a challenging undertaking for low-dose drug products. A particular area of concern is the presence of nondrug-related impurities that can be observed during purity analysis of the low-dose drug product. If these impurities are not identified as nondrug-related, they will be quantitated as drug product degradants, thereby resulting in misleading information. Examples of different types of nondrug-related impurities and strategies to address them are discussed in this section.

10.3.1 Excipient and Packaging-Related Impurities

In the case of Compound B, a tablet dosage strength as low as 0.05 mg was used in clinical studies. The excipients used in the formulation were colloidal silicon dioxide, croscaramellose sodium, lactose, magnesium stearate and microcrystalline cellulose with a drug to excipient ratio of 1 : 2000. In order to assess the purity of these low-dose tablets, it is necessary to composite several tablets into one sample, a common practice for low-dose tablet formulations.[15,16] Although using a composite sample enhances the concentration of the active ingredient for detection, it also increases the concentration of excipients, and excipient-related impurities and degradation products in the sample solution. Since impurities are quantitated relative to the active ingredient, the likelihood of detecting extraneous or nondrug-related materials for low-dose drug products is an issue not normally encountered in higher dose drug products. For example, based on ICH Q3B(R2),[17] a 2.0% impurity for a 0.05 mg tablet represents 1.0 μg of the impurity and is above the reporting threshold (0.1%), identification threshold (1.0%) and qualification threshold (1.0%) for this dose. However, for a 5 mg tablet this same quantity of impurity would be 0.02% of the active ingredient and would be below the reporting (0.1%), identification (0.5%) and qualification (0.5%) thresholds, and may even be below the limit of quantitation (LOQ) of the method. It is therefore important to identify nondrug-related impurities in low-dose formulations so that they are not reported as drug-related impurities. Analyzing a placebo sample that is formulated with the same excipients as the low-dose formulation can aid in identifying excipient-related impurities.[1,16] In addition, as described below, placebo stability testing can help to elucidate excipient-related degradation products and packaging-related impurities, and consequently can be beneficial for judging the quality of the dosage form.

A stability study for 0.05 mg tablets of Compound B was conducted to support use of the formulation in clinical trials. Purity data from the 6-week and 12-week samples showed several impurity peaks above the 0.05% LOQ of the method, which were not present in the initial samples. These degradant peaks were present at higher levels in the stress conditions of 40°C/75% RH and 50°C/20% RH. The amounts of the impurities varied from 0.05 to 2% when quantitated against an external standard of the drug.

In order to identify any excipient- and packaging-related impurities in the formulation, placebo cores and film-coated placebos, were prepared using the same excipients as in the active tablets. The placebo cores and film-coated placebos, as well as active cores and film-coated active tablets were set up on a stability study in high density polyethylene (HDPE) bottles with and without desiccant and in foil–foil blisters. At the designated time intervals, the tablets were tested for purity by gradient HPLC analysis.

The stability study revealed that many of the degradation peaks observed in the active tablet stability program were nondrug-related. Although eight degradation peaks were observed above the LOQ in the accelerated stability study of the 0.05 mg tablets, only two of them were drug-related. The quantity of all degradants was calculated based on the response factors of the drug and hence may have lead to underestimation of the amounts of the nondrug-related degradants in the tablets since the excipient chromophores are usually less strong UV absorbers.

Information on the abundance and origin of the major nondrug-related impurities is summarized in Table 10.2 and example HPLC chromatograms of the placebo stability samples are shown in Fig. 10.2. Only one of the nondrug-related impurities which was present at the highest level of 2%, could be identified. Although five other impurities were present at relatively high levels, 0.6–2%, these levels are relative to the active compound, which is present at 0.05 mg. The actual mass quantity of the impurities is therefore extremely small, making identification of the impurities difficult.

As shown in Table 10.2, the impurity peak at RRT 0.38 was specific to active and placebo cores and film-coated tablets stored with desiccant. An investigation was conducted using desiccant extracts prepared using the sample dissolving solvents.

TABLE 10.2 Major Nondrug-Related Impurities Observed in Placebo and Active Tablets of Compound B

RRT[a]	Impurity	Placebo Cores	Placebo Film-Coated	Active Cores	Active Film-Coated	Maximum Amount
0.31	Unknown	+[b]	+	+	+	0.6%
0.38	Desiccant-related	+	+	+	+	2%
0.39	Unknown	+	+	+	+	0.7%
0.40	Film coating (triacetin)	−[c]	+	−	+	2%
1.38	Unknown	+	+	+	+	1%
3.40	Unknown	+	+	+	+	1.6%

[a]RRT = Relative retention time of the impurity to the drug peak.
[b](+) indicates the presence of the impurity.
[c](−) indicates the absence of the impurity.

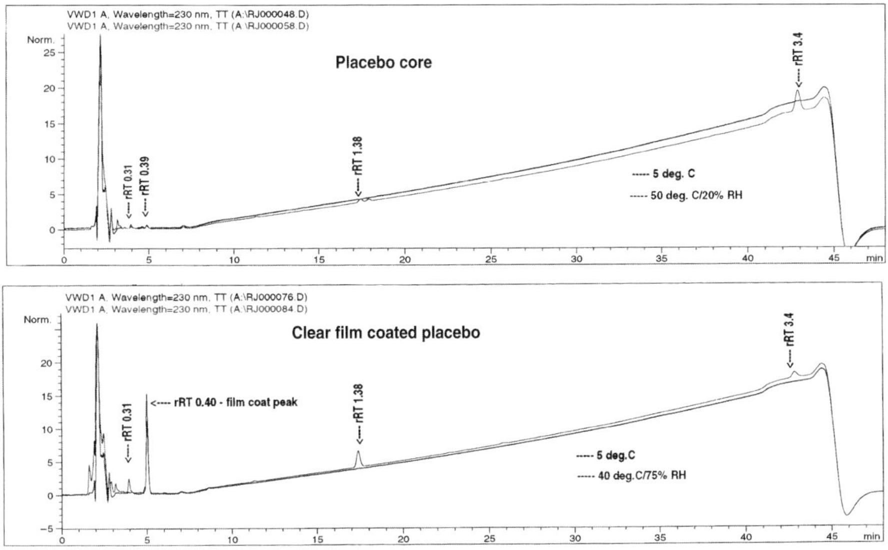

Figure 10.2 Chromatograms of placebo stability samples showing impurity peaks from excipient degradation.

HPLC analysis with photodiode array detection confirmed that retention times as well as the UV spectra of the impurity peak in tablet samples and desiccant extract were identical. Mass spectrometric analysis of the samples for the structural elucidation of this peak was inconclusive.

The impurity peak at RRT 0.40 was observed in all film-coated active and placebo tablets. The structural identification of this peak in the tablet samples was confirmed by both mass spectrometric and UV spectral analyses to be glyceryl triacetate, commonly known as triacetin, a component in the film coating used in these formulations.

The impurity peak at RRT 3.4 was observed in all samples exposed to accelerated conditions. Structural identification of this peak could not be established since this component did not show any response in the mass spectral analysis. The presence of this peak in large amounts in both active and placebo tablets lead to the conclusion that the late eluting impurity observed at RRT 3.4 was indeed a degradation product of one or more of the excipient components present in the tablets. Because of the large amounts of this impurity in the samples, a study using the individual excipients was conducted to identify the source of this degradant. The study lead to the conclusion that the excipients exposed to accelerated conditions in powder form did not produce the degradation product. However, when the same excipients were compressed into pellets and exposed to the same conditions, lactose, microcrystalline cellulose and croscarmellose sodium compacts showed the presence of the peak at RRT 3.4.

Verhaar et al.[18] described the HPLC analysis of reaction mixtures of lactose (oxidation and degradation). In this work, a refractive index (RI) detector coupled with a variable wavelength ultraviolet (UV) detector at 212 nm was used to monitor the degradation products. This suggests that the degradants observed have a λ_{max} of around 212 nm. For the analysis of Compound B and its excipients, the UV spectra obtained for the peak at RRT 3.4 had a λ_{max} approximately between 210 and 220 nm. Glaus et al.[19] discussed the degradation of celluloid materials. The main degradation products of pure cellulose are α-isosaccharinic acid and β-isosaccharinic acid.[19] In this work, a UV detector at a wavelength of 210 nm was used to monitor the degradation products. Since microcrystalline cellulose, lactose, and croscarmellose sodium have similar structural characteristics, it is conceivable that they would follow similar degradation pathways and produce a common degradant at elevated temperatures.

Placebo samples are often analyzed to identify excipient-related peaks and chromatographic interferences in low-dose drug product samples.[1,2,16] The case just described here, however, is an example where analysis of placebo samples alone would not have identified all the nondrug-related peaks in the stability samples. In this case, analysis of placebo stability samples identified several excipient-related degradants and packaging-related impurities. Hence, one should consider the need to analyze placebo samples as well as stressed or stability placebo samples.

10.3.2 Impurities Originating During Sample Preparation

Nondrug-related impurities can be extracted from various components employed in the sample preparation of a low-dose drug product. Classic sources of this type of contamination are glassware,[20] filters, centrifugation tubes, HPLC vials and caps and transfer pipettes.[20] Chemicals from the pH electrode can also be extracted into the sample diluent while adjusting the pH of the solution. In addition, impurities in reagents used in sample preparation[1] can pose issues.

In many cases, diluent with a high organic content is used to extract and dissolve the active ingredient from the dosage form. The extraction/dissolving solvent can potentially extract components from the materials that come in direct contact with the sample solution. To minimize this issue, extreme measures should be taken to clean the glassware prior to sample preparation. Since the unknown peaks are quantified relative to the drug peak, very small amounts of any contamination will be reported at artificially inflated levels when analyzing low-dose drug products.

As an example, tablet samples for a product were prepared in an 85% organic medium and transferred into HPLC vials. An impurity peak was observed in some, but not all, of the tablet samples, blanks and standards. It was suspected that the solution in some of the vials may have come in contact with the HPLC Teflon caps and extracted a component from the cap. To evaluate this possibility, dissolving solvent was transferred into similar HPLC vials. These vials were capped with the Teflon caps and were kept inverted overnight to allow maximum contact of the solvent with the vial caps. A set of control samples were also prepared in which the vials were only filled halfway with dissolving solvent and care was taken not to allow the dissolving solvent to come into contact with the vial caps. These samples were analyzed by HPLC and, as shown in Fig. 10.3, confirmed the origin of the peak in question as being from the vial caps. In addition, the UV spectral analyses of the

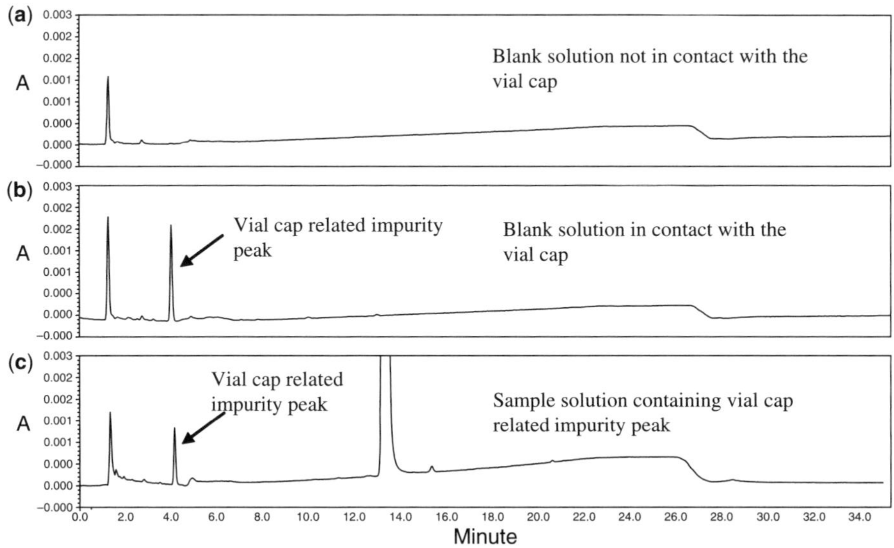

Figure 10.3 (a) Chromatogram showing no impurity peak at 4 min in the control; and chromatograms showing the presence of the impurity peak at 4 min in (b) the dissolving solvent in contact with the vial cap and in (c) an extracted tablet sample.

peaks from the sample and from the blank had similar profiles with absorbance maxima at 256 nm.

In another example related to 0.25 and 0.5 mg tablets of Compound A, an impurity peak observed in dissolution samples was found to be extracted from the rubber plunger stopper from a particular brand of disposable syringes. The syringes were used to filter dissolution samples prior to HPLC analysis. In this case, the impurity eluted close to the peak for the active ingredient and affected the integration of this peak. A syringe from an alternative supplier was identified which did not have the interfering impurity. The method was therefore updated to specify use of this new syringe.

10.3.3 Conclusion

Nondrug-related impurities can lead to inaccurate purity assessments and unnecessary investigations, costing time and resources. When evaluating impurity profiles of low-dose drug products, the excipients and packaging materials should be part of the evaluation. In addition to potential chromatographic interference, nondrug-related peaks may be detected and reported, due to the higher concentration of excipients and reporting the impurities relative to the amount of active ingredient present.

As discussed in the example of Compound B, nondrug-related impurities resulting from several sources were found in sample preparations. In the case of the excipient and packaging-related impurities, six nondrug-related impurities with levels up to 2% were found in stability samples of this formulation. If these impurities had not been identified as nondrug-related, an inaccurate assessment of the tablet stability would likely have been made. Therefore, parallel stability testing of placebo tablets, at similar storage conditions, should be employed to differentiate degradant peaks attributed to the active compound, inactive components, and packaging components. It should be noted that impurities originating from excipients can vary from vendor to vendor,[1,21,22] and the amounts of these impurities can also vary from lot to lot.[21] Hence, conducting a placebo study only one time may not be sufficient over the product's life time. If new unidentified impurities are observed in a drug product batch, it would be valuable to perform an accelerated placebo stability study using the same excipient lot(s) used in the drug product batch to confirm the origin of the new impurities. This will minimize the risk of an inaccurate purity assessment.

Other sources of nondrug-related impurities include packaging components, filters and sample vials/caps. Preparing and analyzing control samples using the sample dissolving solvent can help determine the source of nondrug-related impurities. For example, if the samples are filtered prior to analyses, prepare a dissolving solvent blank using the same type of filter. Similarly, if the samples are centrifuged, use the same centrifuge tubes to prepare the dissolving solvent blanks. Performing a blank analysis using the same lot of filters or centrifugation tubes each time that samples are prepared will account for vendor-to-vendor or batch-to-batch variability of extractable impurities from these devices. Even though manufacturers offer certified deactivated HPLC vials and caps, it is prudent to examine the vial caps for extractables using the solvents that are used in the sample preparation.

10.4 CASE STUDY 3: HPLC PURITY METHOD DEVELOPMENT CHALLENGES FOR A FIXED COMBINATION PRODUCT CONTAINING A LOW-DOSE ACTIVE INGREDIENT AND A HIGH-DOSE ACTIVE INGREDIENT

A number of fixed combination solid oral drug products are currently available on the market. For some of these combination products, one ingredient is present at a significantly lower dose than the second active ingredient.[23] Purity analysis for these fixed combination products can be a challenging endeavor due to the different levels of the two active ingredients. Ideally, one purity method can be developed and validated to detect and quantitate all components of interest to save analysis time. An example of the issues encountered during the development of a single purity method for a fixed combination tablet is described below.

10.4.1 Development of a Purity Method for a Fixed Combination Product

A fixed combination tablet formulation was developed and studied for the treatment of depression. The formulation consisted of two active ingredients in a bilayer tablet, where one active ingredient (i.e., high dose active ingredient) was present at a 25-fold higher quantity than the other active ingredient (i.e., low-dose active ingredient). In addition, the tablet layer with the high dose active ingredient was immediate release and the tablet layer with the low-dose active ingredient was sustained release. Excipients used in the immediate release tablet layer were dibasic calcium phosphate dihydrate, hydroxypropyl cellulose (HPC), magnesium stearate, microcrystalline cellulose, sodium starch glycolate, and a dye; while the excipients present in the sustained release layer were hydroxypropylmethyl cellulose (HPMC), magnesium stearate, pregelatinized starch, and silicon dioxide. Development of a single HPLC purity method for the tablet formulation was challenging due to difficulties resolving all the peaks of interest and due to the fact that the high dose active ingredient and its impurities were present at levels that interfered with the detection and quantitation of the low-dose active ingredient and its degradation products. In addition, extraction of tablet excipients caused interferences with analysis of several peaks of interest.

Method development of a single HPLC purity method with UV detection for the fixed combination tablet formulation began by first evaluating the individual purity profiles of the two active ingredients. The HPLC purity methods for the individual APIs were used as a starting point to develop an HPLC method to resolve the two APIs and their degradants, as well as resolve these from the process-related impurities (PRIs) of the two active ingredients. As shown in Table 10.3, the HPLC methods for each of the two APIs had very little in common other than using a reverse-phase C_{18} column.

Spectral data for the active ingredients and their degradation products were obtained and two viable wavelengths, 230 and 276 nm, were identified for detection. Since the high-dose active ingredient had eight known PRIs and degradation products and the low-dose active ingredient had only three, the high-dose active ingredient method was used as a starting point for development of a single purity method for the fixed combination tablet formulation. Several modifications were made to this method. The first modification to the method was adjusting the mobile phase pH to a lower value due to the solubility of the low-dose API. By using a lower mobile phase pH, however, the method no longer provided the separation of the high dose API impurities that the higher mobile phase pH had provided. At the

TABLE 10.3 Comparison of HPLC Chromatographic Conditions

Parameters	Low-dose API method	High-dose API method
Column	C_{18}	C_{18}
Mobile phase pH	Low pH	High pH
Sample concentration	~0.2 mg/mL	~1.0 mg/mL
Injection volume	50 μL	20 μL
Column temperature	Ambient	40°C
Flow rate	1.2	1.0
Detection wavelength	276 nm	230 nm
Elution mode	Gradient	Isocratic

lower pH, several components co-eluted: one potential degradant co-eluted with the high dose active ingredient, a degradant of the low-dose active ingredient co-eluted with a degradant of the high dose active ingredient, and two PRIs of the high dose active ingredient co-eluted with each other (not considered an issue since PRIs controlled in the API). Seven different C_{18} columns were evaluated and variations of the mobile phase pH (e.g., from a pH of 2–8) and mobile phase composition [e.g., different combinations of organic modifier (tetrahydrofuran–methanol or acetonitrile–methanol) with different aqueous buffers such as triethylamine–phosphate or trifluoroacetic acid] were employed to try to resolve all the necessary components. In addition, chromatography modeling software (e.g., DryLab®, Molnar-Institut für angewandte Chromatographie, Berlin, Germany) was used to evaluate different gradient combinations to improve the separation. The software simulations were able to predict conditions to resolve all the components of interest. When the conditions were tried, it was found that the elution times of all components had been accurately predicted by the software simulations (within 0.5 min). However, when the conditions were run with the active ingredients at their nominal assay concentrations (e.g., high dose active ingredient present at 25 times the concentration of the low-dose active ingredient), the high dose active ingredient peak tailed significantly and caused loss of resolution between it and later eluting PRIs/degradants. In the end, resolution of all the components of interest could not be achieved thorough these efforts.

The low-dose active ingredient purity method was then evaluated. With this method a degradant and a PRI co-eluted with the high-dose active ingredient. Predictions from chromatography modeling software were again used to evaluate modifications to the gradient profile (e.g., changing the starting times of the gradient steps, varying the composition of the organic component during the gradient based) in order to separate this degradant and PRI from the high dose active ingredient and retain separation of all the other known impurities from both active ingredients and from each other. Gradient conditions were identified that resolved all components of interest, however the desired limit of detection (LOD) of 0.05% could not be achieved for the two main degradation products of the low-dose active ingredient at the 230 nm wavelength due to baseline noise. The wavelength of detection was therefore changed to 276 nm in order to achieve the desired LOD of 0.05% for all degradants. The final HPLC purity method conditions are shown in Table 10.4.

10.4.2 Challenges with Excipient-Related Interferences

HPLC method development for the fixed combination tablet formulation became more challenging in the presence of the excipients used in the tablet formulations. HPMC and pregelatinized starch in the sustained release portion of the bilayer tablet caused extraction difficulties and interferences in the HPLC chromatogram.

Tablet sample preparation involved adding methanol to the tablets to extract the low-dose active ingredient from the HPMC. Methanol helped with the disintegration of the HPMC but did not cause the immediate release portion of the tablet to disintegrate. After using methanol, an acetate buffer, pH 4.5, was added to the sample solution to extract the high-dose active ingredient from the immediate release layer of the tablet. The sample solution was centrifuged to separate the larger particles

TABLE 10.4 HPLC Chromatographic Conditions for the Fixed Combination Tablet Purity Method

	Fixed Combination Tablet Method		
HPLC column	C_{18}, 4.6 mm × 25 cm, 5 μm particle size		
Mobile phase	Part A: 900 : 100 : 0.5 (v/v/v) water–acetonitrile–trifluoroacetic acid		
	Part B: 100 : 900 : 0.5 (v/v/v) water–acetonitrile–trifluoroacetic acid		
Elution mode	Gradient		
	Time (min)	% A	% B
	0	80	20
	20	62	38
	30	0	100
	35	0	100
	36	80	20
	41	80	20
Sample concentration	~0.2 mg/mL low-dose active ingredient ~ 5 mg/mL high dose active ingredient		
Injection volume	50 μL		
Column temperature	30°C		
Flow rate	1.2 mL/min		
Detection wavelength	276 nm		

from the filtrate. The sample solution was then filtered through a 0.45 μm glass fiber filter prior to HPLC analysis. Unfortunately, HPMC and pregelatinized starch were also extracted during the sample preparation. The HPMC-related peak interfered with two potential degradation products of the low-dose active ingredient.

Figure 10.4a shows that no excipient-related peaks result from the excipients used in the high dose active ingredient layer of the tablet. Figure 10.4b shows excipient-related peaks (e.g., HPMC and pregelatinized starch) that result from excipients used in the low-dose active ingredient layer of the tablet. In attempts to eliminate the excipient interferences, several different extraction solvents (i.e., different combinations of organic modifiers and aqueous buffers) were tried in an attempt to extract the active ingredients and degradants without extracting and dissolving the problematic excipients. These attempts, however, were unsuccessful.

Different types of syringe filters were then evaluated to try to remove the problematic excipients. Figure 10.4c shows that the use of an Amicon Ultra-4 centrifugal filter (Millipore, Billerica, MA) removed the residual HPMC from the sample solution but did not remove the starch. The Amicon Ultra-4 filter, however, does introduce later eluting filter-related peaks that fortunately do not interfere with any components of interest. Starch was not removed by any of the filters tested. As a result, excipient placebo samples were used as part of the method. These placebo samples were extracted and injected onto the HPLC system to confirm which peaks in the fixed combination tablet samples were excipient-related and these peaks were not quantitated or reported as drug-related degradants.

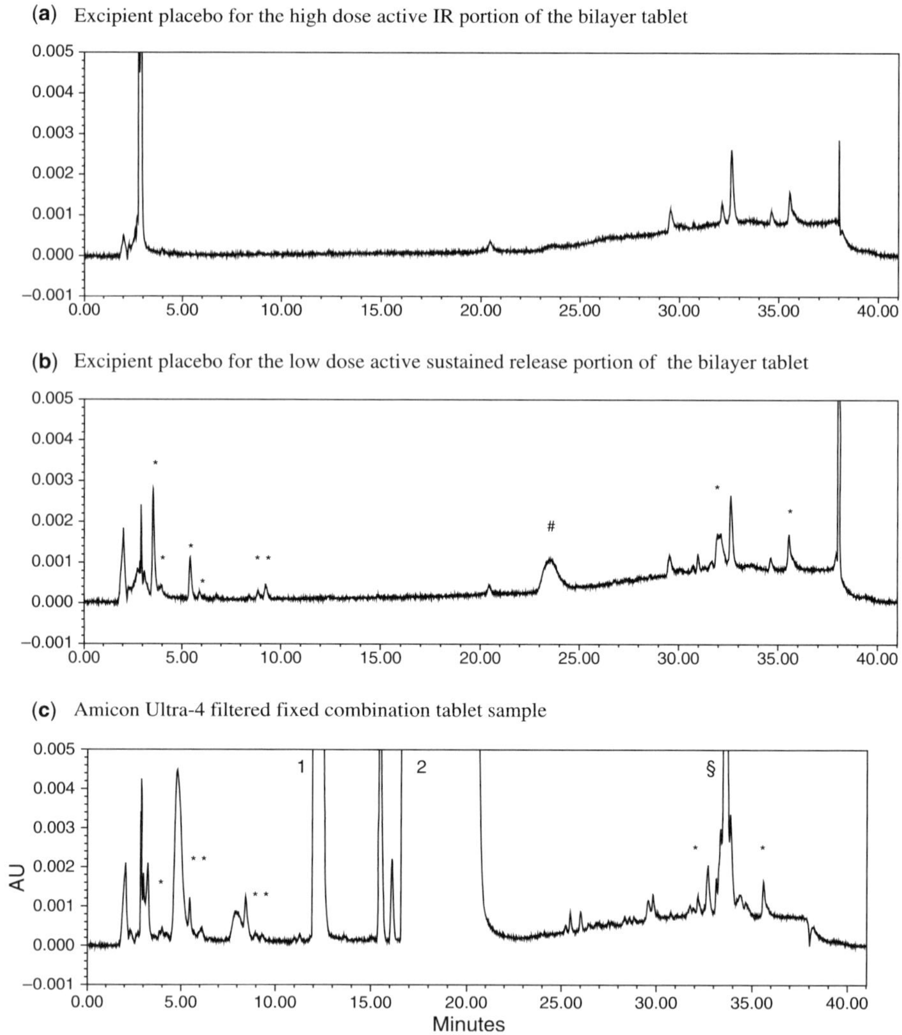

Figure 10.4 Representative HPLC chromatograms: (a) excipient placebo for the high dose active IR portion of the bilayer tablet; (b) excipient placebo for the low-dose active sustained release portion of the bilayer tablet; (c) Amicon Ultra-4 filtered fixed combination tablet sample. Annotation: 1 = low-dose active ingredient; 2 = high-dose active ingredient; * = pregelatinized starch-related peak; # = HPMC-related peak; § = filter-related peaks.

10.4.3 Conclusions

Developing chromatographic purity methods for combination drug products can be challenging, especially when one active ingredient is high-dose and the other is low-dose or when the combination product consists of immediate release and controlled release components. When developing methods for combination drug products, careful screening of all available methods (i.e., active ingredients and drug product chromatographic methods and sample preparation methods) should be evaluated prior to attempting to develop a single purity method for a combination product. In the case study described, the time required to develop an HPLC purity method that resolved all the components of interest was greatly reduced by starting with previously developed methods. Challenges associated with the sample preparation component of the method can include difficulties extracting the active ingredients and degradants, especially if there is an immediate release and a sustained release component to the formulation. As demonstrated in this case study, the extraction of excipients can lead to interferences in the HPLC chromatograms and this issue can sometimes be resolved by use of an appropriate filter. Filter validation, however, should be performed to ensure that the filter also does not remove any peaks of interest or introduce any interfering filter-related peaks. In other cases, the excipient interference cannot be easily removed and use of an excipient placebo sample can be used in the purity method to identify excipient-related peaks.

10.5 CASE STUDY 4: SMALL VOLUME DISSOLUTION TESTING

Dissolution testing of solid oral drug products is typically performed with USP apparatus 1 (baskets) or 2 (paddles) using 500 or 900 mL of dissolution media. For low-dose products, dissolution test samples in 500 or 900 mL media can yield low sample concentrations that are challenging to detect by conventional UV detection. In some cases where HPLC is used to analyze the dissolution samples, larger HPLC injection volumes, up to 1 or 2 mL,[1] or extraction and concentration of the drug in the sample solution[21,24–26] have been used to increase the amount of drug analyzed. Alternative forms of detection, such as fluorescence,[27–32] electrochemical,[33,34] or mass spectroscopy[35] have been used to improve sensitivity for low dissolution sample concentrations. Using multiple tablets in a single vessel can also be used to increase the sample concentration;[36] however, this does not provide information on individual tablets. Another alternative strategy is to use a low-volume dissolution apparatus in order to increase the sample concentration. The use of small volume vessels has been published in the literature.[1,36–39] In addition, there have been publications on the use of other types of low volume dissolution apparatus, including modified flow-through diffusion cells[40,41] and use of USP apparatus 2 with less than 500 mL media.[40] An example of using small volume dissolution vessels and minipaddles for a low-dose drug product is discussed below.

10.5.1 Small Volume Dissolution Apparatus Calibration and Method Development

During development of Compound B, several low-dose tablet formulations were investigated in clinical studies, including 0.05, 0.1, 0.25, and 0.4 mg tablet strengths. With these low-dose tablets, dissolution testing in 500 mL yielded low sample concentrations (0.1–0.8 μg/mL) and the drug could not be adequately quantitated using UV detection for the lower tablet strengths. Alternative forms of detection were considered. Fluorescence detection was not viable without fluorescent labeling of the active ingredient, which was not desired since it would have increased the complexity of the method. Electrochemical detection was an option, but was not pursued due to the difficulties typically associated with this form of detection (e.g., baseline noise, extraneous system peaks, electrode fouling, and the need for long detector equilibration times). Mass spectrometry also was not pursued since the contract laboratory and the manufacturing site which would test this product did not have this instrumentation readily available.

Due to the desire to maintain UV detection to analyze the dissolution samples, the use of small volume dissolution vessels was investigated to increase the sample concentration. Although the contract laboratory and the manufacturing site which would test this product did not have this equipment available, the cost of obtaining this equipment was considered reasonable. Small volume dissolution vessels with minipaddles are commercially available from several vendors (Distek Inc., North Brunswick, NJ; Erweka, Heusenstamm, Germany; Hanson Research, Chatworth, CA; Varian Inc., Palo Alto, CA). In this case, 100 mL vessels with Teflon coated minipaddles (Distek, Inc., North Brunswick, NJ) were used. The 100 mL vessels were covered to minimize evaporation. The paddle height was adjusted so that it was 2.5 cm above the bottom of the vessel. Since the small volume vessels and minipaddles are noncompendial, there is no established calibration or apparatus suitability test for their use. In this case, USP apparatus 2 using standard 1000 mL vessels and standard paddles was calibrated to conform to the dimensions and tolerances specified in USP <711>[42] and apparatus suitability testing was performed as specified in USP <711> using USP calibrator tablets. The standard vessels and paddles were then replaced with the small vessels and minipaddles and USP prednisone calibrator tablets were analyzed. This procedure was performed periodically. The prednisone profile obtained with the small volume vessels and minipaddles over time was compared to the original profile obtained to ensure consistent performance of the small volume vessels and minipaddles.

Based on a dissolution media/agitation screen, a dissolution medium of 0.05 M phosphoric acid, pH 2.0 and a paddle speed of 100 rpm were chosen for the method. The 100 rpm paddle speed was selected because coning was observed at the lower paddle speeds and complete dissolution of the drug was not achieved within 60 min. Using a pipette, 2 mL sample aliquots were manually withdrawn from each vessel from a zone midway between the surface of the medium and the top of the rotating paddle, not less than 1 cm from the vessel wall. These sample solutions were immediately transferred to centrifuge tubes and centrifuged. Centrifugation was used instead of filtration due to the small sample volume. The resulting centrifugates were then analyzed by HPLC to quantitate the amount of drug dissolved. The HPLC method used a 100 μL sample injection in order to achieve adequate sensitivity with UV detection. The small volume dissolution method is summarized in Table 10.5.

TABLE 10.5 Dissolution Method for Tablets of Compound B Using Small Volume Vessels and Minipaddles

	Method Parameters
Apparatus	USP apparatus 2 with 100 mL small volume vessels and Teflon-coated minipaddles
Paddle speed	100 rpm
Dissolution medium	0.05 M H_3PO_4, pH 2.0
Media volume	50 mL for 0.05 mg tablets 100 mL for 0.1, 0.25 and 0.4 mg tablets
Temperature	$37 \pm 0.5°C$
Quantitation method	HPLC analysis with 100 μL sample injection and UV detection

10.5.2 Additional Method Development Studies

Since the small volume vessels and minipaddles were noncompendial, additional studies were performed to confirm the appropriateness of the method parameters selected and the discriminatory ability of the method. The effect of paddle speed, paddle height and sampling zone were evaluated in an experimental design of experiment study. In addition, the discriminatory ability of the method was evaluated using purposefully perturbed or "aberrant" tablets, to model poorly dissolving tablets.

Confirmation of Small Volume Dissolution Method Parameters. A DOE study was performed to assess the effect of paddle speed (50, 75, and 100 rpm), paddle height (2.5, 1.75, and 1.0 cm above the bottom of the vessels) and sampling zone (1 cm below the surface of the media and 2 mm above the paddle height) on dissolution results. The 0.25 mg tablets were used in the study.

As shown in Fig. 10.5, paddle speed was found to be the most influential factor for percentage drug dissolved, with the higher the paddle speed, the more drug dissolved. This is generally true for standard sized dissolution vessels. Paddle height also had an influence on percentage drug dissolved, but not as significant as the paddle speed. Sampling zone did not have a significant impact on percentage drug dissolved.

The results of this study confirmed the appropriateness of the paddle height (2.5 cm above the bottom of the vessel), paddle speed (100 rpm) and sampling zone (midway between the surface of the medium and the top of the rotating paddle, not less than 1 cm from the vessel wall) used in the tablet method.

Evaluation of Discriminating Ability of the Small Volume Dissolution Method. Studies were performed to verify the discriminating power of the dissolution method. The approach used was to evaluate purposefully perturbed or "aberrant" tablets, to model poorly dissolving tablets. These aberrant tablets were

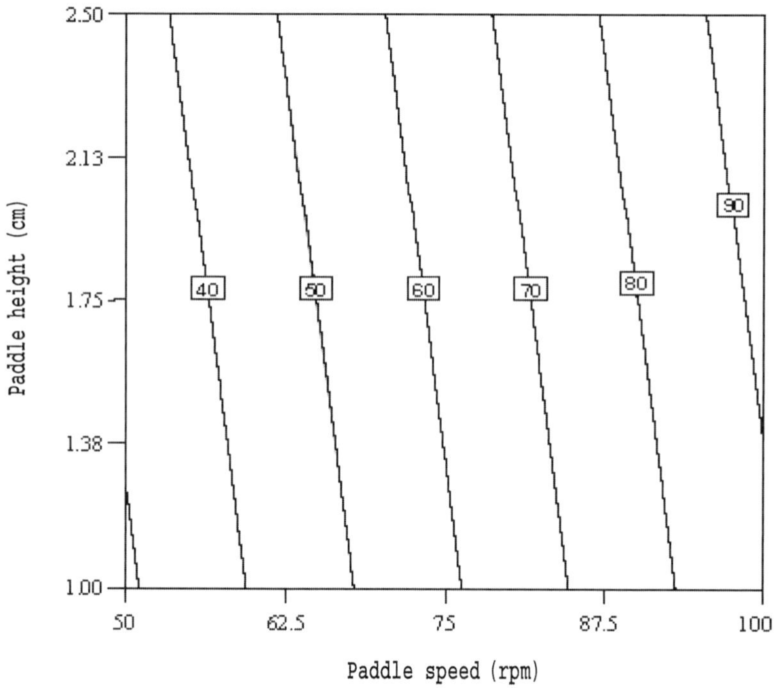

Figure 10.5 Predicted percent drug dissolved at 15 min. Predicted percentage drug dissolved ≈ 62.08 + 27.91 (ps) + 3.58 (ph) at both sampling zones, where ps = paddle speed and ph = paddle height.

purposefully manufactured outside the normal operating ranges to produce tablets that would challenge the discriminatory ability of the test method. By demonstrating that the method could distinguish these aberrant tablets compared to standard target tablets, assurance would be provided that potentially poorly dissolving tablets would be detected.

The immediate release tablets of Compound B are a robust dosage form, consisting of conventional excipients and a drug with acceptable solubility (~4 mg/mL) in the dissolution medium. It is believed that the only significant mechanism to alter the dissolution rate is to prevent disintegration. The perturbations made in the aberrant tablets were targeted to accomplish this. The aberrant tablets studied included the following perturbations for the 0.25 mg tablet strength: omission of the disintegrant; substitution of the diluent; increased tablet hardness; increased level of binder; and increased level of lubricant.

Dissolution testing was performed on the five aberrant tablet formulations ($n = 6$ per formulation) and the target tablet formulation ($n = 6$) using the small volume dissolution method previously described. As shown in Table 10.6 and Fig. 10.6, the dissolution profiles for the aberrant tablet formulations with additional lubricant, diluent substitution, additional binder, and high tablet hardness differ from the profile

TABLE 10.6 Dissolution Results, Reported as Percentage Drug Dissolved, for the 0.25 mg Target Tablet Formulation and Five Aberrant Tablet Formulations

	Formulation					
Time (min)	Target Formulation	Additional Lubricant	Diluent Substitution	Disintegrant Removed	Additional Binder	High Tablet Hardness
15	98	75	48	92	87	74
30	99	75	63	94	91	91
45	100	76	72	95	90	91
60	101	76	76	96	90	92

obtained for the target tablets, demonstrating the discriminatory power of the dissolution method.

10.5.3 Transferability of Small Volume Dissolution Method

The small vessel and minipaddle dissolution method described in Table 10.7 has been extensively used by the originating laboratory. In addition, the method was successfully transferred to several laboratories, demonstrating the method's reproducibility and ruggedness. The data for the analytical method transfer exercise (AMTE) to one of these laboratories is shown in Table 10.7. The AMTE used a bracketing

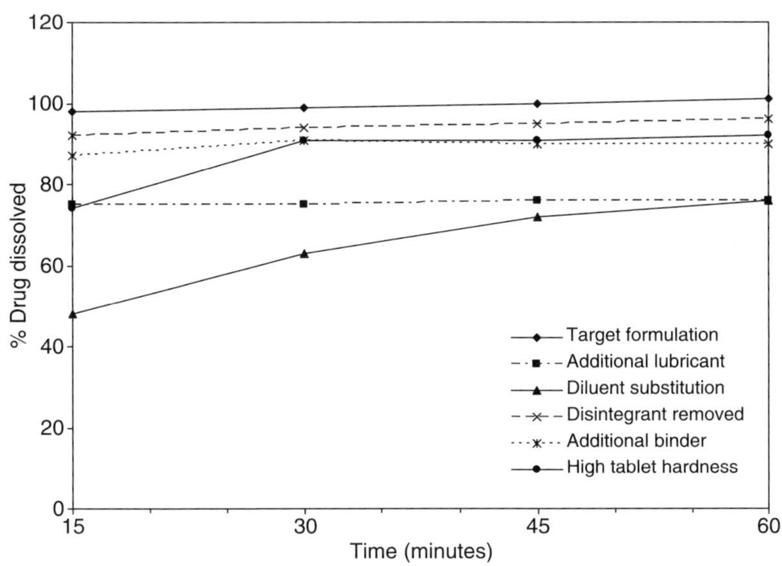

Figure 10.6 Dissolution profiles for the 0.25 mg target tablet formulation and five aberrant tablet formulations.

TABLE 10.7 AMTE Results for Transfer of the Small Volume Dissolution Method Using 0.05 and 0.4 mg Tablets of Compound B. Results Reported as Percentage Drug Dissolved

	0.05 mg Tablets			0.4 mg Tablets	
Sample Number	Originating Laboratory[a]	New Laboratory[a]	New Laboratory[b]	Originating Laboratory[a]	New Laboratory[a]
15 min					
Average	97	95	94	98	97
Range	94–100	92–102	90–97	96–101	94–100
Delta[c]	—	1.5	2.4	—	1.0
30 min					
Average	97	96	95	100	97
Range	95–102	92–103	92–99	98–101	94–102
Delta[c]	—	1.3	2.3	—	2.3
45 min					
Average	98	96	95	100	97
Range	95–101	92–103	89–99	98–102	94–100
Delta[c]	—	2.2	3.2	—	2.9
60 min					
Average	98	96	96	100	97
Range	95–102	92–102	90–99	98–102	94–100
Delta[c]	—	2.0	2.6	—	3.2

[a]Distek dissolution apparatus.
[b]VanKel dissolution apparatus.
[c]Delta = absolute difference of average percentage dissolved compared to the originating laboratory.

strategy for testing the tablet strengths, so only the 0.05 and 0.4 mg tablets were tested during the AMTE. Twelve tablets per lot were tested. In addition, the new laboratory performed the AMTE using dissolution equipment from two different vendors (Distek Inc., North Brunswick, NJ; VanKel, currently Varian Inc., Palo Alto, CA). The dissolution profiles obtained by the new laboratory were similar to the profiles obtained by the originating laboratory and the transfer acceptance criteria (absolute difference of average percentage dissolved at 45 min must be $\leq$6.0%) was met.

10.5.4 Conclusions

Small volume dissolution vessels with minipaddles are a viable option for dissolution testing of low-dose drug products. A discriminating method was developed for several low-dose tablet formulations of a drug development candidate. Paddle speed was found to significantly influence percent drug dissolved, with the higher the paddle speed, the more drug dissolved. Paddle height and sampling zone were found to not significantly affect the dissolution results. The method was successfully transferred to other laboratories. As demonstrated in this case study, a noncompendial small volume dissolution apparatus can be used to develop reproducible, rugged and discriminating dissolution methods for low-dose drug products.

10.6 SUMMARY

Several case studies were discussed which highlighted various challenges associated with analysis of low-dose drug products. Achieving the desired detection limit for the drug and related degradation products in the sample solutions by increasing the drug concentration adds complexity due to the appearance of extraneous nondrug-related peaks in the purity analyses. Drug adsorption, even in small quantities, can have a significant impact on the recovery and assay of the drug when dealing with low-dose formulations. Purity method development for a low-dose product, especially in combination with a high-dose product, can be challenging due to difficulties in the resolving the components of interest and due to potential excipient interferences. Compendial dissolution may not be viable due to the low drug concentration in the sample solution. In addition, as these case studies demonstrate, all aspects of analysis need to be carefully considered and evaluated to ensure accurate results.

ACKNOWLEDGMENTS

The authors would like to thank Vincent Bobin for the solubility data for Compound A. The authors would also like to thank the following individuals for their work on Compound B described in this chapter: Daniel Gierer for manufacture of the placebo tablets; Amy Orce for her work on the extraneous syringe peak; Thomas Sharp, George Horan, and Ronald Morris for their work on impurity identification; and Cheryl Kirkman, Heidi O'Donnell, Britt-Marie Otano, Doreathea Roberts, J. Sean Space, and Gregory Steeno for their work on the small volume dissolution method. In addition, the authors would like to thank Amanda Deal and Kelly Field for their work on the HPLC purity method development for the fixed combination tablet.

REFERENCES

1. Chang Q, Ibrahim R, Veltri J, Weber C, Sesi N. 2005. Low-dose drug products: Analytical challenges and strategies. Presented at AAPS Annual Meeting, Nashville, TN, November 6–10, 2005.
2. Snider R. 2000. Mass balance investigations for low dose pharmaceutical products, presented at the AAPS Annual Meeting, in Indianapolis, IN on October 31, 2000.
3. Yahya AM, McElnay JC, D'Arcy PF. 1998. Drug sorption to glass and plastics. Drug Metab. Drug Interact. 6(1): 1–45.
4. Mitzutani T. 1982. Adsorption of some antibiotics and other drugs on silicone-coated glass surfaces. J. Pharm. Pharmac. 34(9): 608–609.
5. Pinzauti S, La Porta E, Bramanti G, Mazzi G, Mura P. 1980. Storage study on acidic aqueous hexetidine solutions in polyolefinic and glass containers. Boll. Chim. Farm. 119(9): 559–563.
6. Beitz C, Bertsch T, Hannak D, Schrammel W, Einberger C, Wehling M. 1999. Compatibility of plastics with cytotoxic drug solutions-comparison of polyethylene with other container materials. Int. J. Pharm. 185(1): 113–121.

7. D'Arcy PF. 1996. Drug interactions with medicinal plastics. Adv. Drug React. Toxicol. Rev. 15(4): 207–219.
8. Allwood MC. 1983. Sorption of drugs to intravenous delivery systems. Pharm. Int. 4(4): 83–85.
9. Bundgaard H, Illum L. 1983. Kinetics and mechanism of sorption of various drugs by plastics. Acta Pharm. Suecica (Drug-Plast. Interact. Parenter. Drug Adm.) suppl. 3: 68–75.
10. Lindenberg M, Wiegand C, Dressman JB. 2005. Comparison of the adsorption of several drugs to typical filter materials. Dissol. Technol. 12(1): 22–25.
11. Carlson M, Thompson RD. 2000. Analyte loss due to membrane filter adsorption as determined by high-performance liquid chromatography. J. Chromatogr. Sci. 38(2): 77–83.
12. Murphy B. 2004. Glass or deactivated glass vials? Factors to be considered when choosing the proper vial for the application. Lab. Equip. C-17.
13. Guidelines for autosampler vial selection. www.chromspec.com/pdf/e/Guide%20to%20Vial%20Selection.pdf. Accessed March 20, 2007.
14. Vials, caps and septa information. www.chem.agilent.com/Scripts/Generic.ASP?lPage=42735. Accessed March 20, 2007.
15. Jamali B, Lehman S. 2004. Development and validation of a high-resolution capillary electrophoresis method for multianalysis of ragaglitzar and arginine in active pharmaceutical ingredients and low-dose tablets. J. Pharm. Biomed. Anal. 34: 463–472.
16. Nygaard L, Kilde HD, Andersen SG, Henriksen L, Overby VJ. 2004. Development and validation of a reversed-phase liquid chromatographic method for analysis of degradation products of estradiol in Vagifem tablets. J. Pharm. Biomed. Anal. 34: 265–276.
17. ICH Guidance for Industry: Q3B(R2) Impurities in New Drug Products, July 2006.
18. Verhaar LA, Herdriks HEJ, Groeland WP, Kuster BFM. 1991. High performance liquid chromatography of reaction mixtures from the oxidation and degradation of lactose. J. Chromatogr. 549: 113–125.
19. Glaus MA, van Loon LR, Chodura A, Fischer K. 1999. Degradation of cellulosic materials under the alkaline conditions of a cementitious repository for low and intermediate level radioactive waste. Part I . Identification of degradation products. Anal. Chim. Acta 398: 111–122.
20. Strusiak SH, Hoogerheide JG, Gardner MS. 1982. Determination of ethinyl estradiol in solid dosage forms by high performance liquid chromatography. J. Pharm. Sci. 71(6): 636–640.
21. Wasylaschuk WR, Harmon PA, Wagner G, Harmon AB, Templeton AC, Xu H, Reed RA. 2007. Evaluation of hydroperoxides in common pharmaceutical excipients. J. Pharm. Sci. 96(1): 106–116.
22. del Barrio MA, Hu J, Zhao P, Cauchon N. 2006. Simultaneous determination of formic acid and formaldehyde in pharmaceutical excipients using headspace GC/MS. J. Pharm. Biomed. Anal. 41(3): 738–743.
23. PDR® Electronic Library [Internet database]. Greenwood Village, CO: Thomson Micromedex. Updated periodically. www.micromedex.com/products/pdrlibrary/. Accessed March 20, 2007.
24. Jedlička A, Grafnetterovă T, Miller V. 2003. HPLC method with UV detection for evaluation of digoxin tablet dissolution in acidic medium after solid-phase extraction. J. Pharm. Biomed. Anal. 33: 109–115.

25. Nord L, Sundgren M, Torstensson A. 1989. Flow injection extraction applied to dissolution rate studies of felodipine tablets. J. Pharm. Biomed. Anal. 7(4): 421–431.
26. Hirai S, Hussain A, Babhair S. 1980. Sensitive method for determination of ethinyl estradiol in presence of norethindrone. J. Pharm. Sci. 69(7): 857–859.
27. Solich P, Polydorou CK, Koupparis MA, Efstathiou CE. 2001. Automated flow injection fluorimetric determination and dissolution studies of bumetanide in pharmaceuticals. Anal. Chim. Acta 438: 131–136.
28. Ozkan Y, Yilmaz N, Ozkan SA, Birvol I. 2000. High-performance liquid chromatographic analysis of verapamil and its application to determination in tablet dosage forms and to drug dissolution studies. Farmaco 55(5): 376–382.
29. Rogers P, Hailey PA, Johnson GA, Dight VA, Read C, Shinglre A, Savage P, Roche T, Mondry J. 2000. A comprehensive and flexible approach to the automated dissolution testing of pharmaceutical drug products incorporating direct UV–VIS fiber optic analysis, on-line fluorescence analysis and off-line storage options. J. Lab. Rob. Autom. 12: 12–22.
30. Hunt JP, Shah VP, Prasad VK, Schuirmann DJ, Cabana BE. 1981. Dissolution profiles and specifications for dihydroergotoxine sublingual tablets using a new in vitro method. J. Pharm. Sci. 70(7): 796–798.
31. Sonobe T, Hasumi S, Yoshino T, Kobayashi Y, Kawata H, Nagai T. 1980. Digoxin degradation in acidic dissolution media. J. Pharm. Sci. 69(4): 410–413.
32. Konieczny JM, McGonigle E. 1974. Automated fluorescence analysis of perphenazine in dissolution rate testing of tablet formulations. J. Pharm. Sci. 63(8): 1306–1308.
33. Mo J, Dobberpuhl D, Dash AK. 2003. A simple HPLC method with EC detection for the analysis of creatine. J. Pharm. Biomed. Anal. 32: 125–132.
34. Gandhi R, Kaul CL, Panchagnula R. 2000. Validated LC method for in-vitro analysis of azithromycin using electrochemical detection. J. Pharm. Biomed. Anal. 23: 1073–1079.
35. Wang Q, Zhao JG, Ballard JM, Shambor SM, Tsai EW, Ip D. 1999. Application of tandem mass spectrometry to FOSAMAX® dissolution testing, presented at the Mass Frontier Symposium, Purdue University, October 10, 1999.
36. Reisman ME. 1999. Creating a stir in dissolution testing. Pharm. Formul. Qual. 2(6): 16–20
37. Klein S. 2006. The minipaddle apparatus – a useful tool in the early development stage? Experiences with immediate-release dosage forms. Dissol. Technol. 13(4): 6–11.
38. Crail DJ, Tunis A, Dansereau R. 2004. Is the use of a 200 mL vessel suitable for dissolution of low dose drug products? Int. J. Pharm. 269: 203–209.
39. Dissolution Discussion Group. 1999. vol. 1, A user's perspective on dissolution; 50.
40. Khanna R, Agarwal S, Ahuja A. 1996. Preparation and evaluation of bioerodible buccal tablets containing clotrimazole. Int. J. Pharm. 138: 67–73.
41. Owens TS, Dansereau RJ, Sakr A. 2005. Development and evaluation of extended release bioadhesive sodium fluoride tablets. Int. J. Pharm. 288: 109–122.
42. The United States Pharmacopeial Convention Inc. 2006. General Chapter <711> Dissolution in USP29–NF24 Supplement 2.

CHAPTER 11

IN VITRO DISSOLUTION TESTING AND METHOD DEVELOPMENT

VIVIAN A. GRAY
V. A. Gray Consulting Inc., Hockessin, Delaware

JACK Y. ZHENG
Pharmaceutical Sciences R&D, Lilly Research Labs, Eli Lilly and Company, Indianapolis, Indiana

NORMAN N. SESI
Elanco Animal Health, Eli Lilly and Company, Indianapolis, Indiana

11.1 INTRODUCTION

Dissolution testing to measure drug release rate is very important for solid oral dosage forms, since a product must be in solution to be absorbed. The dissolution test can, on a case-by-case basis, link directly to in vivo performance. Of equal importance is that the test can show formulation and/or manufacturing changes. This chapter explores dissolution in the new realm of quality by design (QbD), along with current practices in method development. Compendial and noncompendial equipment and qualification are also covered. The unique challenges in developing and performing dissolution methods for low-dose drug products are discussed, along with a case study.

11.2 OVERVIEW OF DISSOLUTION TESTING

The dissolution test is required for all solid oral dosage forms. It is also required for special dosage forms such as stents, implants, ointments, powders, creams, suppositories, and suspensions. The development of a meaningful test with "clinically relevant specifications" is becoming of primary importance. No longer is the test merely a quality control tool, although understanding the product quality is still a very important attribute of the dissolution test.

Formulation and Analytical Development for Low-Dose Oral Drug Products. Edited by Jack Zheng

There are several FDA guidances and USP general chapters devoted to dissolution and in vitro release testing. The most relevant FDA guidances are listed below:[1–4]

1. Dissolution Testing of Immediate Release Solid Oral Dosage Forms.
2. Extended Release Oral Dosage Forms: Development, Evaluation, and Application of In Vitro/In Vivo Correlations.
3. Waiver of In Vivo Bioavailability and Bioequivalence Studies for Immediate-Release Solid Oral Dosage Forms Based on Biopharmaceutics Classification System.
4. The use of Mechanical Calibration of Dissolution Apparatus 1 and 2 – Current Good Manufacturing Practice (cGMP) (Draft).

The USP General Chapters that contain pertinent information regarding dissolution and drug release testing are as follows:[5–8]

1. Dissolution <711>.
2. Drug Release <724>.
3. In Vitro and In Vivo Evaluation of Dosage Forms <1088>.
4. The Dissolution Procedure: Development and Validation <1092>.

Several recently published books on dissolution testing are also excellent references for pharmaceutical scientists and laboratory analysts:[9–11]

1. *Pharmaceutical Dissolution Testing*, edited by Jennifer Dressman and Johannes Kramer.
2. *Handbook of Dissolution Testing*, 3rd edn, authored by R. Hanson and V. Gray.
3. *Dissolution Theory, Methodology, and Testing*, edited by Anthony Palmieri III.

The scientist can learn much about developing and performing the dissolution test by studying these materials. These resources will allow the scientist to be well-equipped to develop in vitro release tests.

There are two important aspects of the dissolution test: equipment selection and dissolution method development.

11.2.1 Equipment

Compendial Equipment. There are seven USP apparatuses for dissolution testing that are suitable for different dosage forms:

1. USP apparatus 1—rotating basket.
2. USP apparatus 2—paddle.
3. USP apparatus 3—reciprocating cylinder.
4. USP apparatus 4—flow-through cell.

5. USP apparatus 5—paddle over disk.
6. USP apparatus 6—rotating cylinder.
7. USP apparatus 7—reciprocating holder.

USP Apparatus 1 (rotating basket) and 2 (paddle) are the first choices when developing a dissolution method for solid oral dosage forms. Even though the compendial equipment may not be suitable for all low-dose drug products, a brief discussion of these apparatuses is necessary in order to understand the basic operation of dissolution testing.

USP General Chapter <711> Dissolution,[5] describes the basic operation of these apparatuses in detail. The Apparatus section describes the basic parameters or operational qualifications and usually provides tolerances to these operational variables. Operational variables for the basket are the following:

- allowable shaft wobble or "runout";
- basket and basket screen dimensions;
- vessel dimensions;
- shaft and basket materials;
- speed and temperature tolerances;
- the distance from the bottom of the basket to the bottom of the vessel.

The same variables apply to the paddle, with the substitution of the paddle dimensions for basket and the description of the sinker.

The apparatus suitability test described in USP General Chapter <711> Dissolution is equivalent to a performance qualification.[5] The determination of suitability of a test assembly to perform dissolution testing must include conformance to the dimensions and tolerances of the apparatus. In addition, the critical test parameters that have to be monitored periodically include volume and temperature of the dissolution medium, rotation speed (Apparatuses 1 and 2), dip rate (Apparatus 3), and flow rate of medium (Apparatus 4). This test requires that the USP Calibrator Tablets (now known as Performance Verification Standard Tablets) be tested; the dissolution results must be within the ranges stated in the certificate of the calibrator tablets. The performance verification standard tablets include USP Chlorpheniramine Maleate Extended-Release Tablets RS, USP Prednisone Tablets RS, and USP Salicylic Acid Tablets RS.

Carry out the performance verification periodically, as the operational qualification does not include all the variables that can affect the dissolution results. For example, the effects of vibration[12–14] and vessel asymmetry[15–17] are well-known problems that have no mechanical or operational probe.

Modifications are available to Apparatuses 1 and 2 that provide a low-volume vessel to increase the sensitivity of analysis for low-dose drug products. Details of this are discussed in the noncompendial equipment section.

The other compendial apparatuses, especially the flow-through cell (Apparatus 4) and the reciprocating holder (Apparatus 7), can be modified to adapt to small volume cells. For Apparatus 4, there are two sizes of flow through cells: 22.6 and 12.0 mm.[18] There are only a few operational parameters, mainly associated with the pump. The pump has a certain delivery range and must deliver a constant flow and desired pulsation rate. Temperature settings and tolerances are also provided. There currently is no performance verification standard, although a standard is under investigation at the USP. The major advantage of the Apparatus IV for low-dose products is the volume capacity. This compendial equipment can operate using low dissolution media volumes, but very low-dose products (<100 μg) need a very small volume vessel (less than 100 mL, less than a couple of milliliters, or even down to μL). Compendial volumes of dissolution media for Apparatuses 1 and 2 allow for 500 mL in the vessel; when combined with a large HPLC injection volume, the apparatuses can accommodate some low-dose drug products. Therefore, noncompendial equipment or modifications of the compendial equipment are needed for many low-dose drug products.

Noncompendial Equipment. USP General Informational Chapter <1092> The Dissolution Procedure: Development and Validation, contains a statement regarding noncompendial equipment. A noncompendial apparatus may have some utility with proper justification, qualification, and documentation of superiority over the standard equipment. For example, a small volume apparatus with minipaddles and baskets may be considered for low-dose drug products; the rotating bottle or static tubes (jacketed stationary tubes enclosed with a water jacket and equipped with a magnetic stirrer) may also have utility for microspheres and implants; peak vessels may be useful for elimination of coning; and modified flow through cells may be used for special dosage forms, including powders and stents.[8] This statement acknowledges that official apparatuses may not serve the needs of special products.

Some individual monographs already describe and require noncompendial equipment, such as Felodipine extended-release tablets, for dissolution testing.[19] For example, one monograph describes a noncompendial probe inserted into Apparatus 2 as a wafer-like basket to the side of the paddle. Monographs with dissolution tests that require special equipment for low-dose products would most likely use a noncompendial apparatus in this manner. Use of noncompendial equipment should not be an obstacle as long as appropriate justification is provided and necessary qualification of the equipment is performed.

Reducing dissolution vessel volume is one of the simple approaches for equipment manufacturers to help overcome the problem of low drug concentrations for low-dose products. Many apparatuses modified to small volume dissolution vessels are now commercially available. A list of manufacturers for these special apparatuses is provided below:

- Distek, Inc. www.distekinc.com;
- Erweka America, www.erweka.com;
- Hanson Research Corp., www.hansonresearch.com;

- Logan Instruments, www.loganinstruments.com;
- PharmAlliance, www.pharma-alliance.net;
- Pharma Test, www.pharma-test.com;
- pION, Inc. www.pion-inc.com;
- Sotax Corp., www.sotax.com;
- Varian, www.varianinc.com.

When dealing with small volumes, a fairly common approach has been to take the glass vessel and reduce its size to 100–200 mL, and to also scale down the size of the paddle shaft or basket shaft and baskets accordingly (Fig. 11.1). In most cases, the modified and smaller vessels are configured within the standard dissolution tester. Table 11.1 provides a comparison between standard USP dissolution Apparatus 2 and minidissolution assembly. Because the minidissolution assembly is not compendial, chemical and mechanical calibration procedures should be developed for performance verification.

There are also special cells for use with USP Apparatus 4 in a closed-loop configuration. Using a 100 mL bottle, a total volume of dissolution media ranges from 25 to 100 mL. For very low volume assembly, a test tube with a rubber stopper allowing for inlet and outlet tubing can be used. However, with the need for even smaller volumes, internal modifications should be made to the apparatus to minimize the impact on functionality due to a change in the internal tubing volumes. Also, the additional volume of the flow cell must be considered. For example, the implant

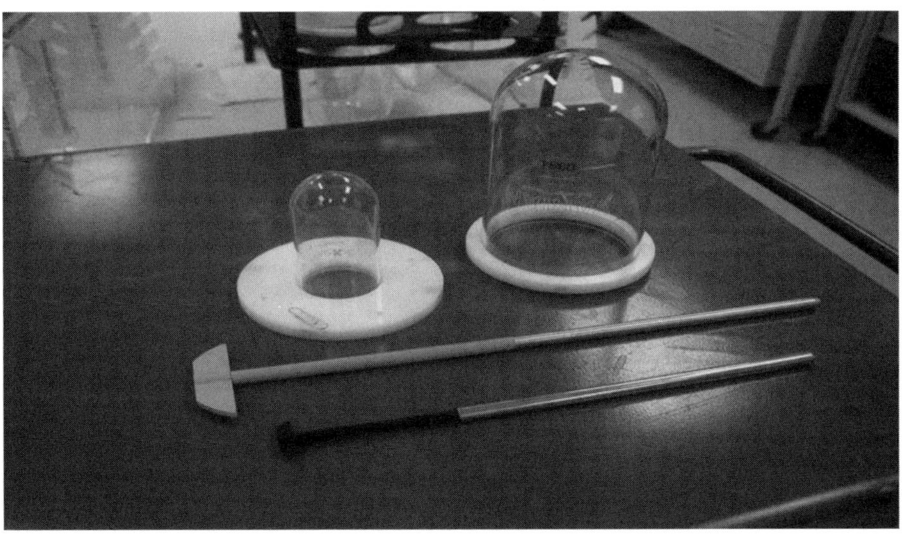

Figure 11.1 Comparison of the USP Apparatus 2 vessel and paddle and small volume conversion kit.

TABLE 11.1 Comparison Between Standard USP Dissolution Apparatus 2 and Minidissolution Assembly

	USP Apparatus 2	Minidissolution Assembly (Paddle)
Vessel volume	0.5, 1, 2, 4 L	100, 200 mL
Compendial	Yes	No
Advantages	• Chemical and mechanical calibration procedure exists • Common and available in most laboratories	• Increase sample concentrations up to 10-fold for low-dose drug products • Standard USP dissolution apparatuses can be easily modified to accommodate minidissolution assembly
Disadvantages	Standard vessel volumes may not be suitable for low-dose formulations due to analyte dilution factors	• Chemical and mechanical calibration procedures do not exist • Equipment may not be available in many laboratories

cell has a volume of approximately 5 mL and total volume of the system will be about 10 mL with the addition of the system tubing volume. Customized cells with specific attributes such as dimensions and orientation can also be made (Fig. 11.2) for a specific dosage form. With the 22.6 mm cell, the cell volume can be minimized by addition of 1 mm glass beads; the sample position can also be controlled. Generally, small volume dissolution assembly with the closed loop set-ups requires lower flow rates, where media turnover through the cell is faster due to the lower volume. Often an in-line spectrophotometer cannot be used for a small volume dissolution apparatus due to analytical sensitivity issues. Development of a small volume autosampler which can allow the collection of samples as low as 100 μL

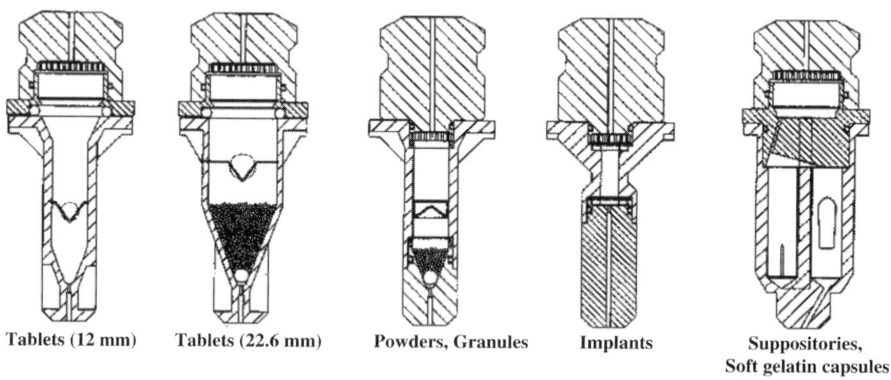

Figure 11.2 Difference cell design for the USP Apparatus 4.

from the closed loop for HPLC analysis has assisted with this problem. As with most of the apparatuses described here, compendial and noncompendial, the setups can be fully automated.

All the noncompendial equipment just mentioned must be qualified in order to generate reportable GMP data. Always justify why compendial equipment is not suitable. This qualification should include the typical operational qualification (OQ) and performance qualification (PQ). For the OQ, look at the adjustable control parameters, and test against the vendor's specifications and tolerances. Establish a baseline for the equipment settings and keep an historical database on the readings obtained. Then develop a regular quality check and set operation limits. Some examples of the critical parameters are temperature, vibration/alignment, volume control and flow rate, dip rate, and agitation rate (i.e., rpm). Other aspects to consider are the reproducibility, transferability, and ruggedness of the equipment. All equipment should have proper documentation of repairs, maintenance, and any out-of-specification dissolution results. These should be recorded in log books and the information is readily retrievable. The hydrodynamics generated by the apparatus, including observations of the fluid flow and any anomalous dissolving properties, should always be noted.

When the PQ is undertaken, always consider calibrator tablets, or a performance verification standard. This standard should be a well-characterized and stable product. The performance qualification should be conducted to evaluate all components of the test, including the analyst, equipment, environment, and method.

11.3 DISSOLUTION METHOD DEVELOPMENT

The current regulatory climate of QbD places an emphasis on clinically relevant specifications and methods for in vitro dissolution.[20] Development scientists should identify dissolution methodology that has been closely examined for its relevance to in vivo performance, as well as for mechanistic information. In other words, the release mechanism of the product should be understood and the dissolution test should be able to detect changes reflecting deviation of the mechanism. There is also the quality control (QC) side of dissolution testing, which, until the process analytical technology (PAT) develops beyond the current capabilities, is very important for stability and end-product release testing.

When developing a dissolution method, the process should begin with a familiarity of the literature on method development. There are many good articles,[21,22] books,[9–11] and the aforementioned new USP Informational General Chapter <1092> The Dissolution Procedure: Development and Validation.[8] Some of the key considerations in dissolution method development are discussed below.

Drug Properties. In keeping with the QbD concept, the physicochemical and biopharmaceutical properties of drug substance should be characterized for a better understanding of *in vivo* and *in vitro* performance of final drug product. Some characteristics of drug substances have a significant impact on development of *in vitro* dissolution method:

- pK_a;
- particle size;
- surface area;
- solubility as function of pH and/or surfactants;
- stability in the chosen media;
- absorptivity (absorbance);
- the drug absorption site;
- drug class in the Biopharmaceutics Classification System;
- polymorphism;
- hydrates;
- amorphous;
- salt forms;
- crystal habit.

With a low-dose drug product, the absorptivity of drug substance is a key property. If it is intense, conventional detection methodology may be viable, typically with a UV-Visible detector using HPLC instrumentation. However, LC/MS may be another option when increased sensitivity is needed.[23]

11.3.1 Drug Product Properties

As the dosage form for commercial production becomes clearer, knowledge of the following attributes becomes important:

- presence of solubility enhancers;
- disintegration properties;
- capsule shell dissolution rate;
- effect of moisture.

Today, there is more emphasis on quality of excipients. For example, some inherent quality variability may occur in the natural products magnesium stearate and sodium starch glycolate. What is the impact of the variability of these excipients on product quality attributes? Also, excipient viscosity, molecular weight, and particle size relative to API particle size could be critical factors to some formulations. An optimal dissolution method can only be developed on the basis of knowledge of the drug product.

11.3.2 Critical Manufacturing Attributes

Although the list of possible critical manufacturing attributes is infinite, some key attributes are shown as follows:

- blend time for lubrication;
- compression force;
- order of addition for formulation compositions;
- drying method;
- coating method;
- equipment capabilities;
- granulation method;
- amount of water used in wet granulation;
- impeller speed during high-shear wet granulation.

These processing parameters could have a significant impact on *in vitro* dissolution of drug product. They should be understood and controlled for critical parameters.

11.3.3 Dissolution Media

The choice of media is a very critical aspect of the dissolution test. When the API has no solubility issues in the typical pH range of acid, neutral, and basic solution, the typical media choices would be 0.1 M hydrochloric acid, pH 4.5 acetate buffer, or pH 6.8 phosphate buffer. However, there are many special considerations for poorly water-soluble drugs. The use of surfactants should especially be considered to achieve "sink conditions." Establishing and maintaining sink conditions during the dissolution test are important criteria for a good dissolution method. Sink conditions are needed when the true dissolution rate can be measured without an overlap in the area of equilibrium. As the solution into which the API is dissolving becomes more concentrated, the dissolution rate will decrease. The quantity of medium used should be not less than three times that required to form a saturated solution of the drug substance, as stated in USP General Chapter <1088> In Vitro and In Vivo Evaluation of Dosage Units.[7] Therefore, addition of a surfactant in the dissolution media is necessary to increase the dissolution rate for poorly water soluble compounds. Some commonly used surfactants in dissolution testing are listed below:[24]

- polysorbates (Tween™);
- sodium dodecyl sulfate (sodium lauryl sulfate);
- lauryl dimethyl amine oxide;
- cetyltrimethylammonium bromide (CTAB);
- polyethoxylated alcohols;
- polyoxyethylene sorbitan;

- octoxynol (Triton X100™);
- *N*,*N*-dimethyldodecylamine-*N*-oxide;
- hexadecyltrimethylammonium bromide (HTAB);
- polyoxyl 10 lauryl ether;
- Brij 721™;
- bile salts (sodium deoxycholate, sodium cholate);
- polyoxyl castor oil (Cremophor™);
- nonylphenol ethoxylate (Tergitol™);
- lecithin;
- methylbenzethonium chloride (Hyamine™).

Concentrations range from very low levels (less than 1%) to upwards of 7% or even 10% when products are dissolved in oil.

11.3.4 Sampling Timepoints

For immediate release, the sampling timepoints will typically be 15, 30, 45, and 60 min. The 5 and 10 min timepoints may be considered if disintegration is rapid; otherwise, the results for those early timepoints could be highly variable. However, these early timepoints may be important in suspension formulations or where extra timepoints are needed for f_2 calculation as follows:[1]

$$f_2 = 50 \log \left\{ \left[1 + \frac{1}{n} \sum_{t=1}^{n} (rt - Tt)^2 \right]^{-0.5} \times 100 \right\}$$

where R = reference formulation, T = test formulation, Rt and Tt = the percent dissolved at each time point for the reference and test products, respectively.

An f_2 value between 50 and 100 suggests that the two dissolution profiles are similar, indicating the test formulation is bioequivalent to the reference formulation.[1] There are a minimum of three timepoints in extended release dosage forms: an early timepoint that detects dose dumping, a middle point, and a not-less-than (NLT) 80% point. More points may be added, especially for very long drug release testing periods.

11.3.5 Apparatus

Available apparatuses for low-dose drug products were discussed earlier in this chapter. Any of the equipment mentioned, including compendial and noncompendial, can be considered as long as there is proper justification for its use and proof that the equipment is qualified according to GMP regulations. There are also references for small volume apparatuses that may be helpful in understanding this issue.[24–27]

During dissolution method development, the speed, dip rate, or flow rate can be adjusted to produce the optimal dissolution rate. The optimal dissolution rate is typically one that gives at least a three-timepoint profile that allows calculating the f_2 similarity factor. To determine bioequivalence and/or to develop a discriminating test, a good dissolution profile is important. This means that the dissolution rate should be somewhat gradual, and not too rapid (e.g., 100% drug dissolved in 10 min). For bioequivalence comparisons the f_2 factor should be calculated from at least three timepoints. Therefore, a profile that has at least three timepoints (preferably below 85% drug released) is ideal. A good profile is also needed so that any change can be detected from one condition/formulation/critical attribute to another.

11.3.6 Variability

An important aspect of the method development is selecting a method that generates less variable data. There is no regulatory definition of unacceptable variability, except in the concept of f_2 and the recommendations from USP General Chapter <1092>. In both sources the data may be considered highly variable if the relative standard deviation (RSD) is greater than 20% at timepoints 10 min or earlier and greater than 10% RSD at later timepoints. If the variability is higher, identify and control the root cause. The two most likely causes are the formulation itself or artifacts associated with the test procedure (e.g., coning or tablets sticking to the vessel wall). Visual observations are important for understanding the source of the variability and determining whether the dissolution test conditions are contributing to the variability. Variable test results can occur any time the dosage contents do not disperse freely throughout the vessel. Depending on the observed artifact, some ways to solve the problem include changing the apparatus and/or speed of agitation; improving the deaeration method; examining sinker type; or changing the media. Large variability can also result from the formulation and manufacturing process. However, the main problem for low-dose drug products could stem from poor sensitivity when measuring small quantities. Also, poor content uniformity, process inconsistencies, and excipient interactions or interference could be prevalent with these low-dose formulations, especially when the excipient-to-API ratio is extremely high.

11.4 DISSOLUTION METHOD DEVELOPMENT FOR LOW-DOSE ORAL DRUG PRODUCTS

There are four basic steps in the development (excluding validation) of a dissolution method for low-dose drug products: (1) selection of dissolution apparatus; (2) selection of a suitable analytical technique to quantify analyte release; (3) selection of dissolution medium; and (4) selection of dissolution apparatus operating conditions.

11.4.1 Selection of Dissolution Apparatus

For a low-dose drug product, the ability to maximize the detected analyte response during dissolution testing becomes a critical factor. For an immediate release, oral drug product ranging in capsule strength from 10–100 μg, the analyte concentration

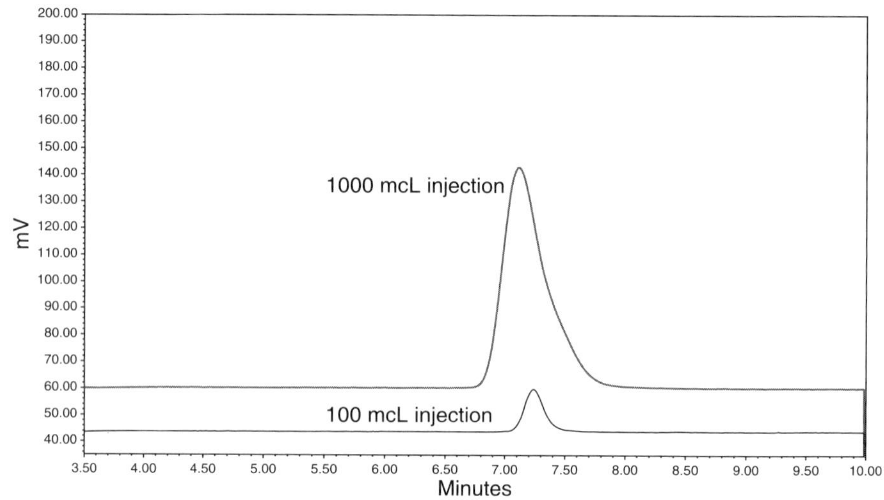

Figure 11.3 HPLC chromatograms of dissolution sample solution for 10 μg Compound X capsules using large volume injection.

of the lowest strength capsule in a standard dissolution vessel containing 1000 mL of medium would be approximately 10 ng/mL (assuming 100% dissolved). Using the common quantification approach of high-performance liquid chromatography (HPLC) with ultraviolet detection, the analyte in a 10 ng/mL sample would be difficult to detect (0.1 mL injection volume × 10 ng/mL = 1 ng on column). The bottom trace in Fig. 11.3 shows a chromatogram of a 100 μL injection of a 1000 ng/mL solution. Clearly, an analyte at the 10 ng/mL level (100 times lower concentration) would not be detected in the chromatogram. However, by decreasing the vessel volume to 100 mL, a 10-fold increase in sensitivity can be obtained relative to the use of "standard" 900–1000 mL dissolution volumes (analyte concentration in smaller 100 mL volume would be 100 ng/mL). The use of small dissolution volumes to enhance the analytical signal also requires the use of noncompendial dissolution equipment. In this case, the use of minivessels and associated minipaddles are justified.

11.4.2 Selection of Quantification Approach

For a low-dose drug product, the ability to clearly distinguish the analyte signal from the background is a significant consideration. Depending on the characteristics of the drug molecule, there are several inherently sensitive analytical techniques. These techniques include mass spectrometry, fluorescence spectrometry, and electrochemical detection, to name just a few. However, these detection techniques are specialized and may not be commonly found in many quality control laboratories. The use of UV detection is still the primary detection approach for a majority of HPLC methods. To enhance the analyte signal, the use of large volume injection HPLC (injecting milliliter quantities of sample onto the HPLC vs 10–100 μL) provides a simple and inexpensive solution. Standard HPLC-UV injection volumes normally go up to the 100 μL range. However, injecting a larger volume of sample (e.g., 1–2 mL) yields a correspondingly bigger signal (Fig. 11.3). The chromatographic response for a 1000 μL injection of a 100 ng/mL solution (concentration obtained for a 10 μg drug product dissolved in 100 mL of volume) is equivalent to the chromatogram displayed in the bottom trace of Fig. 11.3 (100 μL × 1 μg/mL = 1000 μL × 0.1 μg/mL). The gain in signal strength by using large volume injection is obvious.

11.4.3 Selection of Dissolution Medium

Three primary factors that influence the selection of the dissolution medium are physiological relevance, drug solubility and drug recovery. In general, dissolution testing is carried out under conditions that mimic the gastrointestinal environment. Commonly accepted dissolution media include dilute hydrochloric acid (e.g., 0.1 M), pH 4.5 acetate buffer, and pH 6.8 phosphate buffer; prepared as directed in the pharmacopeia. The use of surfactants and simulated gastric or intestinal fluids (with or without enzymes) are also acceptable, with appropriate justification. Sink conditions of the drug in the medium are also desirable, but not necessarily a requirement, to ensure the dissolution results more adequately reflect the properties of the dosage form rather than the inherent kinetic rate of solubility of the drug substance.[1,8,28] Table 11.2 lists the solubility of a potent, low-dose drug substance in several dissolution media. This drug substance was formulated into capsules ranging in strength from 10 to 100 μg. To ensure sink conditions of at least three times the drug strength tested, a measured solubility of at least 0.3 and 3 μg/mL for the 10 and 100 μg strengths, respectively, is needed. Based on the results in Table 11.2, an appropriate dissolution medium for this low-dose drug product would be pH 6.8 phosphate buffer (solubility of 7 μg/mL). Although the surfactant-containing medium also demonstrated comparable sink conditions to the pH 6.8 buffer, the use of a surfactant is not an accepted approach without adequate justification.[1,8,28] However, in the case of the drug product just noted, using the pH 6.8 medium resulted in approximately 115% recovery being obtained for a drug product placebo spiked with 50 ng/mL of analyte; equivalent to 50% release for the 10 μg dosage strength in 100 mL. An investigation into the higher-than-expected recovery

TABLE 11.2 Dissolution Medium Selection—Solubility of Active Component

Medium	Solubility (μg/mL)
0.1 M HCl	0.1
pH 2.0 phosphate buffer	0.1
pH 4.5 acetate buffer	0.2
pH 6.8 phosphate buffer	7
1% surfactant in water (sodium dodecyl sulfate)	9

10 μg/100 mL = 0.1 μg/mL.
100 μg/100 mL = 1 μg/mL.

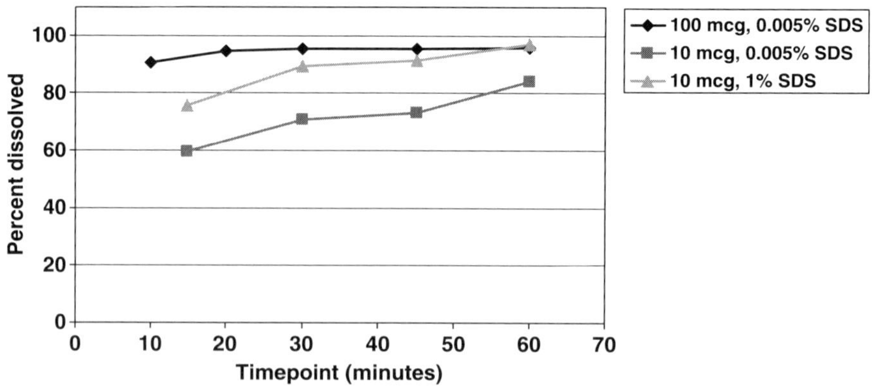

Figure 11.4 Effect of sodium dodecyl sulfate (SDS) on dissolution profiles of Compound X capsules using minidissolution assembly in pH 6.8 phosphate buffer, 100 mL.

results revealed the problem to be loss of analyte to various surfaces of the instrument setup. The placebo contained about 1–2 mg of sodium dodecyl sulfate (SDS) as a wetting agent in the formulation but the standard solution was prepared in pH 6.8 phosphate buffer without any surfactants. The presence of the SDS surfactant in the placebo prevented the analyte from adsorbing to the various glass and plastic surfaces of the instrument setup. Since the standard solution did not contain SDS, analyte adsorption occurred and resulted in a lower than expected standard signal and thus higher measured recoveries. This information formed the justification for why a surfactant was needed in the dissolution medium. However, accepted industry and regulatory guidance[1,8,28] also require the concentration of surfactant in the dissolution medium to be justified as well. The least amount of surfactant needed to be effective should be used. Consequently, several experiments were performed to determine the lowest amount of surfactant needed in the dissolution medium to prevent adsorption of the active. Figure 11.4 shows the effect of surfactant concentration on drug product release (measured by near 100% release at the 60 min time point) for two different dosage strengths (10 and 100 μg). As might be expected, the lower strength requires the dissolution medium to contain more surfactant to prevent analyte adsorption. A small absolute loss of analyte from a low strength dosage form results in a larger relative percentage loss vs a higher dosage strength.

11.4.4 Selection of Dissolution Apparatus Operating Conditions

The use of a noncompendial dissolution apparatus (in this case, 100 mL vessels with minipaddles) requires the operating conditions to be justified because accepted settings for compendial apparatuses are generally not appropriate. In the case of a "miniapparatus 2," the key operating parameters to examine include paddle height and paddle speed. Figure 11.5 compares the dissolution profiles of a 100 μg drug product using various miniapparatus operating conditions (paddle height and speed) relative to those of standard USP apparatus 2. For this particular drug

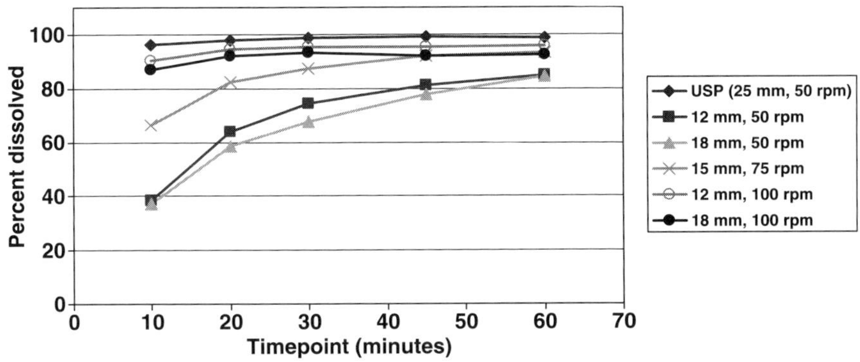

Figure 11.5 Effect of miniassembly paddle height and speed on dissolution profiles using 100 mL vessels. The 100 μg strength drug product was examined in a dissolution medium consisting of pH 6.8 phosphate buffer with 0.005% sodium dodecyl sulfate.

product, paddle height using the miniapparatus does not significantly impact dissolution rate. Furthermore, the miniapparatus is more discriminating than the standard USP apparatus 2 as seen by the more defined dissolution profiles obtained at the lower miniapparatus paddle speeds. To more closely mimic the standard USP apparatus 2, the miniapparatus requires the use of higher paddle speeds (100 rpm vs the standard 50 or 75 rpm for USP apparatus 2). If correlation to accepted pharmacopeial dissolution conditions is needed, the use of higher paddle speeds with the miniapparatus can certainly be justified.

Drug dissolution testing is not only a fundamental part of drug product development and manufacturing, it is also a quality control tool to monitor batch-to-batch consistency of drug release from a commercial product. However, when dose strength is very low, especially less than 100 μg, concentrations of testing samples can be extremely low when using a conventional dissolution apparatus. Obviously, two significant challenges in dissolution method development are (1) detection sensitivity of selected analytical method and (2) recovery of trace amounts of drug substance from the formulation matrix and testing system. An example was used in this section to illustrate a scientific and practical approach to overcoming the method development challenges.

11.5 SUMMARY

The pharmaceutical industry conducts dissolution testing of solid oral dosage forms to serve many purposes, including:

- as a quality control tool to demonstrate that a given manufacturing process results in final product consistent with previous batches;
- as a guide for the product development scientist in the development of new formulations;

- as a prognostic tool in the prediction of the in vivo performance of a dosage form.

Many compendial and noncompendial dissolution apparatuses are commercially available for different dosage forms. The key issues for low-dose drug products are (1) to analyze dissolution samples containing extremely low concentrations and (2) to have a good recovery of drug substance from the formulation matrix and testing system. These challenges may be overcome by the following solutions:

- a minidissolution assembly modified from USP Apparatus 2;
- large-volume injection HPLC;
- multiple dosage units in one single vessel;
- addition of surfactant in dissolution media.

A combination of these approaches has utility for better characterizing the dissolution profile of low-dose solid oral drug products.

REFERENCES

1. U.S. Food and Drug Administration. 1997. Guidance for industry: dissolution testing of immediate release solid oral dosage forms.
2. U.S. Food and Drug Administration. 1997. Guidance for industry: extended release oral dosage forms: development, evaluation, and application of in vitro/in vivo correlations.
3. U.S. Food and Drug Administration. 2000. Guidance for industry: waiver of in vivo bioavailability and bioequivalence studies for immediate-release solid oral dosage forms based on biopharmaceutics classification system.
4. U.S. Food and Drug Administration. 2007. Guidance for industry: the use of mechanical calibration of dissolution apparatus 1 and 2—current good manufacturing practice (cGMP).
5. USP General Chapter <711> Dissolution. USP 30, Volume 1, 2007, 277–284.
6. USP General Chapter <724> Drug release. USP 30, Volume 1, 2007, 285–289.
7. USP Informational General Chapter <1088> In vitro and in vivo evaluation of dosage forms. USP 30, Volume 1, 2007, 532–538.
8. USP Informational General Chapter <1092> The dissolution procedure: development and validation. USP 30, Volume 1, 2007, 579–584.
9. Dressman J, Krämer J. 2005. Pharmaceutical dissolution testing. Boca Raton, FL: Taylor and Francis.
10. Hanson R, Gray V. 2004. Handbook of dissolution testing, 3rd ed. Hockessin, DE: Dissolution Technologies.
11. Palmieri A. 2007. Dissolution theory, methodology, and testing. Hockessin, DE: Dissolution Technologies.
12. Collins CC. 1998. Vibration: what is it and how might it effect dissolution testing. Dissolution Technol. 5: 16–18.
13. Thakker K, Naik N, Gray V, Sun S. 1980. Fine tuning of the dissolution apparatus. Pharm. Forum 6: 177–185.

14. Crist B, Spisak D. 2005. Evaluation of induced variance of physical parameters on the calibrated USP dissolution apparatus 1 and 2. Dissolution Technol. 12: 28–34.
15. Scott P. 2005. Geometric irregularities common to the dissolution vessel. Dissolution Technol. 12: 18–21.
16. Cox DC, Wells CE, Furman WB, Savage TS, King AC. 1982. Systematic error associated with apparatus 2 of the USP dissolution test II: effects of deviations in vessel curvature from that of a sphere. J. Pharm. Sci. 71: 395–399.
17. Liddell MR, Deng G, Huack WW, Brown WE, Wahab SZ, Manning RG. 2007. Evaluation of glass dissolution vessel dimensions and irregularities. Dissolution Technol. 14: 28–34.
18. Singh I, Aboul-Enein HY. 2006. Advantage of USP apparatus IV (flow-through cell apparatus) in dissolution studies. J. Iran. Chem. Soc. 3(3): 220–222.
19. USP Monograph Felodipine Extended-Release Tablets. USP 30, Vol. 2, 2007, 2114–2116.
20. Zhang H, Xu L. 2004. Dissolution testing for solid oral drug products: theoretical considerations. Am. Pharm. Rev. 7(5): 26–31.
21. Rohrs BR. 2001. Dissolution method development for poorly soluble compounds. Dissolution Technol. 8: 6–12.
22. Brown CK, Chokshi HP, Nickerson B, Reed RA, Rohrs B, Shah PA. 2004. Dissolution testing of poorly soluble compounds. Pharm. Tech. 28: 56–43.
23. Barroso MB, Alonso RM, Jimenez RM. J. 1996. Liquid Chromatogr. Relat. Technol. 19(2): 179–186.
24. Crail DJ, Tunis A, Dansereau R. 2004. Is the use of a 200 mL vessel suitable for dissolution of low dose drug products? Int. J. Pharm. 269: 203–209.
25. Klein S. 2006. The minipaddle apparatus-a useful tool in the early development stage? Experiences with immediate release dosage forms. Dissolution Technol. 13: 6.
26. Chang Q, Ibrahim R, Veltri J, Weber C, Sesi N. 2006. Low-dose drug products: analytical challenges and strategies. Oral presentation in American Association of Pharmaceutical Scientists Annual Meeting, Nashville, TN.
27. Reisman ME. 1999. Creating a stir in dissolution testing. Pharm. Form. Qual. Cover Story. 1: 1.
28. Noory C, Tran N, Ouderkrik L, Shah V. 2000. Steps for development of a dissolution method for sparingly water-soluble drug products. Dissolution Technol. 7(1): 16–19.

CHAPTER 12

ANALYSIS OF PHYSICAL TRANSFORMATION OF API DURING MANUFACTURE AND STORAGE

GREGORY A. STEPHENSON
Pharmaceutical Sciences R&D, Lilly Research Laboratories, Eli Lilly and Company, Indianapolis, IN 46285

12.1 INTRODUCTION

Low-dose drug formulations present a different set of challenges to the formulator relative to higher strength doses. The prominent properties of disentigration, wettability of compound, friability of tablet, etc. become much less of a challenge due to the lack of the pharmaceutical's physical properties impacting the behavior of the macroscopic formulation due to its lower drug loading. On the other hand, flow properties of the bulk active pharmaceutical and its morphology may have an impact on issues with content uniformity. Many of the components added to tablet formulations enable better disintegration, improve wet ability of the pharmaceutical, and increase rate of dissolution. Invariably the greatest chemical instability is observed at the lowest dosage strengths. Frequently no instability will be observed for many years when stored as a pure bulk active pharmaceutical. ingredient. The complexity of the tablet formulation adds a lot of potential chemical reactions and physical interactions. Often, the property an excipient imparts on the tablet performance is also responsible for its tendency to interact. Excipients are often amorphous, enabling better compressibility and tablet formation, unfortunately often carrying with them increased mobile water molecules. The extreme hygroscopic nature of disintegrants such as sodium croscarmellose, the property responsible for its rapid volume expansion when it comes into contact with water, also makes it ideally suited for interaction. Wetting agents are surface active and can lead to increased molecular mobility. Other agents may carry with them free radicals. It is highly probable that the majority of the instability observed in such formulations is the result of the interaction of these

Formulation and Analytical Development for Low-Dose Oral Drug Products. Edited by Jack Zheng

agents with an amorphous region or domain within the active pharmaceutical – even if it is present at undetectable levels initially. The initial interaction may generate a defect structure that propagates throughout the crystal rendering what initially may have been predominantly crystalline drug an amorphous product. Advances in analytical technologies have enabled us to better look at formulations at concentration levels far lower than in the past; however still at times direct quantification or even detection can be problematic in low-dose tablet formulations.

In the following pages, an attempt will be made to describe many of the properties of the solid state that come into play and need to be considered when formulating low-dose pharmaceuticals. The solid forms may be broadly classified as crystalline and amorphous and then describe the solid-state techniques used in their characterization. Many of the quantitative aspects and their respective advantages and disadvantages will be described. Finally, a few approaches will be described that may be used to investigate the effect of formulation on the low-dose active ingredient in the tablet.

12.2 DISCUSSION OF SOLID-STATE FORMS

Pharmaceuticals may exist in numerous solid forms which may feature different physical and chemical properties. These solid forms may be classified broadly as being crystalline or amorphous. Crystallographic forms are often termed as demonstrating a greater "long range order" than amorphous forms. Crystalline forms have a basic packing arrangement of matter (the pharmaceutical; its counter-ion, if a salt; and solvent molecule, if it is a solvate or hydrate) collectively in a specific three-dimensional arrangement with respect to one another comprising the "short-range order" of the crystalline structure. Using the three-dimensional coordinates that describe the arrangement of the atoms that compose this smallest unit of the structure (the asymmetric unit) in combination with the space group and its symmetry operations (including translations), the entire crystallographic structure can be described and makes the unique properties associated with having the "long-range order" of the crystal lattice. There are only a limited number of space groups or ways in which molecules can arrange themselves and fill space in such an orderly fashion. This space filling property minimizes void space within the solid structure and allows for greater interaction between molecules, thereby lowering the free energy of the system.

Crystals, however, are not always so perfectly ordered. Atomic mobility exists within the crystal lattice; however, it is greatly reduced relative to the amorphous state. Partial loss of solvent from the lattice can result in static disorder within the lattice where the atomic positions of a given atom can deviate slightly within one asymmetric unit of the unit cell relative to another. Lattice strain and defects occur for many reasons. Solvents can be present within channels of the lattice in sites not described by the symmetry of the crystal structure itself, resulting in disordered solvent molecules or incommensurate structures and potentially nonstoichiometric solvates or hydrates.

Amorphous forms in many ways are even more complex to describe than crystalline materials. Amorphous forms are usually not completely disordered in that they possess some average short-range order or organization of molecules. The intermolecular distances in amorphous states are generally longer and they possess greater molecular mobility. Such materials have greater free volume or void space resulting in what is generally higher free energy. The positive aspect of a higher free energy is the enhanced solubility and rate of dissolution and specific surface area. The negative aspect is the potential for such forms to establish a more orderly organization and crystallize to a dramatically less soluble form. Furthermore and perhaps more importantly for low-dose pharmaceuticals is that such forms tend to be chemically less stable. Decreased stability may arise from increased surface area and the greater accessibility of gases such as oxygen or water, leading to increased oxidation or hydrolysis rates. Greater instability may result from the greater degree of molecular contact between solid components of the tablet with the active ingredient leading to common drug—excipient interactions. Inevitably, the greatest practical problem facing the solid-state pharmaceutical scientist who hopes to ensure the chemical stability of a chemically unstable compound is to detect and control the amount of amorphous component within the tablet formulation. Quantification of low levels of amorphous component is a challenge even in the pure active pharmaceutical ingredient, let alone in a low-dose tablet. This problem has been known and has existed for decade(s) and is yet to be adequately resolved.

If a compound is known to have chemical stability issues and is going to be administered in low dose, the best prevention is to ensure the highest degree of crystallinity of the bulk active ingredient delivered to the formulation and maintain it in the state with the highest ratio of drug to excipient possible.

12.3 MONITORING PROCESSING STEPS

Many processing steps could potentially impact the integrity of the crystal form introduced into the low-dose tablet. Recrystallization of the active pharmaceutical itself can be a point where control should be investigated. While quantitatively it is easy to assess by any of a variety of methods whether or not the correct form is produced. The degree of crystallinity can vary depending on the compound and the conditions used in its crystallization. Crystallizations are stochastic in nature and their outcome can vary merely based upon the degree of super-saturation in which the compound spontaneously nucleates relative to its equilibrium solubility. The crystallization rate can impact what crystallographic form nucleates and possibly its degree of crystallinity. After the API is recrystallized and dried, it is typically milled to a specific particle size by pin milling, ball milling, slurry milling, or jet milling operations, dependent upon material properties and the desired particle size for the API. The milling process can generate significant amounts of heat and shear stress. As a consequence, phase transformations and amorphous components can be generated. Wet granulation involves mixing the active ingredient and possibly some excipients in a mixer. A binder is typically added in the dry mix state or dissolved in the fluid used for granulating. The granulating solution or suspension is added to the dry powders in the mixer and mixed until the desired characteristics are achieved. This usually produces a granule that is of suitable characteristics for producing tablets with adequate hardness, dissolution, content uniformity, and other physical characteristics. After the wet granulation step, the product is most often dried and then milled after drying to get a major percentage of the product within a desired size range. The dry granulation is then processed to get an acceptable size range by first screening with a sieving device, and then milling the oversized particles. For normal compressed tablets, the broad particle size range produced by this method is usually satisfactory. It is important to understand the physical factors that influence phase conversions that occur during processing and the unit processes where they might be encountered; see Table 12.1. By profiling the process, one can determine which phases dissolve and then recrystallized upon drying. If the API dissolves, it is important to understand whether it recrystallizes or remains amorphous, or if it forms a hydrate or different polymorph. Certainly if it dissolves and recrystallizes, its particle size will differ from that of the API introduced into the dry blend of the formulation. All of these factors can impact the chemical stability of the drug product, and potentially its bioavailability or tablet disintegration. Figure 12.1 shows a profiling of a formulation that is predominantly composed of lactose monohydrate, a smaller amount of anhydrous lactose and a small concentration of a water-insoluble drug when the dry blend is formed. After adding the granulating solution, the lactose is exclusively converted to the monohydrate form. As drying process proceeds, most of the lactose monohydrate is converted to anhydrous lactose after 2 h of drying. Throughout this process, due to the drug's low solubility, the API remains in the same crystalline state as it was first introduced into the formulation. Sometimes crystalline compounds become amorphous during wet granulation steps, in particular if the drug is highly water-soluble. Other times, the final step has been used to stabilize the active pharmaceutical and increase the drug's interaction with a particular stabilizing ingredient. Analysis of some of the angiotensin-converting enzyme (ACE) inhibitors indicates

TABLE 12.1 Physical Factors Considered in Unit Operations of Solid Oral Dosage Forms

	Solvent	Moisture	Temperature	Stress
API				
Recrystallization	√	√	√	
Drying		√	√	
Milling		√	√	√
Storage		√	√	
Formulation				
Wet granulation		√		
Drying		√	√	√
Tableting		√	√	√
Film coating	√	√		
Storage		√	√	

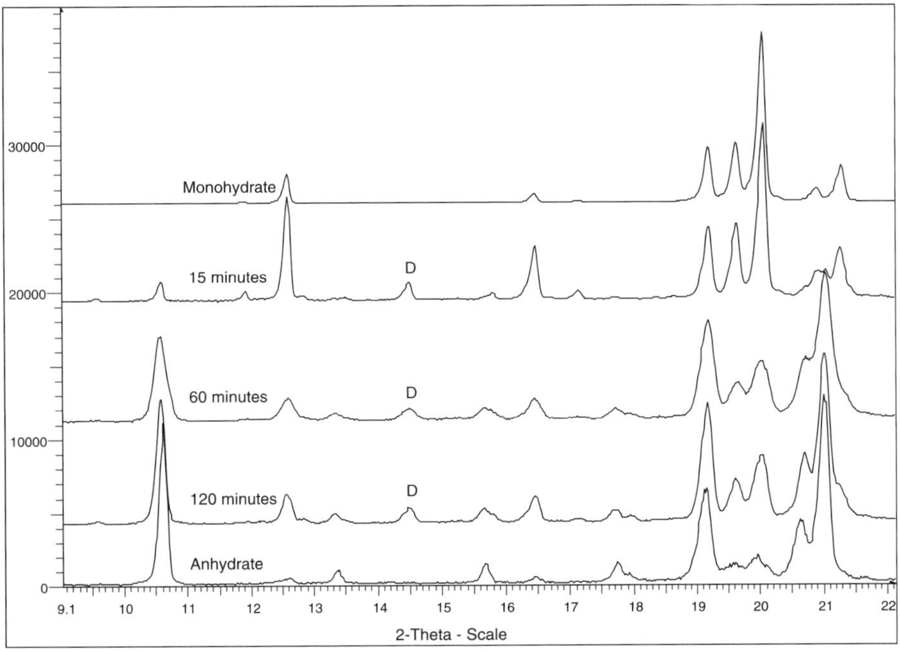

Figure 12.1 Characterization of changes occurring during drying of a wet granulated formulation. The top trace is of lactose monohydrate. The middle three are of the formulation composed of a mixture of hydrated and anhydrous lactose, as well as the drug at 15, 60, and 120 min (top to bottom). The lower trace shows a diffraction pattern of anhydrous lactose.

that the pharmaceutical itself is highly crystalline as a pure API; however in the formulation the pharmaceutical is essentially amorphous due presumably to its wet granulation with a stabilizing agent that acts to "buffer" the solid formulation at a pH that reduces the rate of decomposition via diketo piperazine, rendering a more stable product.

12.4 MEASURING TRANSITIONS AND SOLID-FORM TRANSFORMATIONS IN THE LOW-DOSE TABLET

There are a number of approaches that can be used to better understand the state of the solid in the tablet formulation. One common approach is to modify the formulation by increasing the amount of pharmaceutical in the tablet formulation until it is possible to detect or quantify any phase transitions that occur within the tablet. If the tablet maintains approximately 10% drug by weight, one can usually determine within a reasonable degree of certainty any phase transformation occurring within the tablet. One can do such analysis with a goal of detecting the form after processing or upon storage under stability indicating conditions. One can also use any of a number of the quantitative methods discussed later in this chapter. Another approach that can be used is nuclear enrichment of the sample and its subsequent analysis by solid-state NMR. Since the natural abundance of ^{13}C is approximately 1%, if a ^{13}C labeled intermediate is used to form the final product, ^{13}C NMR can be readily be used to analyze the formulation at very low drug loadings. The enriched carbon signal will appear dramatically enhanced relative to the rest of the carbon resonances. It is important that the labeled site be one that is sensitive to the different chemical environment in the solid forms being analyzed, thereby having well resolved resonances that occur in regions that are not obscured by excipient. Figure 12.2 illustrates this approach being applied to enhance the detection of the crystal form present in a low-dose formulation of a pharmaceutical used for hormone replacement therapy.[1] The active, OD14, was present in tablets ranging in strength ranging from 0.5 to 2.5% by weight. The compound is polymorphic, having at least two crystalline forms. The two forms could be differentiated by pronounced differences throughout their spectra when pure active was present. Due to dilution by the excipients, determination of which form was present in the actual

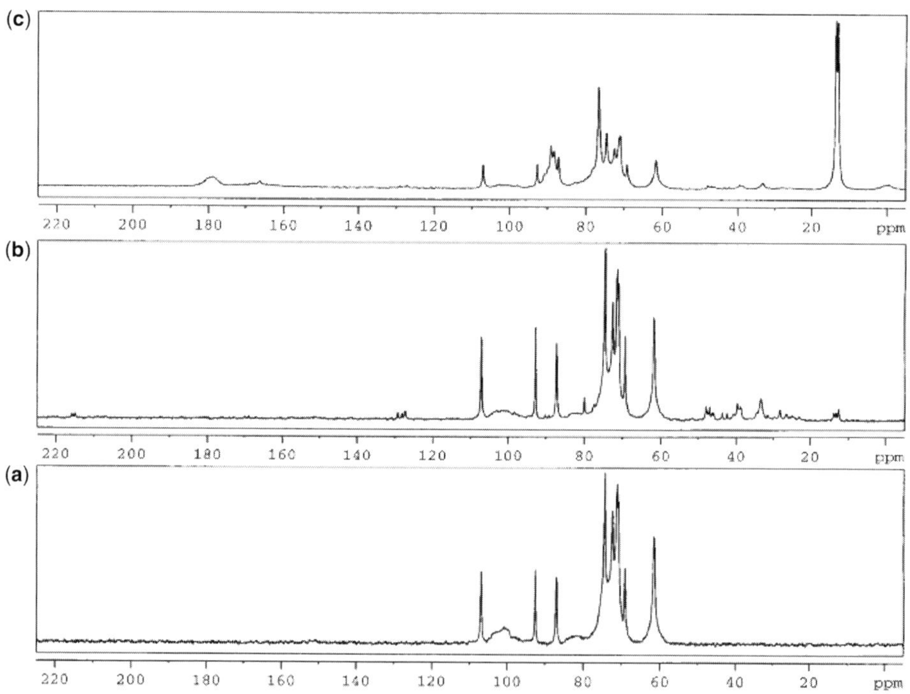

Figure 12.2 (a) ^{13}C CPMAS spectrum of a crushed placebo tablet showing the signals of the excipients only. (b) ^{13}C CPMAS spectrum of a crushed tablet containing 2.5 w/w% unlabeled Org OD 14. The ^{13}C signals of Org OD 14 are only just detectable. (c) ^{13}C CPMAS spectrum of a crushed tablet containing 2.5 w/w% Org OD 14 ^{13}C labeled at the 19- and 20-ethynyl and the 21-methyl carbons. The vertical scale in (a) and (b) has been expanded about three times relative to (c) to allow visualization of the unlabeled Org OD 14 ^{13}C resonances.

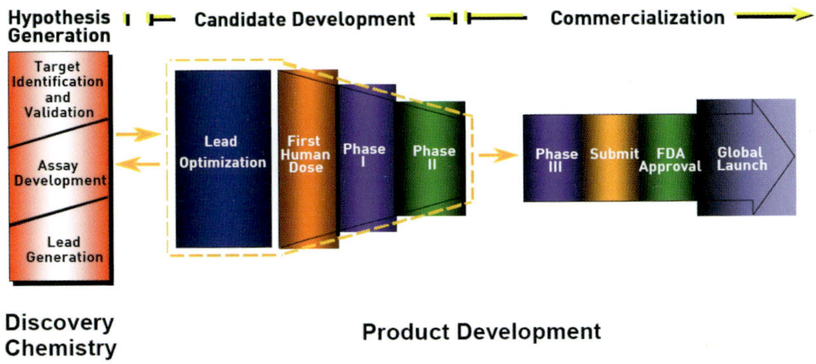

Figure 1.1 New drug discovery and development process.

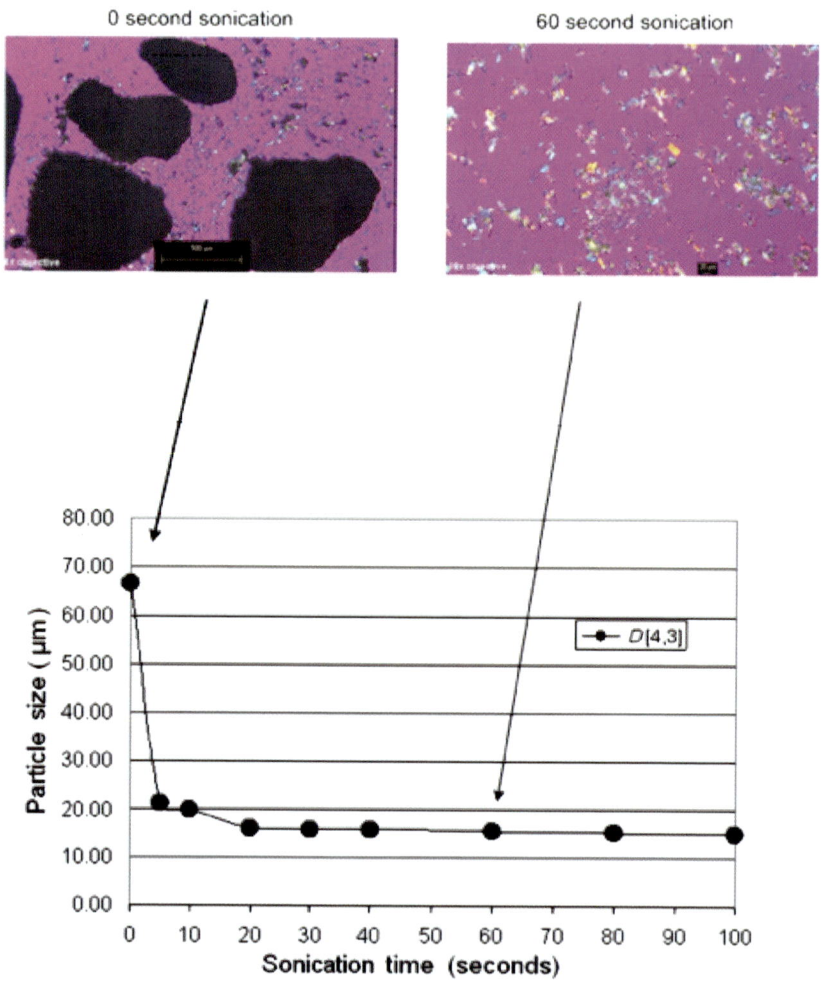

Figure 6.4 Effect of sonication time on API particle size in terms of *D*[4,3].

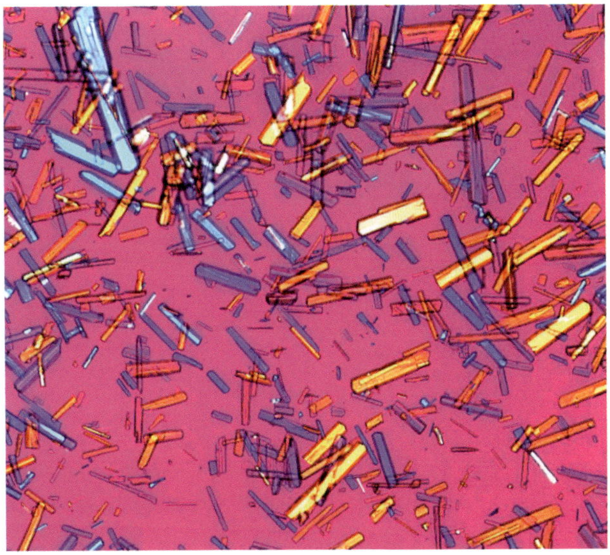

Figure 13.1 Optical micrograph of a typical drug substance that would be used in a low-dose solid oral formulation.

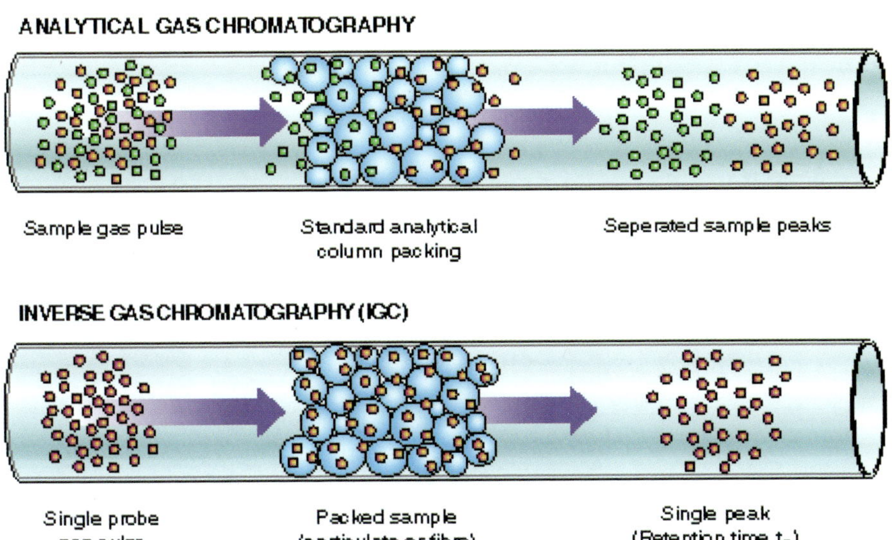

Figure 13.6 Schematic showing a comparison of conventional GC and IGC (courtesy of SMS, Inc.).

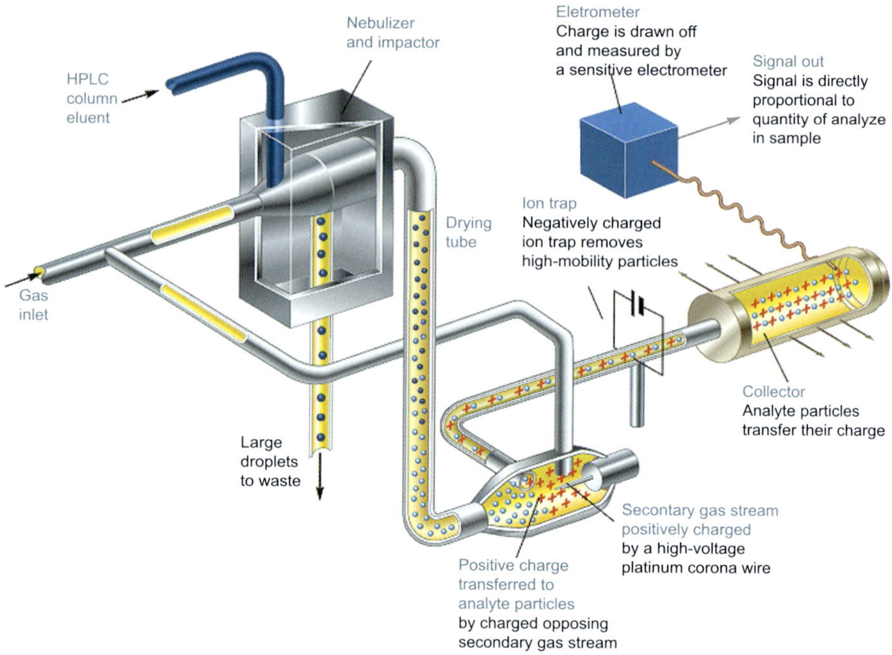

Figure 15.5 Instrument schematic of the CAD™ (charged aerosol detection). (Reproduced with permission from ESA Bioscience.)

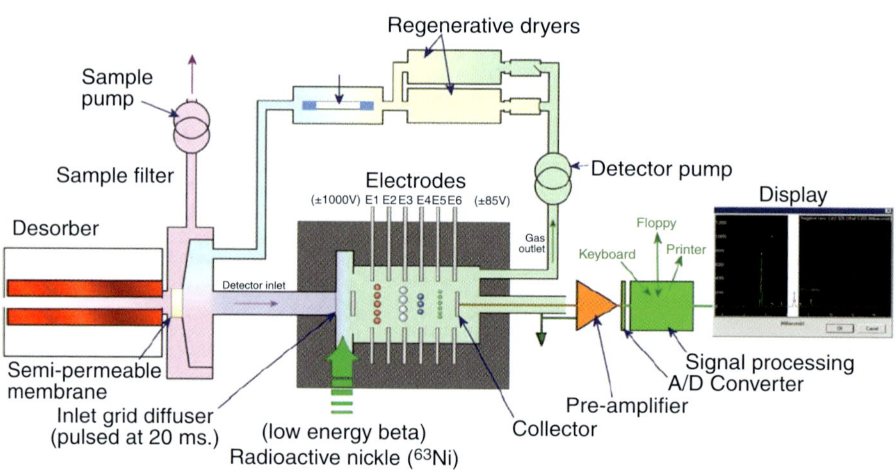

Figure 15.6 Instrument schematic of GE ITMS. (Reproduced with permission from GE Sensing.)

formulated product after processing proved challenging. Three sites of the molecule were isotopically labeled. Since isotopic natural abundance of ^{13}C is only 1.1%, when the molecule is labeled, its abundance is effectively increased to 100%, thereby enhancing the carbon signal by 100 times its original intensity. Methyl carbon 21 of OD14 readily distinguished the two forms, with form I having two resonances, one at 13.4 and another at 14.0 ppm, since its crystal structure contains two independent molecules in its asymmetric unit. Form II has a single resonance at a chemical shift of 13.3 ppm. Figure 12.2c shows the dramatically increased signal of the two resonances of form I relative to the natural abundant spectrum of the tablet containing naturally abundant ^{13}C. This approach enabled the scientists to determine that no phase transition occurred during processing or upon storage for extended periods of time at accelerated stability conditions.

This serves as an example of the extremes one can go if one truly wants to better understand the process and the form of the compound in the product. This approach is less important for detecting polymorphic form conversion in the solid state, since polymorphic solubility typically varies by less than a factor of two and tablets at very low strength would generally be classified as a type one by the biopharmaceutical classification system. In addition, polymorphs rarely have pronounced differences in chemical stability. On the other hand, if a compound is somewhat unstable and significant amount of amorphous material is potentially present, this approach can be used to determine if it is responsible for drug instability in the tablet formulation. In any event, this reference serves as a very good example of the strength of a powerful approach that has not been widely applied in our industry.

12.5 COMMON METHODS USED FOR EXAMINATION OF SOLID FORMS

There are numerous analytical methods that can be used to characterize the physical state of the pharmaceutical in the pure active ingredient as well as in the formulated tablet. Each technique has its own strengths and weaknesses and in most cases one must choose the appropriate technique based on the specific physical property of concern and the sensitivity required. It is nearly impossible to predict a priori which technique will be most sensitive and it is best practice to use a variety of techniques initially to determine which one method will be most suited for assessment of the particular attribute of interest. For instance, Raman spectroscopy is particularly well suited for examination of crystal form of drug present within an excipient matrix, since the organic drug molecule is relatively nonpolar, highly polarizable and "good Raman scatterer," whereas many excipients such as lactose or celluloses tend to be relatively polar and "poor Raman scatterers." On the other hand Raman spectroscopy is subject to limitations of sample fluorescence and may not be suitable at all for analysis of a particular drug molecule. Perhaps the best approach is to consider the property that ones wishes to characterize, or the form that one wishes to distinguish, and try a number of potentially suitable techniques until one arrives at the optimal technique. Table 12.2 provides a list of commonly employed techniques, the

TABLE 12.2 Common Solid-State Techniques and Approximate Sensitivities to Physical Forms

Physical Form	X-ray Powder Diffraction	LOD LOQ (%)	Solid-State NMR Spectroscopy	LOD LOQ (%)	IR/Raman Spectroscopy	LOD LOQ (%)
True polymorphs	Unique diffraction peaks. Useful for determination of phase purity and percentage crystallinity	0.5–2	Unique chemical shifts. Useful for determining phase purity, molecular mobility	0.5–5	Characteristic spectra, sensitive to H-bonding	5–10
Solvates (hydrates)	Same as for true polymorphs	0.5–2	Unique solvent resonances, shifted drug resonances, solvent mobility may be assessed	0.5–5	Solvent bands and shifted absorption bands due to H-bonding interactions	5–10
Isomorphic desolvates	Substantial overlap of diffraction pattern (poorly distinguished)	0.5–2	Solvent resonances disappear. Drug resonances shift significantly relative to X-ray	0.5–5	Solvent bands disappear, drug bands shifted, highly similar to "parent solvate" spectra	5–10
Amorphous solids	No diffraction peaks poor sensitivity	~10	Broadened spectra	2–10	Broadened spectra	5–10
Polymorphic mixtures	Composite pattern of crystalline components	0.5–2		0.5–2	Composite spectrum of each absorbing component	5–10

type of solid characteristic that it is sensitive to and some of its limitations. There are many other techniques that may be employed in assessing the effects and physical state of the pharmaceutical in low-dose formulations; however only the ones most commonly employed in our laboratories for examination of phases in formulations at low dose are discussed in detail.

12.5.1 X-ray Powder Diffraction

In determining whether a compound is crystalline or amorphous, often the first instrumental technique applied is typically X-ray powder diffraction (XRPD). XRPD enables the direct determination of the presence of different crystalline forms of a compound. XRPD is often referred to as the gold standard for determination of the existence of drug polymorphism. In the powder method, crystals to be examined are reduced to a fine powder and placed in a beam of monochromatic X rays. Each tiny crystal is oriented at random with respect to the incident beam. The crystal diffracts X rays similarly to a diffraction grating. The three-dimensional crystal functions like a series of plane gratings stacked one above the other, giving rise to diffraction of electromagnetic ray whose wavelength approximates the atomic spacing in the crystal lattice.[2] The wavelength of the X rays, λ, is related to the angle of incidence, θ, and the interatomic distance, d, by the Bragg equation;

$$n\lambda = 2d \sin(\theta) \tag{12.1}$$

where n is the order of the diffraction, 1, 2, 3, etc.

The analogy of planes in a crystal owes its existence to the repetition of molecules packed in the crystal lattice, since diffraction occurs as the result of the interaction of the radiation with the electrons of the atoms. The planes are separated by an interplanar spacing of atoms, d, commonly termed the d-spacing. Constructive interference occurs when the path difference of the two rays travels an integral number of wavelengths before they constructively recombine. When the "Bragg condition" is fulfilled, a peak is detected that is representative of the interplanar spacing of the symmetry equivalent sets of Miller planes. Figure 12.3 provides an illustration of cones of diffraction that emanate from a powdered sample when a beam of X rays strikes the crystalline sample. The position that the diffracted radiation intersects with the detector, in this case a piece of photographic film, is characteristic of the material.

The peak positions of the unit cell reflect its size and angular relations of the crystal system. The intensity detected is a function of the atoms that make up the crystal and their scattering factors, a function of the electron density surrounding the atoms comprising the sample, as well as the location of the atoms within the unit cell. As a consequence, the diffraction pattern provides a unique characterization of a crystalline substance representing both its crystallographic packing and its unit cell contents. Each substance scatters the beam in a particular diffracting pattern, producing a unique fingerprint for each crystal form. Amorphous forms, however, scatter

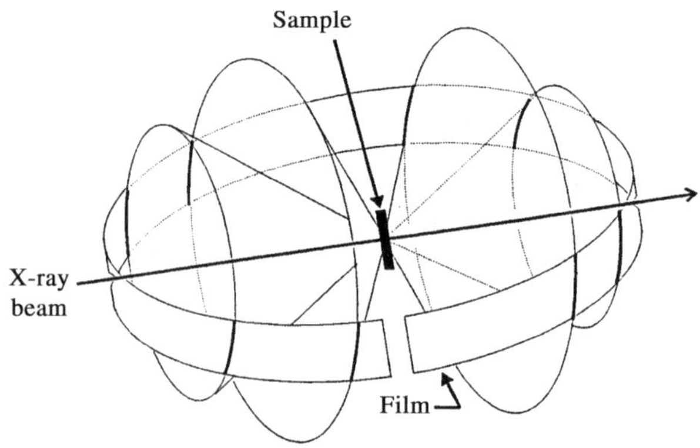

Figure 12.3 Illustration of the cones of diffraction produced by an X-ray beam striking a crystalline powder sample (reproduced with permission).

in an incoherent fashion owing to their lack of long-range three dimensional molecular order. Many amorphous materials and even some forms of liquid crystals will have a characteristic, albeit less defined, pattern owing to the less defined molecular spatial relationships within the solid. This distribution of molecular positions gives rise to a more diffuse pattern. As a consequence, X-ray powder diffraction is much less sensitive to amorphous solids than crystalline materials.

12.5.2 Quantitative X-ray Powder Diffraction

X-ray powder diffraction has been used extensively for quantitative analysis of mixtures of crystal forms and to a lesser extent the determination of the degree of crystallinity. There are two primary methods for quantification: using either individual peaks or the whole patterns to establish the relationship between phase composition and the intensity of individual peaks or of patterns of the phases being quantified. The basic elements of quantitative analysis of powder mixtures and the mathematical relationships between pattern intensity and composition were first outlined by Klug and Alexander in 1948.[3] The primary assumptions of the diffraction method rely on the particle size to be sufficiently small that extinction and micro-absorption effects are negligible. Furthermore, accurate quantification relies heavily on our ability to minimize the effects of preferred orientation. With inorganic samples, this is typically accomplished by grinding of the sample. With organic compounds, this may not be so readily accomplished. The potential of phase inter-conversion while reducing particle size is of major concern. Frequently crystalline samples can be made amorphous, solvates can desolvate, and metastable phases convert to more thermodynamically stable forms. This problem is particularly troublesome during the earliest stages of development when only limited amounts of unmilled material are available and lot sizes are smaller. Obtaining a nonpreferentially oriented powder diffraction pattern representative of the pure metastable phase can be particularly problematic. There are numerous methods used to generate standards of smaller particle sizes, the most common being grinding the sample using an analytical mill or mortar and pestle. In our laboratory we have found that sonication is a good method for maintaining less stable phases in its native state during particle size reduction. By this approach, a solvate can be stabilized by using its solvent of crystallization. If the form is nonsolvated, one can suspend the drug in a liquid in that the compound is not soluble. The nonsolvent reduces the potential for phase inter-conversion to the more stable form by minimizing the rate of solvent-mediated transformations. An additional method of overcoming preferred orientation is to mix the sample with an inert amorphous component, as was proposed in the first quantitative pharmaceutical X-ray powder diffraction method published.[4] This is highly convenient in the pharmaceutical industry since many of the commonly employed excipients are amorphous. There are numerous other methods for generating powder patterns free of preferred orientation. Furthermore, if the crystal structures of the components being analyzed are available, the success of eliminating preferred orientation can be determined by comparison of the relative intensities of the phases being quantified in the experimental powder patterns to their respective calculated powder patterns.

The general expression underlying quantitative diffraction analysis was presented by Alexander and Klug:[3]

$$I_1 = \frac{K_1 x_1}{\rho_1 [x_1(\mu_1^* - \mu_M^*) + \mu_M^*]} \tag{12.2}$$

where I_1 is the intensity; K_1 is a function of a number of physical constants – the dimensions of the diffractometer (slit size, goniometer radius), Lorentz-polarization factors, and reflection multiplicity of the phase of interest; ρ_1 is the analyte density; x_1 is the weight fraction of the analyte in the sample matrix; and $\mu_1{}^*$ and $\mu_M{}^*$ are the mass absorption coefficients of the analyte and the sample matrix, respectively. In the special case of a mixture of polymorphic forms of a substance, the mass absorption coefficient of the polymorph being quantified is the same as the sample matrix, that is $\mu_1{}^* = \mu_M{}^*$. The intensity of a given peak is directly proportional to its concentration such that linear analysis can be made directly by a plot of intensity vs concentration. When the absorption coefficient of the phase of unknown composition differs from that of the matrix, that is $\mu_1{}^* \neq \mu_M{}^*$, the more general Eq. (12.2) needs to be considered to accurately quantify crystal forms in the formulation or in mixtures of solvates and nonsolvated forms. The concentration vs weight fraction of the analyte will deviate from linearity. In purely organic systems, the deviation from linearity is not as severe as with inorganic systems,[5] since their mass absorption coefficients are relatively low and such samples generally do not have as large of a range of mass absorption coefficients.

In the pharmaceutical industry, typically one will examine the previously defined API either as mixture of polymorphic forms or as a mixture of crystalline and amorphous phases (both having a simple linear intensity proportionality to concentration). Alternatively one may encounter a mixture of hydration or solvation states, in which cases the intensity would not necessarily be directly proportional to concentration. Figure 12.4 demonstrates the deviation from linearity resulting from differences in

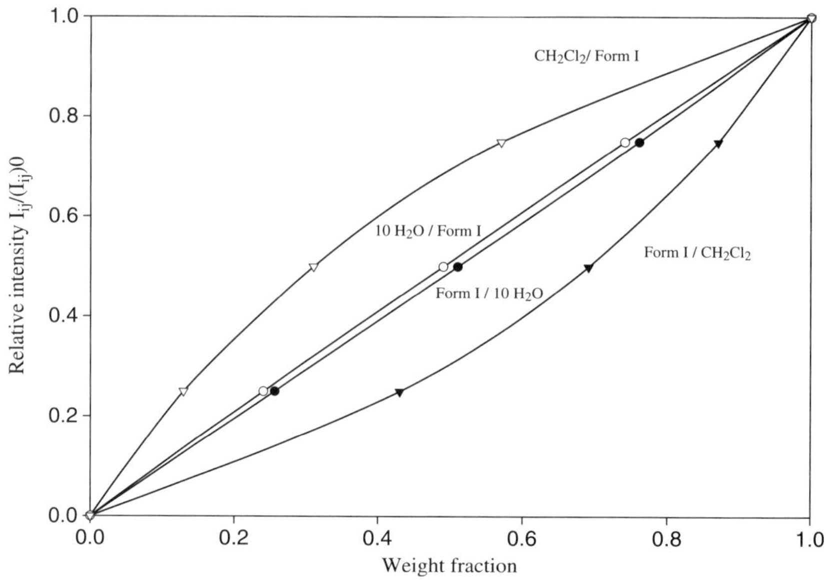

Figure 12.4 Theoretical intensity-concentration curves for several mixtures of the pentahydrate form of cromolyn sodium vs anhydrate form I (and vice versa) demonstrate the minor impact of hydration state on quantification. In contrast, the theoretical intensity of a "hypothetical" methylene chloride solvate of a cromolyn sodium vs anhydrate composition (and vice versa) shows significant deviation from linearity as a result of differences in mass absorption coefficient.

mass absorption coefficients between the analyte and the sample matrix. In the example, the mass absorption coefficient of the pentahydrate form of cromolyn sodium was calculated and a theoretical intensity vs concentration curve was generated for it as a mixture with an anhydrous form. Since this represents a highly hydrated system, this indicates that, in general, hydrates will not result in a significant deviation from linearity due to a difference in mass absorption coefficients (despite it not being a truly polymorphic system). Neglecting to account for the difference in mass absorption coefficient will introduce a relatively small error compared to other errors influencing the accuracy of quantitative measurement. In contrast, curves calculated based on a hypothetical methylene chloride solvate mixed with the anhydrous crystals would result in significant inaccuracy if the different mass absorption coefficient of the analyte was not accounted for. Similar considerations apply if one were to quantify the amount of a pharmaceutical salt vs its unionized form; it is always best to account for the difference in mass absorption coefficient. In formulations where excipients are mixed with the API, linear relationships between intensity and concentration are encountered; however, a constant amount of the intensity of the API peaks, and therefore the range of quantification, will be reduced. As a result of the constant excipient-to-API ratio, the intensity of the API will be reduced, thereby influencing the range of quantification; however the linear intensity/concentration relationship will still exist for polymorphic systems and will be approximately correct for mixture of hydrates (solvates) with nonsolvated forms.

There are numerous variants to quantitative analysis by X-ray powder diffraction. Some methods use direct analysis of an individual phase concentration based upon the intensity of single peak relative to its pure phase intensity. Other methods reference the analyte's intensity to an internal standard, while still others rely on a change in diffraction response as a result of spiking or dilution of the sample. The best approach to use is dependent upon many factors. These approaches may be developed using single peaks representative of the individual phases comprising the sample or they may use the entire diffraction pattern. Single line methods generally require less knowledge about the phases to be quantified than whole pattern methods. They will often be the most sensitive approach, since the method may be developed to quantify based on the intensity of only the most intense peak of the diffraction pattern. Single peak methods will suffer greater variability due to the influence of factors such as preferred orientation. Such methods are the least sophisticated and are often ideally suited for long-term quality control applications after particle size specifications are made.

Most whole pattern methods require a greater level of knowledge about the phases to be analyzed than the single peak methods. Two exceptions would be the whole pattern approaches such as factor-based partial least squares (PLS) or the whole pattern method described by Smith et al. Factor-based PLS is a multivariate method that has found widespread analytical application.[6] Such methods involve establishing a calibration set that is used to derive a predictive model for analysis of future data sets. The calibration set should contain as many sources of sample variation as possible. In doing so, one might expect to be able to empirically correct for (or at least partially compensate for) the influence of preferred orientation.[7] Such methods require no more information than single peak methods because they rely on empirically derived correlation of intensity/composition through training sets.

The program *GMQUANT*, developed by Smith et al., uses a whole powder pattern approach that does not require indexation of the individual components of the mixture.[8] Indexation of pharmaceuticals can be highly problematic due to their low symmetry and commonly large unit cell axes. This requirement is perhaps the greatest limitation to the utility of the whole powder pattern approaches described later. *GMQUANT* uses least squares minimization of the difference between the digitized experimental pattern of a mixture and that of a convolution of the digitized pattern of the individual phases related by weighting factors. This approach represents perhaps the most easily applied whole pattern method and is suitable for quality control applications, since it requires minimal interaction of the analyst. Fortunately, a number of programs have been developed that adopt similar approaches; *FULLPAT* uses a whole pattern fitting least-squares approach and is distributed freely.[9] There are also a number of recently marketed vendor-softwares that incorporate this approach.

Whole Powder-Pattern Decomposition Methods (WPPD). In WPPD the integrated intensity parameters, unit-cell parameters, and the peak profile parameters are refined by least squares fitting procedures along with an overall scale-factor relating the individual phases (or even amorphous background). The intensity of the diffraction pattern profile intensity, Y, at individual steps, i, of 2θ is decomposed

$$Y(2\theta_i) = B(2\theta_i) + \sum_{k=1}^{N} S_k \Sigma_j I_{jk} P(2\theta_i)_{jk} \tag{12.3}$$

where $B(2\theta_i)$ is the background function, $P(2\theta_i)$ is the profile function and S_k is the scale factor. There are a number of different background functions and profile functions that describe the diffraction profile.[10]

Toraya's Method. The WPPD as implemented by Toraya et al.[11] decomposes the peak profiles and background functions to obtain the best fit to the experimental powder pattern of the individual pure phase data by least-squares refinement. The integrated intensities of the pure phases are then stored with the other refined parameters, such as the profile parameters and the unit-cell parameters of the phases to be quantified. During quantification step, the integrated intensity of the phase being quantified is scaled, as defined in Eq. (12.4), such that the total of the scale factors for the component phases sum to unity. The scale factors of the individual components are then refined by least-squares methods until a best fit is observed with respect to the pattern of unknown composition.

$$S_y = \sum w_i [Y(2\theta_i) - Y(2\theta_{ci})]^2 \tag{12.4}$$

where the weighting function is $w_i = 1/Y(2\theta_i)$. If an amorphous phase is present, its composition can be determined by addition of a known quantity of a crystalline standard:

$$S_{\text{amorphous}} = 1 - \sum_{k=1}^{n-1} S_k^{\text{crystalline}} \tag{12.5}$$

Rietveld's Method. In the Rietveld method, essentially the same approach is used as in Toraya's method except a structural model (typically from a crystallographic determination) is used to calculate the intensities of the individual phases, as shown in Eq. (12.6):

$$Y_{ci} = S_y \sum_K L_K |F_K| P_{\text{Bragg}}(2\theta_i - 2\theta_K) PO_K A + Y_{\text{background}} \tag{12.6}$$

where Y_{ci} is the intensity calculated at an individual point, i, in the diffraction pattern, s is a scale factor, L_K contains the Lorentz, polarization, and multiplicity factors, K represents the individual Miller indices, h, k, l for the reflection, F_K is the structure factor for the Kth Bragg reflection, P_{Bragg} is the peak profile function, PO_K a function describing the sample's preferred orientation, A is an absorption factor, and $Y_{\text{background}}$ is the intensity of the background. The function minimized is based on the difference (residual) in intensity between the experimental pattern of the mixture and the scaled ratio of the calculated powder patterns of the phases being quantified.

Toraya's WPPD approach is quite similar to the Rietveld method; it requires knowledge of the chemical composition of the individual phases (mass absorption coefficients of phases of the sample), and their unit cell parameters from indexing. The benefit of this method is that it does not require the structural model required by the Rietveld method. Furthermore, if the quality of the crystallographic structure is poor and contains disordered pharmaceutical or poorly refined solvent molecules, quantification by the WPPD approach will be unbiased by an inadequate structural model, in contrast to the Rietveld method. If an appropriate internal standard of known quantity is introduced to the sample, the method can be applied to determine the amorphous phase composition as well as the crystalline components.[9] The Rietveld method uses structural-based parameters such as atomic coordinates and atomic site occupancies are required for the calculation of the structure factor, in addition to the parameters refined by the WPPD method of Toraya. The additional complexity of the Rietveld method affords a greater amount of information to be extracted from the data set, due to the increased number of refinable parameters. Furthermore, the method is commonly referred to as a standardless method, since the structural model serves the role of a standard crystalline phase. It is generally best to minimize the effect of preferred orientation through sample preparation. In certain instances models of its influence on the powder pattern can be used to improve the refinement.[12]

There seems to be an endless number of approaches to quantification by X-ray powder diffraction, some of which have been briefly discussed herein. When deciding what approach to use, there are many considerations one must take into account: Are you developing a method to guide the development of a process? Are you developing a method that will ultimately serve as a quality control application? Many factors influence the laboratory-to-laboratory or instrument-to-instrument transferability of a diffraction method. For instance, it might not be advisable for one to transfer a Rietveld method to a quality control laboratory since the success of quantification relies heavily on obtaining a global minimum from a nonlinear least squares refinement process. The robustness of such a methodology is highly dependent upon the skill level of the analyst and may not be readily automated. Since organic compounds may decompose with time, consideration must be given to the long-term availability of standards if standard curves are to be used. When instruments are changed or upgraded over time, many of the geometrical factors that influence K in Eq. (12.2) may be affected. Standard curves will need to be regenerated even when changing X-ray tubes for most methods other than the "standardless" methods. Development of a good quantitative method requires careful consideration of many factors and oftentimes depends on trade-off between ease and sophistication of approach.

12.5.3 Spectroscopy

Spectroscopic methods are nondestructive and can be used in conjunction with other solid-state techniques (TGA, microscopy, DSC, XRD) for the quantitative analysis of pharmaceutical solids. Once suitable spectral features, which arise from observed crystallographic differences, are identified, they can be used to develop methods for the quantitative analysis of one polymorph (or solvate) in the presence of the other.[13] One advantage of spectroscopic methods over diffraction methods for quantitative analysis is that these methods are often superior for the quantitative analysis of crystallinity, since Raman, IR, or SSNMR spectra of amorphous phases give specific, albeit broadened signals. The nondestructive nature of spectroscopic methods renders these techniques superior to thermal methods of analysis in most cases.

NMR Spectroscopy. Solid-state NMR spectroscopy may also be used for the quantitative analysis of pharmaceutical solids. The advantage of this technique over other spectroscopic techniques lies in its high degree of spectral resolution. Several solid-state NMR experiments are available for quantitative analysis, depending on the nature of the sample. Recent advances in multiple pulse sequences have made it possible to collect solid-state ^{1}H NMR spectra; however these measurements are hardware-intensive and difficult. Furthermore, because the isotropic chemical shift range of ^{1}H is only 12 ppm, solid-state ^{1}H NMR spectra are overwhelmed by peak broadening effects of proton–proton dipolar interactions that span several ppm, effectively limiting even qualitative applications of ^{1}H NMR spectroscopy. The significantly larger isotropic chemical shift range of ^{13}C is better suited for quantitative analysis, since highly resolved solid-state ^{13}C NMR spectra are possible. Hayes,[14] and later Harris,[15] have provided excellent descriptions of the quantitative aspects of high resolution solid-state NMR spectroscopy. The quantitative aspects of ^{13}C NMR spectroscopy are reviewed here as they apply to problems of pharmaceutical interest. This discussion can be extended to other nuclei, such as ^{31}P or ^{15}N, which also give high resolution spectra.

To obtain high resolution solid-state ^{13}C spectra, strong $^{1}H-^{13}C$ dipolar interactions and the chemical shift anisotropy (CSA) of the ^{13}C nuclei must be overcome. The CSA pattern arises from the simultaneous observation of chemical shifts for each and every orientation of a molecule with respect to the applied magnetic field. A combination of magic angle spinning (MAS),[16] which averages the CSA to zero, and high-power proton decoupling, which reduces strong $^{1}H-^{13}C$ dipolar interactions (MAS also helps to reduce $^{1}H-^{13}C$ dipolar interactions), is used to obtain high resolution solid-state ^{13}C spectra. Because high spinning speeds are often required to collect high-resolution SSNMR spectra, metastable forms which may undergo phase transitions may not be amenable to characterization by this technique. In cases where MAS can be used for quantitative analysis, the magic angle *must* be precisely set to $54^{\circ}44'$,[17] since deviations will cause line broadening and intensity deviations proportional to the CSA of each nucleus.

One complication of magic angle spinning is the appearance of spinning sidebands, which arise from insufficient sample spinning rates relative to the shielding anisotropy of the nucleus. Spinning sidebands, which are separated from the centerbands, that is, isotropic peaks, by the spinning rate (in Hz) and therefore may be readily identified as the peaks which shift in spectra acquired at different spinning speeds, are particularly significant at high magnetic fields or using low spinning rates. MAS not only affects the distribution of sidebands, but also their relative intensities. Therefore, in cases where spinning sidebands are significant and the relative peak intensities do not appear to be sensible, the entire spinning sideband manifold must be considered. For quantitative analysis, peak *areas* should be used as opposed to peak heights in adding back the signal intensity of the sidebands into the centerband intensity. Eliminating spinning sidebands by TOSS[18] (total suppression of spinning sidebands) or improving baselines of MAS spectra by spin echo sequences is generally not recommended for quantitative work.[15]

The key to developing a quantitative NMR method (solution or solid state) is to ensure that experimental conditions are selected, such that the integrated NMR signal is proportional to the number of nuclear spins producing it. For accurate integrations, the recycle time between successive pulses must be properly set to allow for the net magnetization (M_z) to return to its equilibrium state (M_o) after the R_f-induced spin transition. The choice of recycle delay will depend on the pulse sequence used for quantitation, which in turn is determined by the nature of the sample. Single pulse magic angle spinning (SP/MAS) experiments, using normal 90° pulses (or lower pulse angles) and high power proton decoupling, are recommended for mobile systems (with very short $T_{1\rho H}$). If SP/MAS is to be used for quantitative analysis, T_1 values should be precisely determined for the carbons of interest using inversion recovery pulse sequences[19] and recycle delays of $5T_{1C}$ then selected to allow for complete relaxation. If cross polarization magic angle spinning (CP/MAS) is used for quantitative analysis, as is generally recommended for rigid, proton-containing samples (with long T_{1C}), the recycle time will depend on the magnetization transfer process and relaxation behavior of the protons, not the carbons. The net result is that the recycle delay will be shorter, on the order of that of the proton T_1, that is, a few to tens instead of hundreds of seconds.

Cross polarization was introduced by Pines, Gibby, and Waugh to address the low sensitivity associated with collecting NMR spectra of dilute spin-1/2 nuclei, such as ^{13}C.[20] The basic CP pulse sequence is shown for $^{13}C-(^{1}H)$ in Fig. 12.5. Polarization transfer between ^{1}H and ^{13}C will occur by transferring the proton magnetization to the x'-axis with a 90° pulse, phase shifting the magnetization to the y' axis by an on-resonance spin locking pulse, and then applying an on-resonance pulse to the ^{13}C spins of precise magnitude so as to achieve the Hartmann–Hahn matching condition ($\gamma_H B_{1H} = \gamma_C B_{1C}$). Because the rare spin (^{13}C) takes on the magnetization and relaxation behavior of the abundant spin (^{1}H), not only is the sensitivity of the ^{13}C experiment enhanced by use of the CP pulse sequence, but as mentioned earlier, the recycle delay (which depends on the magnetization transfer process and the ^{1}H spin–lattice relaxation time) is also significantly reduced.

To understand how the CP/MAS experiment can be applied to quantitative analysis, the magnetization transfer and relaxation processes, which directly affect the signal intensity, must be considered. Cross polarization is mediated by $^{1}H-^{13}C$ dipolar interactions, so the magnetization buildup will occur at different rates for different types of carbons. In general, the cross polarization rate (T_{CP}^{-1}) increases with the degree of protonation.[21,22] That is, T_{CP} is generally shorter for methylene and methine carbons than for quaternary carbons, Fig. 12.6. Motional modulation

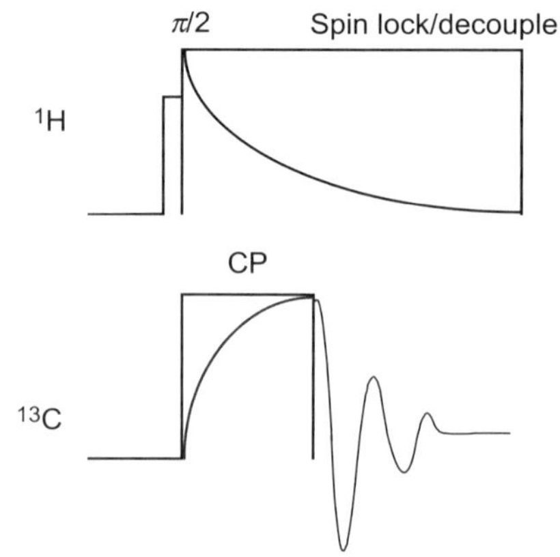

Figure 12.5 The cross polarization pulse sequence.

of the $^{13}C-^{1}H$ dipolar interaction, however, can significantly attenuate the magnetization buildup. Thus, for mobile methyl groups, the static dipolar interactions that allow for cross polarization start to average out, and longer contact times are required for full polarization.[14]

At the same time the proton magnetization is being partially transferred to the carbon spins (T_{CP}), it relaxes to the lattice ($T_{1\rho H}$, proton spin lattice relaxation in the rotating frame). The net result of the competing relaxation and polarization

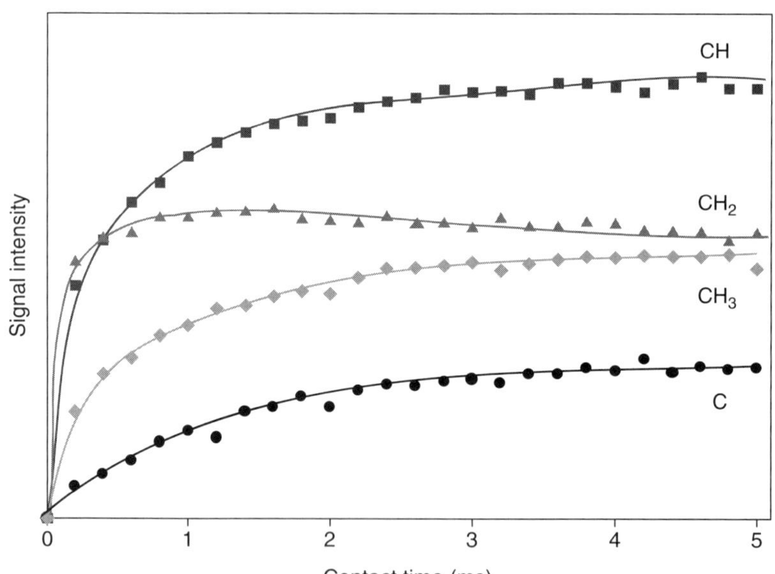

Figure 12.6 Signal intensity of several ^{13}C resonances of a developmental drug substance as a function of the contact time in a CP experiment.

transfer processes is that ^{13}C magnetization reaches a maximum. Once the ^{1}H and ^{13}C spins reach a common spin temperature, both spins relax to the lattice at a rate of $T_{1\rho H}^{-1}$. The exponential rise and decay of ^{13}C magnetization of a single species as a function of contact time is given by:[23]

$$I(\tau) = \frac{M_0\left(\frac{\gamma_H}{\gamma_C}\right)\left[\exp\left(-\frac{\tau}{T_{1\rho H}}\right) - \exp\left(\frac{\tau}{T_{CH}}\right)\right]}{1 - \frac{T_{CH}}{T_{1\rho H}}} \tag{12.7}$$

where $I(\tau)$ is the peak intensity at variable contact time, τ. The main requirement for efficient cross polarization is that the contact time (τ) is larger than T_{CP}, but smaller than $T_{1\rho H}$.

For homogeneous solids, all protons have identical relaxation times due to proton spin diffusion, which is mediated by homonuclear dipolar coupling. Spin diffusion is not fast enough, however, to average the proton relaxation times of materials with spatially distinct regions greater than 1 nm across.[24] As a result, heterogeneous materials may have multiple proton relaxation times associated with the different regions. Different relaxation behavior is evident from the signal decay of the CP curves of different crystal forms of a developmental drug substance (Fig. 12.7). For these samples, both the cross polarization rates and proton relaxation times in the rotating frame must be considered for each component to ensure that the signal

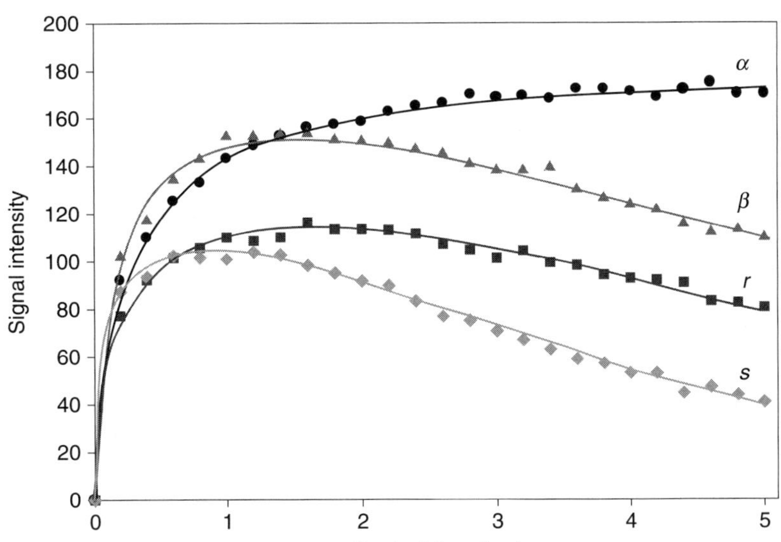

Figure 12.7 Signal intensity of a diagnostic ^{13}C resonance in the SSNMR spectra of several crystal forms of a developmental drug substance as a function of the contact time during the CP experiment.

is truly proportional to the amount of species present. It is also important to recognize that $T_{1\rho H}$, which is sensitive to mobility in molecular solids, may change drastically with variations in temperature. Therefore, sample temperature must be carefully selected and controlled to ensure quantitative results.

Clearly, in order to correctly apply CP pulse sequences for quantitative analysis (or even qualitative analysis), many relaxation processes (T_{1C}, $T_{1\rho H}$, T_{1H}, T_{CP}) must be considered and spectral acquisition parameters appropriately set. While a CP spectrum may be obtained when $T_{1C} > T_{1H}\,{}^{3}T_{1\rho H} \gg T_{CP}$, a quantitative CP spectrum requires that the recycle delay is sufficient (on the order of T_{1H}) for the protons to be uniformly relaxed at the beginning of the contact time,[25] all proton magnetization spin locked in the rotating frame decays at the same rate ($T_{1\rho H}^{-1}$), and the contact time is sufficient to allow complete cross polarization (at least 5 times the longest T_{CP}).[26] Except when relative peak intensities are constant and appear to be correct, single contact time measurements should be avoided. Instead, ^{13}C spectra *and* ^{1}H relaxation times should be measured and complete magnetization curves analyzed.

To correct the signal intensities in CP/MAS spectra for T_{CP} and $T_{1\rho H}$, complete magnetization curves should be constructed by varying the contact time and plotting the log of the signal intensity as a function of contact time. For homogeneous solids (with full spin diffusion for T_{1H} and $T_{1\rho H}$), the correct signal intensity may be obtained by simply extrapolating the signal to zero contact time.[15] Rethwisch et al. recommends collecting 10–15 spectra with ~75% of the data at contact times greater than $5T_{CP}$ for determining correct signal intensities by this method.[27] An approximate T_{CP} can be obtained by analysis of the initial rise in intensity, that is, at short contact times, while an approximate $T_{1\rho H}$ value can be obtained from the exponential decrease in intensity at long contact times.[2] For heterogeneous samples with complex spin diffusion (multiexponential $T_{1\rho H}$) and regions of different T_{CP}, line fitting of the CP curves may be required to obtain the correct signal intensity, as well as $T_{1\rho H}$ and T_{CP} values.[28] To improve the quantitative reliability of CP/MAS NMR spectra in cases where overlapping peaks (with different polarization and relaxation time constants) prevent the signal intensities from being corrected directly, a mathematical correction to $T_{1\rho H}$ may also be applied.[28]

Vibrational Spectroscopy [Infrared (mid-IR, NIR), Raman]. In contrast to X-ray powder diffraction, which probes the orderly arrangement of molecules in the crystal lattice, vibration spectroscopy probes differences in the influence of the solid state on the molecular spectroscopy. As a result, there is often a severe overlap of the majority of the spectra for different forms of the pharmaceutical. Sometimes complete resolution of the vibrational modes of a particular functional group suffices to differentiate the solid-state form and allows direct quantification. In other instances, particularly with near-infrared (NIR) spectroscopy, the overlap of spectral features results in the need to rely on more sophisticated approaches for quantification. Of the spectroscopic methods which have been shown to be useful for quantitative analysis, vibrational (mid-IR absorption, Raman scattering, and NIR) spectroscopy is perhaps the most amenable to routine, on-line, off-line, and quality-control quantitation.

Diffuse reflectance IR spectroscopy has become an attractive alternative to mulls with the introduction of DRIFT cell by Griffiths,[29] later modified by Yang.[30] Since materials are dispersed in a nonabsorbing medium and not subjected to thermal or mechanical energy during sample preparation, DRIFT spectroscopy is especially suitable for the qualitative/quantitative analysis for polymorphs, which are prone to solid-state transformations. The Kubelka–Munk (K–M) equation,[31] which is analogous to Beer's law for transmission measurements, is used to quantitatively describe diffusely-reflected radiation:

$$F(R_\infty) = \frac{(1 - R_\infty)^2}{2R_\infty} + \frac{2.303ac}{s} \tag{12.8}$$

where $F(R_\infty)$ is the K–M function, R_∞ the absolute reflectance of an "infinitely thick" sample ratioed to that of a nonabsorbing reference, a is the molar absorption coefficient, c is the molar concentration of the analyte, and s is the scattering coefficient. Clearly for a linear relationship between intensity and concentration to exist, the scattering coefficient must be constant. At low analyte concentrations, the scattering coefficient will depend on the nonabsorbing dispersant, while at higher concentrations, the linearity of the DRIFT analysis may be limited by the analyte. To minimize the effects of the analyte on the scattering coefficient, that is, to maximize the linear calibration range, care must be taken to control sample homogeneity, bulk density, particle size and shape. Specular reflectance must also be negligible.

In developing a quantitative method based on vibrational spectroscopy, measures must be taken to ensure homogeneous sample mixing, particle size, and instrument variability and reproducibility.[32] Roston et al. recommend grinding a spectroscopic-grade dispersant, for example, KCl, for 2 min in a laboratory mixer to ensure uniform, consistent particle size, a prerequisite for run-to-run and day-to-day consistency.[33] Unique spectral features must be identified and calibration studies must be performed on samples of known composition using peak areas determined by integration. Multivariate calibration methods (e.g., PLS) or regression analysis are typically required.

Near-infrared reflectance analysis (NIRS) shares many of the same advantages as DRIFT; however, the need to dilute the sample is eliminated. This is due to the relatively weak molar absorptivities of the peaks found in the near-infrared region, which are typically two or more orders of magnitude less intense than those found in the mid-infrared region. Absorbance peaks in the NIR region arise from combination bands (1900–2500 nm), harmonic overtones (1500–2000 nm, first overtone; 1100–1600, second overtone; and 700–1100, third overtone) and are weak due to the fact that, in a quantum mechanical sense, they are forbidden transitions of the simple harmonic oscillator. They arise only because of the deviation of the actual system from the harmonic oscillator (anharmonicity), causing a slight overlap of the energies (wave functions) of the initial and final states. As one might expect, the absorptivities of the second overtones are much weaker than first overtones, and the third weaker than the second. As a consequence, this weak interaction of light in the 700–1500 nm region affords a greater depth of penetration into the sample. Thus, instruments are now commercially available that can record a transmission spectrum through a tablet several millimeters thick, as demonstrated by Jee et al. for 500 mg paracetamol tablets, 4 mm thick.[34] With powder samples, scattering, which is also wavelength-dependent, competes with absorption. The combination of the effects of scattering and absorption determine the depth of penetration of the light into the sample, and thereby the effective sample size. For microcrystalline cellulose powder samples, depth of penetration was found to vary from tenths of millimeters (1500–2500 nm range) to a few millimeters (700–1100 nm range), as reported in paper by Berntsson et al., which also included a rigorous discussion of reflectance theory using the radiative transfer equation.[35]

One limitation of NIRS is that the absorbance peaks in the NIR region arise primarily from hydrogen to heteroatom bonds. This is simply due to the fact that the frequencies of these vibrations, because of the large mass difference of the atoms, are high enough for their overtones and combinations to fall outside the mid-IR region. The frequencies of the combinations and first overtones of other IR active bonds for atoms closer in mass (e.g., C—O, C—N) fall within the IR region, and are obscured by the stronger, primary absorbance peaks. Therefore, NIR is ill suited to compounds that do not contain hydrogen. At the same time, water absorbs strongly in the NIR region, and its peaks are resolved from alcohols and amines, making NIR ideal for analysis of hydrates.

Compared to spectra obtained in the mid-infrared region, NIR spectra contain fewer, less resolved, peaks. Due to scattering and other effects, a set of NIR spectra on similar samples often exhibits constant baseline offsets from one to the next. To eliminate these baseline offset differences, reduce (but not eliminate) scattering effects, and increase the resolution of neighboring peaks, first- or second-derivatization is often applied to NIR spectra prior to their use in calculations. Other preprocessing techniques, such as standard normal variate (SNV) or multiplicative scatter correction (MSC), may be applied to more effectively reduce scattering effects that arise from particle size differences among samples.[36]

When developing quantitative calibrations, it is important to understand that, since a single compound typically absorbs at many different wavelengths, the absorbance values in a given spectrum are highly collinear. Thus, multivariate calibration is often utilized to relate spectral information to some analytical property (chemometrics). Some of the most popular approaches include multiple linear regression (MLR), principle components analysis (PCA) and partial least-squares; for an excellent description of the basis for these approaches, see the textbook by Martens and Naes.[37] Given the large number of data-points in a spectrum, the chances of finding random spectral information in a set of spectra that correlate to any analytical property are quite good. Thus one must carefully validate calibration models by testing them with spectra that are completely independent from the spectra used to develop the calibrations.

Once a valid calibration has been established, the calibration curve is stored in computer memory for ongoing usage. Modern NIR instruments are highly stable with respect to sensitivity drift, and extensive calibration and diagnostic test procedures have been developed which may be routinely applied to ensure this stability.[38] Thus, a compelling advantage of NIRS analysis is the possibility of quantitative analysis without daily standardization or sample manipulation. When using an instrument equipped with a fiber-optic probe, samples may be analyzed without any preparation steps. This can afford both a rapid, and a precise measurement, since preparation steps (such as dilution and mixing with KBr for DRIFTS) that introduce variation have been eliminated. The ability to record spectra through a glass sample container is another major advantage of NIRS, especially for hygroscopic substances, where handling and manipulation could cause a form conversion and/or change water content.[39] Spectra may even be recorded through polymeric films such as bags or packaging materials. A multivariate calibration can be developed that is not affected by the contribution of polymer absorbance, or a transparent spectral region may be found. Also, the sensitivity of reflectance analysis to changes in sample particle size may be exploited for additional selectivity in identification testing. Using an instrument equipped with a fiber-optic probe, O'Neil, et al. have successfully developed NIRS calibrations for the median particle diameter of a number of powdered drugs and excipients.[40]

Raman spectroscopy is similar to DRIFT in the sense that it is a surface technique, where particle size is an important parameter to control. The smaller bandwidths in Raman (relative to IR) make this method more powerful for differentiating polymorphs than IR, and therefore potentially more powerful for quantitative analysis. No sample preparation is required (sampling can be done through containers), however, because of the small excitation range used in Raman spectroscopy, sample homogeneity must be considered. Bugay recommends either of two approaches, (1) a slurry technique utilizing a standard sample accessory[32] or (2) using a Step-n-Repeat sampling accessory to acquire spectra of several regions of a sample.[41] Langkilde, et al. reported sample rotation method ($\sim$1 mm diameter of sample is typically excited by a Raman laser) to address sample inhomogeneity concerns of quantitative Raman spectroscopy and was able to achieve linear concentration curves (1–15%).[42] To ensure a rugged assay, Bugay recommends concurrent method development using another analytical technique.[41]

12.6 CONCLUSIONS

Many things must be considered during the development of an active pharmaceutical that may alter the performance of the drug product. Solid-state techniques themselves are much less sensitive than their solution-state counterparts. Furthermore, quantitative analysis by such methods provides an even greater challenge. As a consequence, analysis of physical form composition of low-dose pharmaceuticals is particularly challenging. In many respects, due to the lower dosage strength, the influence of solid form on the bioavailability of the product is of less concern than with high dose drugs, considering the biopharmaceutical classification system. On the other hand, the influence of physical form on chemical stability is extremely important and can be exacerbated by the inherently low drug-to-excipient ratio. The choice of which analytical technique best suited for the task of monitoring the physical phase present at different stages of processing and in the final product requires consideration of the sensitivity of the method to the solid-state form and the composition of the sample to be analyzed. There are cases where it may not even be possible to analyze the physical form of the drug in a formulation, however through careful assessment of risk, choice of composition, processing steps and conditions, one can usually ensure that a consistent, stable product is produced.

REFERENCES

1. Booy K-J, Wiegerinck P, Vader J, Kaspersen F, Lambregts D, Vromans H, Kellenbach E. 2005. The use of ^{13}C labeling to enhance the sensitivity of ^{13}C solid-state CPMAS NMR to study polymorphism in low dose solid formulations. Pre- and early clinical development. J. Pharm. Sci. 94(2): 458–463.
2. Bragg WL. 1913. The structure of crystals as indicated by their diffraction of X-rays. Proc. R. Soc. Lond. A 89: 248–277.
3. Alexander LE, Klug HP. 1948. Basic aspects of X-ray absorption in quantitative diffraction analysis of powder mixtures. Anal. Chem. 20: 886–894.
4. Christ CL, Barnes RB, Williams EF. 1948. Organic quantitative analysis using the Geiger counter X-ray spectrometer. Anal. Chem. 20(9): 789–795.
5. Shell JW. 1963. X-ray and crystallographic applications in pharmaceutical research II. J. Pharm. Sci. 52(1): 24–29.
6. Thomas EV. 1994. A primer on multivariate calibration. Anal. Chem. 66(15): 795A–804A.
7. Artursson T, Hagman A, Bjork S, Trygg J, Wold S, Jacobsson SP. 2000. Study of preprocessing methods for the determination of crystalline phases in binary mixtures of drug substances by X-ray powder diffraction and multivariate calibration. Appl. Spectrosc. 54(8): 1222–1230.
8. Smith DK, Johnson GG Jr, Scheible A, Wims AM, Johnson JL, Ullmann G. 1987. Quantitative X-ray powder diffraction method using the full diffraction pattern. Powder Diffr. 2(2): 73–77.
9. Chipera SJ, Bish DL. 2002. FULLPAT: a full-pattern quantitative analysis program for X-ray powder diffraction using measured and calculated patterns. J. Appl. Cryst. 35: 744–749.
10. Young RA. 1995. The Rietveld method. Oxford University Press: New York.
11. Toraya H, Tsusaka S. 1995. Quantitative phase analysis using the whole-powder-pattern decomposition method. I. Solution from knowledge of chemical compositions. J. Appl. Cryst. 28: 392–399.
12. Dollase WA. 1986. Correction of intensities for preferred orientation in powder diffractometry: application of the March model. J. Appl. Cryst. 19: 267–272.
13. Brittain HG. 1997. Spectral methods for the characterization of polymorphs and solvates. J. Pharm. Sci. 86: 405–412.
14. Hays GR. 1982. High resolution carbon-13 solid-state nuclear magnetic resonance spectroscopy. Analyst 107: 241–252.
15. Harris RK. 1985. Quantitative aspects of high-resolution solid-state nuclear magnetic resonance spectroscopy. Analyst 110: 649–655.

16. Andrew ER. 1981. Magic angle spinning. Int. Rev. Phys. Chem. 1: 195–224.

17. Frye JS. 1982. Maciel GE. Setting the magic angle using a quadrupolar nuclide. J. Magn. Reson. 48: 125–131.

18. Dixon WT. 1982. Spinning-sideband-free and spinning-sideband-only NMR spectra in spinning samples. J. Chem. Phys. 77(4): 1800–1809.

19. Farrar TC, Becker ED. 1971. Pulse and fourier transform NMR. New York: Academic Press; 20–22.

20. Pines A, Gibby MG, Waugh JS. 1973. Proton-enhanced NMR of dilute spins in solids. J. Chem. Phys. 59: 569–590.

21. Alemany LB, Grant DM, Pugmire RJ, Alger TD, Zilm KW. 1983. Cross polarization and magic angle sample spinning NMR spectra of model organic compounds. 1. Highly protonated molecules. J. Am. Chem. Soc. 105: 2133–2141.

22. Alemany LB, Grant DM, Pugmire RJ, Alger TD, Zilm KW. 1983. Cross polarization and magic angle sample spinning NMR spectra of model organic compounds. 2. Molecules of low or remote protonation. J. Am. Chem. Soc. 105: 2142–2147.

23. Mehring M. 1983. Principles of High Resolution in Solids. Berlin: Springer, Chapter 4.

24. Zumbulyadis N. 1983. Selective carbon excitation and the detection of spatial heterogeneity in cross-polarization magic-angle-spinning NMR. J. Magn. Reson. 59: 486–494.

25. Havens JR, Koenig JL. 1983. Applications of high-resolution carbon-^{13}C nuclear magnetic resonance spectroscopy to solid polymers. Appl. Spectrosc. 37: 226–249.

26. Lindberg JJ, Hortling B. 1985. Cross polarization–magic angle spinning NMR studies of carbohydrates and aromatic polymers. Adv. Polym. Sci. 66: 1–22.

27. Rethwisch DG, Jacintha MA, Dybowski CR. 1993. Quantitation of ^{13}C in solids using CPMAS-DD-NMR spectroscopy. Anal. Chim. Acta 283: 1033–1043.

28. Collazo-Lopez H, Koch M, Cooper WT. 1993. Mathematical correction for variable $T_{1\rho H}$ relaxation of overlapping signals in solid state ^{13}C cross polarization NMR spectroscopy. Comput. Chem. 17: 73–79.

29. Fuller MP, Griffiths PR. 1978. Diffuse reflectance measurements by infrared fourier transform spectrometry. Anal. Chem. 50: 1906–1910.

30. Yang SS, Guillory JK. 1972. Polymorphism of sulfonamides. J. Pharm. Sci. 61: 626–640.

31. Kubelka P, Munk F. 1931. Ein beitung sur optik der farbanstriche. Z. Tech. Phys. 12: 593–601.

32. Bugay DE, Newman AW, Findlay WP. 1996. Quantitation of cefepime 2HCl dihydrate in cefepime 2HCl monohydrate by diffuse reflectance IR and powder X-ray diffraction techniques. J. Pharm. Biomed. Anal. 15: 49–61.

33. Roston DA, Walters MC, Rhinebarger RR, Ferro LJ. 1993. Characterization of polymorphs of a new anti-inflammatory drug. J. Pharm. Biomed. Anal. 11: 293–300.

34. Eustaquio A, Graham P, Jee RD, Moffatt AC, Trafford AD. 1998. Quantification of paracetamol in intact tablets using near-infrared transmittance spectroscopy. Analyst 123: 2303–2306.

35. Berntsson O, Burger T, Folestad S, Danielsson LG, Kuhn J, Fricke J. 1999. Effective sample size in diffuse reflectance near-IR spectrometry. Anal. Chem. 71(3): 617–623.

36. Blanco M, Coello J, Iturriaga H, Maspoch S, de la Pezuela C. 1997. Effect of data preprocessing methods in near-infrared diffuse reflectance spectroscopy for the determination of the active compound in a pharmaceutical preparation. Appl. Spectrosc. 51(2): 240–246.

37. Martens H, Naes T. 1989. Multivariate calibration. New York: John Wiley, Chapter 5.
38. General Information Chapter ⟨1119⟩ Near-Infrared Spectrophotometry. 1998. Pharmacopeial Forum 24(4): 6463–6473.
39. Zhou X, Hines P, Borer MW. 1998. Moisture determination in hygroscopic drug substances by near infrared spectroscopy. J. Pharm. Biomed. Anal. 17: 219–225.
40. O'Neil AJ, Jee RD, Moffat AC. 1998. The application of multiple linear regression to the measurement of the median particle size of drugs and pharmaceutical excipients by near-infrared spectroscopy. Analyst 123: 2297–2302.
41. Findlay WP, Bugay DE. 1998. Utilization of fourier transform-raman spectroscopy for the study for pharmaceutical crystal forms. J. Pharm. Biomed. Anal. 16: 921–930.
42. Langkilde FW, Sjoblom J, Tekenbers-Hjelte L, Mrak J. 1997. Quantitative FT-Raman analysis of two crystal forms of a pharmaceutical compound. J. Pharm. Biomed. Anal. 13: 687–696.

CHAPTER 13

PHYSICAL CHARACTERIZATION TESTS FOR DRUG SUBSTANCES USED IN LOW-DOSE FORMULATIONS

RONALD G. IACOCCA
Analytical Sciences R&D, Lilly Research Laboratories, Eli Lilly and Company, Indianapolis, IN 46285

13.1 GENERAL ISSUES IN THE PHYSICAL CHARACTERIZATION OF MICRONIZED POWDERS USED IN LOW-DOSE FORMULATIONS

With the advances in pharmaceutical sciences and the ever-increasing complexity in the therapeutic pathways for drug substances, the need for accurate and robust physical characterization continues to increase. The need for this information has been further emphasized by regulatory agencies that have established the concept of quality by design.

In low-dose formulations using highly potent synthetic molecules, the ability to obtain a thorough physical characterization data package is often limited by tangible physical constraints. Unlike with other analytical assays such as purity and potency, where the methods are designed around the properties of the molecule itself, the physical control strategy for any drug substance must be designed to fit the attributes of the powder, as well as how the powder will interact with drug product manufacturing components. These tasks can be further complicated by the fact that, in low-dose formulations, the amount of drug substance can be extremely limited because very little is needed for therapeutic effect. Thus, the physical property control strategy must be designed to give meaningful data while meeting these constraints.

13.2 PARTICLE SIZE ANALYSIS

13.2.1 Introduction

Regardless of the technique that is chosen for particle size analysis, there are several overarching issues that must be considered when performing these measurements.

Formulation and Analytical Development for Low-Dose Oral Drug Products. Edited by Jack Zheng

Perhaps the largest single consideration is the availability of drug substances to develop the necessary testing conditions that produce reliable, accurate, robust data. Optical microscopy and image analysis, for example, require very little material, while laser diffraction with a large capacity liquid dispersing cell will require substantially more powder. For low-dose compounds in early phases of development, material availability may be a challenge.

Second, the highly potent nature of the molecule must also be considered when selecting an appropriate particle sizing technique and dispersion method. Laser diffraction particle size analysis, for example, can be accomplished by dispersing the powder in either a moving liquid or gas. Liquids are the preferable dispersion medium since they can contain the powder and minimize environmental contamination. Dispersion in air or nitrogen significantly increases the risk of accidental exposure to the operator. If optical microscopy and image analysis were the preferred technique for particle size determination, the use of appropriate containment hoods and personal protective equipment would help ensure the safety of the analyst.

Third, in selecting a particle sizing technique, one must consider the size of the material itself. Most techniques have effective upper and lower limits of detection. Laser diffraction, for example, can measure particles from approximately 0.01 μm to several millimeters. With optical microscopy and image analysis, it becomes very difficult to resolve features that are smaller than a 0.3 μm because of the wavelength of light used in conventional optical microscopes.[1]

13.2.2 Particle Size Analysis via Laser Diffraction

Fundamentals. When considering the available platforms for particle size analysis, laser diffraction is one of the dominant techniques because it adequately addresses the aforementioned considerations, and is widely available on numerous commercial platforms. A simplified version of the basic fundamentals behind the technique is quite easily described. A beam of polarized light (i.e., a laser beam or polarized light from another source) impinges on an ensemble of particles that are dispersed in a carrier fluid, that can be a liquid or a gas (diluent). Upon intersecting the particles, the light is scattered. The angle and intensity of the diffracted light is monitored by a series of photo sensitive detectors. Using sophisticated mathematical algorithms, these signals are then converted to particle size distributions. The type of light source and the position of the detectors are dictated by the size of the particles. Typically, several light sources and an array of detectors are available in most commercially available instruments, enabling the dynamic range previously quoted for laser diffraction. More specific information on the fundamentals of laser diffraction can be found in the literature.[2–7]

Although the mathematics required to transform the scattered light patterns into a particle size distribution are complicated, it is beneficial to examine the basic scattering equation of light by a single particle, as certain optical properties of the powder must be known to obtain accurate sizing information:

$$I(\theta) = \frac{I_o}{2\kappa^2 a^2}\left\{[S_1(\theta)]^2 + [S_2(\theta)]^2\right\} \tag{13.1}$$

where $I(\theta)$ = the intensity of the scattered light as a function of angle, θ; I_o = the intensity of the incident light beam; κ = the wave number; a = the distance from the scattering object to the detector; $S_1(\theta)$ and $S_2(\theta)$ = complex scattering functions describing the scattering of light in a 360° surface.

Gustav Mie was able to solve this equation for $S_1(\theta)$ and $S_2(\theta)$ using a rigorous mathematical solution, assuming the scattering objects were spheres.[8] To apply Mie's solution to the scattering equation, as most laser diffraction instruments do, the refractive index of the material must be known (both the real and imaginary component) The refractive index is expressed as:

$$N_p = n_p - ik_p$$

where N_p = the refractive index of the particle; n_p = the real component of the refractive index; and ik_p = imaginary component of the refractive index, representing absorption of light.

Real refractive index information on particles can be measured using refractive oils having precise optical properties[9] or by referring to handbooks for more common materials.[8] The imaginary component of the refractive index refers to the ability of the powder to absorb light, rather than diffracting it. The absorption of light is a function of both the material and its size. For most materials, one does not have to consider the imaginary component of the refractive index above 10 μm. For some powders, the imaginary component can have an impact at a particle size of 50 μm. The effect of this imaginary component must be determined on a case-by-case basis by adjusting the refractive index and monitoring its effect on the particle size distribution. Additional information on this topic can be found in the literature.[2,5,6,10,11]

Powder Dispersion. Low-dose formulations require a very small particle size to ensure dose content uniformity.[12] This can create logistical challenges when particle size information is required. Small particles dissolve more quickly than larger ones; therefore, if a liquid is used for a dispersing medium, the compound should be insoluble or nearly insoluble in that medium.

Small particles also have a greater tendency to flocculate because of the increased role of Brownian motion over gravitational settling. This requires a thorough investigation of dispersing conditions including: surfactants, mechanical agitation, and sonication. With all three scenarios, the challenge is to provide adequate dispersion without dissolving the powder or without breaking the primary particles, both of which will produce spurious results.

With surfactants, two specific aspects must be considered: (1) does the chemical provide adequate dispersion; and (2) does the surfactant increase the solubility of the powder in the diluent such that it dissolves. If there is sparing solubility of the drug substance in the diluent/surfactant solution, the diluent can be saturated with the compound itself prior to performing the measurement. If there are material availability constraints, one may then have to consider another liquid system for dispersion. For many compounds, hexane (or hexanes) with Span 80 as a dispersant work well; however, this should not be taken as an absolute for all drug substances.

Mechanical agitation can further aid in the dispersion of powder. All sample cells for laser diffraction instruments are capable of delivering varying degrees of mechanical agitation, either through mechanical pumps or stirring devices. Additionally, during sample preparation, one can also stir the powder in the diluent prior to introducing it into the measurement cell. In general, this will facilitate the dispersion of weakly bonded particles. Should the material be strongly aggregated, mechanical agitation, either internal or external to the instrument, is insufficient to break apart agglomerates.

The use of sonic energy provides further energy to aid in dispersion. Laser diffraction instruments are often equipped with sonic energy sources. Additional dispersion can be achieved by using external sonic energy baths or probes. The cavitation that results from the use of these devices produces sufficient stress to break apart strongly aggregated material, allowing the analyst to measure the particle size of the primary particles in the aggregate. If taken to excess, however, sonication can also fracture these primary particles, thereby producing spurious results in the particle size distribution. Sonication also causes a temperature rise in the diluent, which may increase the solubility of the drug substance. This will produce a particle size distribution that is devoid of small particles as they will dissolve in the liquid.

Powders that have particle sizes ranging from a few micrometers to less than a micrometer, can be dispersed by knowing the zeta potential of the particles. The theory behind this measurement came into existence with the development of the Stern double layer.[13] Particles, when placed in a polar liquid, will develop an atmosphere of charged molecules (or ions) around it. By applying a scanning electric field and measuring the velocity of the particles created by this electric field, the electrophoretic mobility of the particle can be determined, which can then be used to calculate the charge of the particles with respect to the liquid medium. Once this charge, or more accurately, distribution of charge is known, the pH of the liquid medium can be adjusted by adding acid or base such that either the surface charges are all positive, or all negative. Practically, the median charge on the particles should have an absolute value of 30 mV or greater to ensure complete repulsion of the particles.

The surface charge of particles in a liquid medium can also be adjusted through the selective use of surfactants. Whether through the use of pH adjustment or surfactants, one must always ensure that the solubility of the powder does not increase, thereby dissolving the particles. Commercial instruments are readily available for this technique. The same apparatus often performs particle size measurements using photon correlation spectroscopy, which is discussed in a following section.

Practical Measurement Considerations

(A) Particle Shape: Evenwith a proper dispersion technique and adequate information about the optical properties of the material, several other considerations

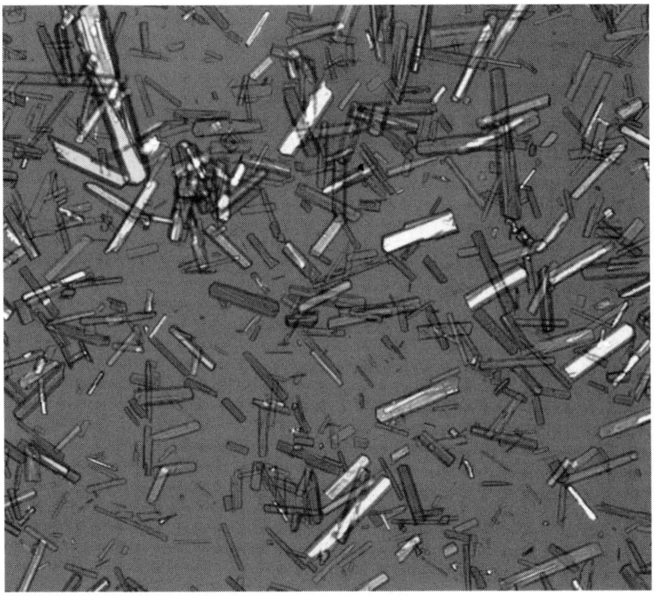

Figure 13.1 Optical micrograph of a typical drug substance that would be used in a low-dose solid oral formulation. (See color insert.)

exist when using laser diffraction as a technique for low-dose drug substances. Figure 13.1 shows a typical optical micrograph of a powder (unmilled) that would be used in a low-dose formulation. From the micrograph, it is evident that these particles are prismatic in shape, thereby violating the fundamental assumption of spherical particles. When analyzing several lots of this material via laser diffraction, the following particle size distributions are obtained (Fig. 13.1).

From the particle size distributions shown in Fig. 13.2 combined with the shape information provided in the optical micrograph (Fig. 13.1), it is difficult to make any clear conclusions about the differences observed in the distributions. Because of the high aspect ratio of the material, the distributions are multimodal. Additionally, it cannot be stated that the differences in the distributions are due to size alone. It is quite probable that observable differences are created by variations in particle shape.

The distributions shown in Fig. 13.2 represent unmilled material. It could be asserted that these data are not germane because, after passing through the mill, the aspect ratio will be reduced significantly. Mathematical milling models are often developed to predict the final size of the milled drug substance and particle size of the unmilled material is frequently used as input data for the model. Although the unmilled material will not appear in the final drug product, its particle size is a valuable process parameter that is required to produce the final drug substance.

Unfortunately, this is not an atypical situation. APIs frequently exhibit rod- or needle-like morphology. Using laser diffraction instruments, particle size distributions of these materials appear as multimodal, making it difficult to assert that

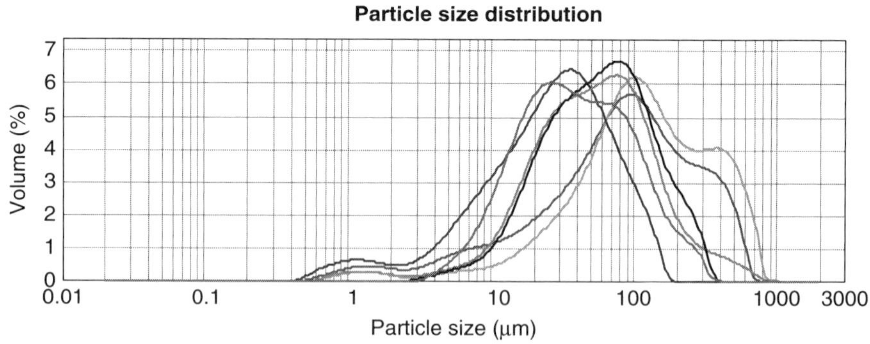

Figure 13.2 Laser diffraction particle size distributions obtained from several lots of an API used in a low-dose formulation (API is unmilled).

apparent size differences are not impacted by particle shape considerations. Investigators have proposed that it is possible to deconvolute the particle size and shape information obtained by laser diffraction.[14–18] This a daunting task when considering the computer codes used for laser diffraction instruments are confidential, a variety of light sources and detector arrays are used to gather the scattered light, and no single solution exists for all instruments. When the aspect ratio of the particle is greater than 5, consideration must be given to selecting an alternate particle sizing technique such as dynamic image analysis.

(B) Particle Aggregation: The consideration of particle shape can be further exacerbated when the drug substance particles do not exist as discrete particles, but rather as aggregates of particles, as shown in Fig. 13.3. Because the primary particles are

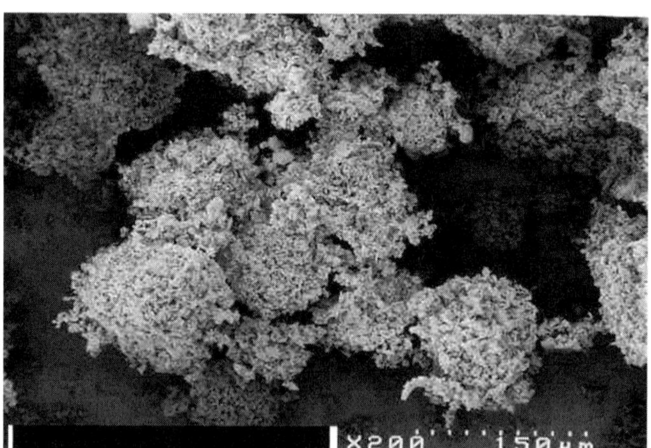

Figure 13.3 Scanning electron micrograph of a highly aggregated drug substance (unmilled).

strongly bonded to each other, it is necessary to mill drug substances such as this prior to being introduced into the drug product process. Even when milled, however, it is highly unlikely that all of the aggregates will be disintegrated. Thus, to obtain a representative particle size distribution on the milled material, dispersion of this material prior to measurement becomes a critical issue, particularly around the use of sonication. The dispersion strategy should be designed to either preserve the size of the aggregates during the measurement, or to provide sufficient energy to completely disperse the primary particles without fracturing them. The latter scenario is very difficult to achieve. Usually, the particle size distribution exhibits multiple modes for the material shown in Fig. 13.3 after being exposed to sonication. Because of incomplete disintegration of the aggregates, neither the primary particle size nor the initial aggregate size can be deconvoluted from the above distribution.

These practical issues of particle shape and dispersion are not intended to cast aspersions on the laser diffraction technique; rather, these factors have been discussed to bring awareness around the analytical results that are obtained when these factors are present. Laser diffraction has proven itself to be a reliable, robust technique for particle size analysis. When the assumption of nonaggregated spherical particles is violated, there are clear manifestations in the calculated particle size distribution. When analyzing drug substances that are used in low-dose solid oral formulations, the impact of these manifestations can be particularly impactful as there is often a limited number of API lots to be used for method development. Therefore, the analyst must be aware of these issues prior to the commencement of method development to avoid these pitfalls. In addition to the information contained in ISO 13320, Snorek et al. have written a summary around the general practices of laser diffraction measurements in the pharmaceutical industry.[19]

(C) Parameters for Laser Diffraction Measurements: The previous discussion has focused on the information that is required to obtaining meaningful particle size information via laser diffraction. For low-dose formulations, there are some basic ranges for instrument parameters and sample preparation that can be followed as one begins to develop a particle sizing method. Theses are basic starting points, and must be in greater detail for each compound.

- *Carrier fluid*: The API should be insoluble in the liquid. Hexane(s) is a good liquid to start with.
- *Dispersion*: Sonication of the sample should be avoided if at all possible. Dispersion should be accomplished through the selection of an appropriate surfactant and the mechanical agitation that is available with the stirring and pump settings on the laser diffraction instrument.
- *Optical concentration of API in the carrier liquid*: For particles less than 10 μm, the optical concentration will fall within the 5–15% range for obscuration (85–95% transmittance). Concentrations that greatly exceed this range will result in spurious data as multiple scattering will occur within the sample, causing the material to appear smaller than it actually is.

- *Circulation and stirring conditions*: This must be done on an individual basis. If the particles in the API exist as single crystals, aggressive settings should be avoided to prevent particle fracture.

13.2.3 Photon Correlation Spectroscopy

Photon correlation spectroscopy (PCS), also referred to as dynamic light scattering, is a technique that is used to measure particles in the size range of 1–0.001 μm. Unlike particle sizing by laser diffraction, the sample, dispersed in a diluent, is not circulated, stirred, or sonicated during the measurement. The technique is dependent upon a stable suspension of particles that are in constant random motion due to collisions with molecules of the suspending liquid.

The instrument design is less complicated as compared with laser diffraction. A stable suspension of particles is placed in a transparent cell, where a laser beam impinges on the particles. As the light is scattered from the randomly moving particles, interference patterns are created. Using suitable mathematical algorithms, these patterns are converted into particle size distributions. This technique is not well suited for material that exhibits a multimodal particle size distribution. One should not use this technique to obtain particle size distributions because of the assumptions that are needed to convert the interference patterns into usable information. The technique should be used to assess average particle size only. Additional information on this technique can be found in the literature.[2,6,13]

Adequate dispersion must be obtained for the measurement to be successful because the technique is based upon the Brownian motion of the particles in a liquid medium. If the particles should flocculate in the liquid, gravitational settling will occur, thereby removing the particles from the measurement zone in the sample cell. For this measurement to be successful, the refractive index of the material, both the real and the imaginary component, must be known. In the particle size regime where PCS can be employed, the refractive index has a very significant effect on the measured average particle size.

13.2.4 Image Analysis

Static Image Analysis. Image analysis, unlike laser diffraction and PCS measurements, is a direct measurement of particle size because, in using a microscope (either optical or transmission electron microscope), the images that are obtained are not a deconvolution of a light-scattering pattern or an electronic recreation of the particles (such as encountered in a scanning electron microscope). It is considered one of the fundamental techniques used for accurate particle size measurement because of this. Additionally, image analysis is a particle counting technique, where a measurement exists for every particle that is analyzed.

The process of image analysis begins with obtaining microscopic images of the desired particles. Typically, the powder is dispersed in a liquid to create a suspension. The concentration must be low to prevent the particles from overlapping when deposited on a microscope slide. Each particle should exist as a discrete entity to facilitate accurate measurement. Although particles are three dimensional structures, the images must be two-dimensional silhouettes. Computer software does exist that analyzes three-dimensional structures but, for practical purposes, two dimensions are sufficient to obtain necessary information about particle size and shape.

One must ensure that a sufficient number of particles is counted. The required number is a function of the polydispersity of the sample (e.g., the size difference between the largest and smallest particles). ISO standard 13322-1 is an excellent source to consult for determining the number of particles that must be measured for various size parameters.[20]

For particles that are too small to be resolved by a light optical microscope (sub micrometer or nano-sized), transmission electron microscopy can be used to obtain the images. Materials in this size range will flocculate easily because of their high mobility in liquids; therefore, in most instances, the particles will have to be separated using image analysis software. Once the digital images are obtained, measurements can be made using a number of commercial software packages. The benefit and drawback of size measurements obtained by image analysis lie in the variety of measurements that can be obtained. Unless the particles are perfectly spherical, no single number can represent the size of a particle (for spheres, this value is the diameter/radius). Any other geometric shape requires two or more values to describe its size. For this reason, a number of parameters have been identified such as the maximum chord length, the minimum chord length, the average chord length, Ferret's diameter, Martin's diameter, and so on. References[21–26] contain detailed information about the shape/size parameters that can be used in characterizing particles via image analysis.

The parameters mentioned above for shape analysis are straightforward to obtain. As computing technology has advanced, so have the descriptors that have been used to describe particles. Kaye proposed the use of fractal dimensions in describing particulate solids.[27] Leurkins proposed the application of the morphological variational principle to describe particle shape that states:[25]

> A mathematical representation of a particle or surface may be derived by finding a normalized boundary function which causes the surface integral to take on stationary values.

Using functions of R, θ, Z (radius, angle, height), Leurkens proposed surface integrals that could be used to describe three dimensional shapes. In a simplified space described by R and θ, a trace of the particle perimeter produces a plot that can be analyzed using Fourier analysis. Leurkins extends the theory to describe particles with three-dimensional complex shapes.

Perhaps one of the most complicated techniques that has been suggested is to look at moment models to describe particle shape.[28] Although these models present interesting scenarios to describe particle shape, the information cannot be easily automated and incorporated into a usable format for routine analysis.

Scanning electron microscopy (SEM) can provide a wealth of information about particle morphology; however, it is not well suited for quantitative image analysis.

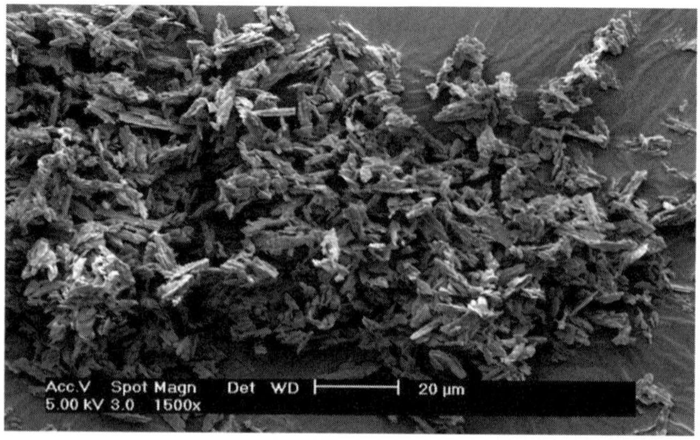

Figure 13.4 Scanning electron micrograph of a typical API used in a low-dose formulation.

When a gray scale digital image of the desired particles is obtained, the image must be turned into a binary image, where the typically the particles are converted to black, and the background is turned to white. This process, referred to as thresholding, is maximized when there is sufficient contrast between the particles and their background. This is easily obtained with optical and transmission electron microscopy; however, scanning electron microscopy does not provide this delineation. Figure 13.4 shows a typical scanning electron micrograph of a pharmaceutical powder. In converting this image to a binary rendition, it would be very difficult to select a gray scale region where the particle silhouette would be captured adequately. Either the edges of the particle would be eroded, or the background would be included as belonging to the particle. This produces error in the measurement. Additionally, scanning electron micrographs are intended to capture the three-dimensional nature of particles. Quantitative image analysis requires representative two-dimensional silhouettes, which are not provided using a scanning electron microscope.

Dynamic Image Analysis. With advances in digital imaging technology, image analysis has been transformed from a microscopic platform to real-time video capturing instruments. Referred to as dynamic image analysis, particles in a moving fluid are passed through a beam of light. Particle silhouettes are captured using high-speed cameras. The binary black and white images are stored as the raw data, allowing reanalysis of the images after the experiment is completed. Figure 13.5 shows a typical image produced by these instruments. As with static image analysis, numerous parameters can be selected to describe particle size and shape. The data report must include the parameter used and the basis (number or volume) employed to plot the data.

Since image analysis techniques are not as widely used as laser diffraction techniques, the common tendency is to compare all size data back to laser diffraction

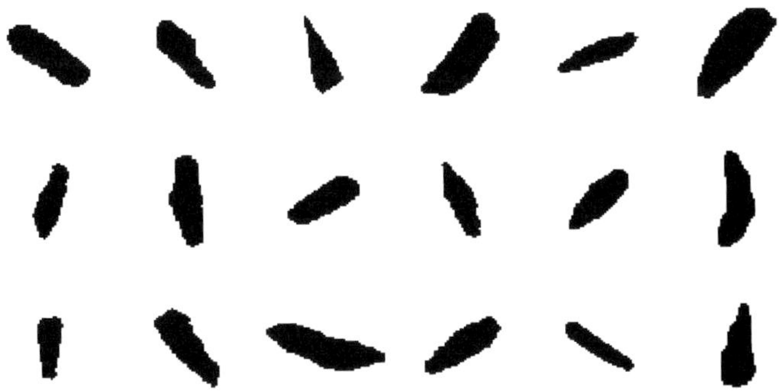

Figure 13.5 Binary digitized images of particles obtained by dynamic image analysis (courtesy of Sympatec GmbH).

particle size distributions. To perform this comparison, assumptions must be made to re-plot the data on either a volume or number basis. The errors created by these assumptions are often larger than any real differences between two sets of data. Rather than trying to converge all particle size data to a common basis, the data in

TABLE 13.1 Comparison of Particle Sizing Techniques for Active Pharmaceutical Ingredients

Technique	Advantages	Disadvantages
Laser diffraction	• Measures hundreds of thousands of particles per analysis • Provides robust and reproducible data • Powder can be dispersed in various fluid media (gases and liquids)	• For small particles, information must be known about the real and imaginary components of the refractive index • Information about particle shape cannot be obtained • Assumes spherical particles
Image analysis	• Information about particle size and shape can be obtained • The technique is one of the few direct methods of obtain particle size/shape information • With enough particle counts, particle size distributions can be obtained • Using computer software, many different parameters can be selected to measure particle size	• Without automation, the process can be slow • Inaccurate data particle size distributions will be obtained if insufficient particle counts are performed. • Images must be properly thresholded to avoid spurious results.

its native form should be examined for unique information, realizing the given platform has an impact on the data.

The challenge for dynamic image analysis is to obtain particle silhouettes that are in focus. As particle size decreases, so must the field of vision and the depth of field for the sample cell. This limits the number of particles that can be imaged in a single field. Statistically significant particle size distributions are obtained by utilizing longer measurement times to ensure an adequate number of images are captured and measured.

13.2.5 Comparison of Techniques

Each of the aforementioned techniques is capable of measuring powder that would be used in low-dose, solid oral dosage formulations. The technique must be compatible with the drug substance, and must be capable of producing the information that is needed. For example, if the particle size distribution is needed to ensure dose content uniformity, photon correlation spectroscopy can only provide an average particle size. In this instance, laser diffraction or image analysis would be more suitable techniques. Table 13.1 contains a comparison of the techniques that have been discussed.

13.3 SPECIFIC SURFACE AREA ANALYSIS

13.3.1 Gas Adsorption—BET Method

As one might surmise from the previous section on particle size analysis, a single physical characterization test does not produce absolute, singular values. For example, it is possible to have many different particle size distributions that possess the same average (median) particle size (x_{50}). Other orthogonal tests that are based upon different analytical techniques can be performed to confirm the results. Specific surface area (SSA) provides an excellent compliment to particle size analysis, particularly when the material is milled or micronized. Surface area measurements do not have the number of underlying assumptions that particle sizing techniques require (e.g., spherical smooth particles, no effect of particle color). The principle behind the measurement is rather elegant. Using a gas of known molecular/atomic radius (either N_2 or Kr), a powder is exposed to a known amount of the gaseous probe molecule. An empty cell is exposed to the identical dose. The gas will adsorb on to the surface of the powder, producing a lower pressure than the empty sample cell. Using a mathematical relationship, this pressure difference is converted into a surface area, knowing the diameter of the gas. The gas molecules are modeled at "hard spheres" that cover the surface of the powder. Because atoms/molecules of both of these gases have very small dimensions and are very fast diffusers, most of the available surface can be accessed by these gases.

For this technique to be effective, the adsorbing surface must be free from all impurities such as moisture, solvents, and other contaminants. Prior to measurement, the sample is outgased under either vacuum or high purity nitrogen, with or without the application of heat. All unwanted adsorbed species must be removed at this time. Should this not occur, spurious results will be produced in the analyses that will be obvious to the analyst.

Several different mathematical relationships (referred to as isotherms) have been developed to describe the relationship of fractional surface coverage with respect to the adsorbing species. Work by Langmuir, Freundlich, Tempkin, and others have attempted to describe the above mentioned pressure differential to fractional surface coverage. The most widely used and accepted isotherm is the BET equation, named after its orignators, Brunauer, Emmett, and Teller, and is as follows:[29]

$$\frac{p/p^{o}}{n^{a} * (1 - (p/p^{o}))} = \frac{1}{n_{m}^{a} * C} + \frac{(C-1) * (p/p^{o})}{n_{m}^{a} * C}$$

where p/p° = relative pressure; n^{a} = amount of gas adsorbed, mol/g; n_{m}^{a} = monolayer capacity of sample, mol/g; C = BET constant.

The BET isotherm, like the isotherm developed by Langmuir (the first person to develop a rigorous model for gas adsorption), assumes that the adsorbing surface is energetically uniform, and that only one molecule could adsorb at each surface site. The BET isotherm is a generalized form of the Langmuir equation to account for multilayer adsorption, and assumes that after the adsorption of the first layer, the heat of condensation is equal to the heat of evaporation, and that the rates of adsorption for the second adsorbed layer and beyond are the same.[29–31] From a practical perspective, variables in the equation must have specific values for the BET model to be valid, namely the y-intercept and BET constant, C, must be positive. Several excellent reviews of surface area measurement and gas adsorption can be found in References.[6,32–34]

13.3.2 Selection of Adsorbing Gas

In most applications, measurement of specific surface area is synonymous with the use of nitrogen and the BET isotherm. For most commercial surface area instruments, at least 1 m^2 of surface area must be present in the sample cell for the measurement to be repeatable. This requires that a significant mass of material ($>$1 g) must be present in the sample cell for low surface-area materials. When these conditions cannot be met due to material availability, an instrument that uses krypton as the adsorbate should be utilized. Krypton allows specific surface area measurement with as little as 0.1 m^2 present in the sample.

13.3.3 Inverse Gas Chromatography

Inverse gas chromatography (IGC) is another technique that can be used to measure the specific surface area of a particulate material, as well as to measure a number of surface thermodynamic properties of powders. Such instrumentation operates on a different principle than traditional nitrogen/krypton adsorption using the BET isotherm.

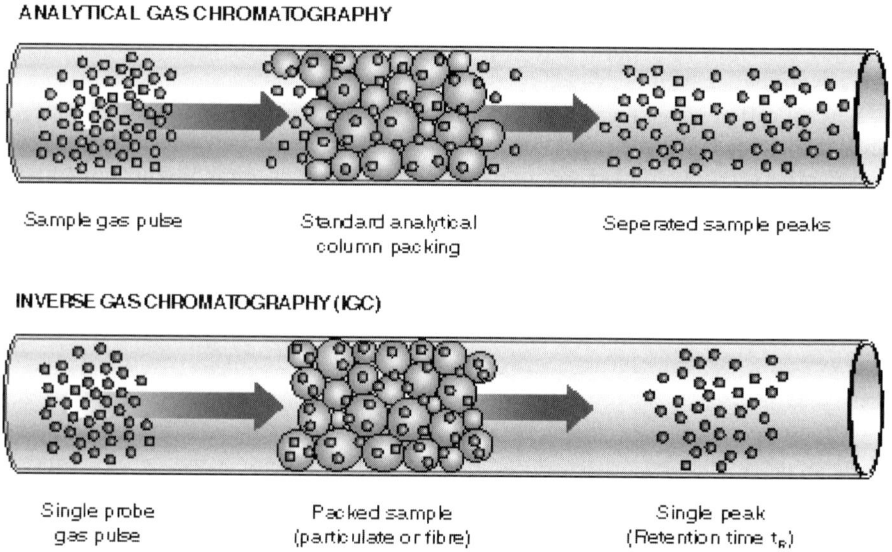

Figure 13.6 Schematic showing a comparison of conventional GC and IGC (courtesy of SMS, Inc.). (See color insert.)

Figure 13.6 shows a schematic for IGC operation. "Inverse," in this instance, refers to the observation that the powder is the "unknown" material, and the vapor that is injected into the column is known, which is "inverse" to the conditions that exist in traditional gas chromatography. After the initial injection of the known gas probe, the retention time and volume of the probe are measured as it passes through the packed powder bed. The gas probes range from a series of alkanes, which are nonpolar in nature, to polar probes such as chloroform and water. Using these different probes, the acid–base nature of the compound, specific surface energies of adsorption, and other thermodynamic properties are calculated. The governing equations for these calculations are based upon fundamental thermodynamic principles, and reveal a great deal of information about the surface of powder with a relatively simple experimental setup (Fig. 13.6). This technique has been applied to a number of different applications. IGC has been used to detect the following scenarios:

- polymorphs of crystalline compounds;[35,36]
- the presence of amorphous materials;[36]
- surface impurities on APIs and excipients;[37]
- lot-to-lot differences of powders;[38,39]
- the ability of liquids to wet powders;[40,41]
- surface connected porosity;[42]
- acid–base nature of surfaces;[43–45]
- phase transitions.[46]

TABLE 13.2 Advantages and Disadvantages of IGC for the Measurement of Surface Area

Advantages	Disadvantages
• Sample does not have to be tested at liquid N_2 temperatures. • Different molecular probes can be used to measure surface area • Additional information on the surface properties can be obtained simultaneously	• SSA not widely obtained via IGC • Cost of equipment is higher • Limited number of vendors

As stated previously, IGC can also be used to measure the specific surface area of a given powder. The adsorbate gas is not restricted to N_2 and Kr; rather, the same probes that are used to characterize the surface thermodynamic properties of the powder can be used as probe to measure its specific surface area. Table 13.2 contains a comparison of specific surface area measurements via traditional N_2/Kr adsorption vs IGC.

For low-dose solid oral formulations, there may be considerable advantages to using IGC to measure the surface area of drug substances because the probe molecule can be tuned for the specific compound, and additional information can be obtained about surface chemistry.

13.4 SUMMARY

The techniques discussed here are a brief subset of the physicochemical testing that can be performed on drug substances for low-dose solid oral formulations. They serve as a foundation for the testing that should be done rather than as a restrictive recipe. Chemical imaging techniques such as X-ray mapping, imaging vibrational spectroscopy (IR, NIR, terahertz imaging, etc.), and time-of-flight secondary ion mass spectroscopy (TOF-SIMS) are new technologies that provide key linkages between physical and chemical characterization. With the advances that are occurring in therapeutic areas, what once was considered "specialized" testing will become more routine as the information obtained from such testing continues to add value and answer complex analytical questions in pharmaceutical development.

REFERENCES

1. Friel J, et al. 2000. Practical guide to image analysis. Metals Park: ASM International; 290.
2. Xu R. 2000. Particle characterization: light scattering methods. Dordrecht: Kluwer Academic; 397.
3. Kerker M. 1969. The scattering of light and other electromagnetic radiation. Physical Chemistry, Lobel EM, editor, Vol. 16, 1st ed. New York: Academic Press; 666.

4. Van de Hulst HC. 1957. Light scattering by small particles. New York: Wiley; 470.
5. Bohren CA, Huffman DR. 1983. Absorption and scattering of light by small particles. New York: Wiley Interscience; 530.
6. Allen T. 1997. Particle size measurement, 5th ed. Powder Technology Series. In: Scarlett B and Jimbo G, editors. New York: Chapman and Hall.
7. Jillavenkatesa A, Dapkunas SJ, Lum HLS. 2001. Special Publication 960-1: Particle size characterization. Washington, DC: NIST; 165.
8. Mie G. 1908. Beitrage zur Optik trüber Medien speziell kolloidaler Metallösungen. Ann. Phys. 25: 377–445.
9. ISO 489: Plastics—Determination of Refractive Index, 1999.
10. Zhang HJ, Xu GD. 1992. The effect of particle refractive index on size measurement. Powder Technol. 70: 189–192.
11. Hand J. 2002. Comparisons of aerosol properties measured by impactors and light scattering from individual particles: Refractive index, number and volume concentrations, and size distributions. Atmos. Environ. 36: 1853–1861.
12. Rohrs BR, et al. 2006. Particle size limits to meet USP content uniformity criteria for tablets and capsules. J. Pharm. Sci. 95(5): 1049–1059.
13. Barth HG. 1984. Modern methods of particle size analysis. Chemical analysis: a series of monographys on analytical chemistry and its applications. In: Elving PJ, Winefordner JD, editors. New York: Wiley Interscience; 309.
14. Heffels C, et al. 1996. Correction of the effect of particle shape on the size distribution measured with a laser diffraction instrument. Part. Part. Syst. Charact. 13: 271–279.
15. Munlenweg H, Hirleman ED. 1998. Laser diffraction spectroscopy: Influence of particle shape and a shape adaptation technique. Part. Part. Syst. Charact. 15: 163–169.
16. Ma Z, et al. 2000. New developments in particle characterization by laser diffraction: Size and shape. Powder Technol. 111: 66–78.
17. Ma Z, Merkus HG, Scarlett B. 2001. Extending laser diffraction for particle shape considerations: technical aspects and application. Powder Technol. 118: 180–187.
18. Yamamoto H, Matsuyama T, Wada M. 2002. Shape distinction of particulate materials by laser diffraction powder analysis. Powder Technol. 122: 205–211.
19. Snorek S, et al. 2007. PQRI recommendations on particle-size analysis of drug substances used in orgal dosage forms. J. Pharm. Sci. 96(6): 1451–1467.
20. ISO 133322-1:2004 Image Analysis Methods—Part I: Static image analysis methods. 2004, ISO; 1–39.
21. Podczek F. 1997. Shape factor to assess the shape of particles using image analysis. Powder Technol. 93(1): 47–53.
22. Kohlus R, Bottlinger M. 1993. Particle shape analysis as an example of knowledge extraction by neural nets. Part. Part. Syst. Charact. 10: 275–278.
23. Drescher S, Heidenreich E. 1990. Technologically relevant particle shape analysis. Part. Part. Sys. Charact. 7: 30–35.
24. Laitinen N, et al. 2002. Visualization of particle size and shape distributions using self-organizing maps. Chemomet. Intell. Lab. Syst. 62: 47–60.
25. Leurkens DW. 1991. Theory and application of morphological analysis: fine particles and surfaces. CRC Series on Fine Particle Science and Technology. In: Beddow JK, editor. Boca Raton, FL: CRC; 282.

26. Heywood AE. 1993. The shape of powder-particle outlines. Materials science and technology, Greenwood GW, editor, Vol. 1. Taunton: Research Studies Press Ltd. 150.
27. Kaye B. 1993. Fractal dimensions in dataspace; New descriptor for fineparticle systems. Part. Part. Sys. Charact. 10: 191–200.
28. Diemer RB, et al. 2005. Interpretation of size reduction data via moment models. Powder Technol. 156: 83–94.
29. Braunauer S, Emmett PH, Teller E. 1938. Adsorption of gases in multimolecular layers. J. Am. Chem. Soc. 60: 309–319.
30. Langmuir I. 1932. Vapor pressures, evaporation, condensation, and adsorption. J. Am. Chem. Soc. 54: 2798–832.
31. Langmuir I. 1939. Molecular monolayers. Proc. R. Soc. A170(940): 1–39.
32. Dabrowski A. 2001. Adsorption—from theory to practice. Adv. Colloid Interface Sci. 93: 135–224.
33. Webb PA, Orr C. 1997. Analytical methods in fine particle technology, 1st ed. Norcross: Micromeritics Inc.; 301.
34. Lowell S, et al. 2004. Characterization of porous solids and powders: surace area, pore size and density. Dordrecht: Kluwer Academic; 347.
35. Grimsey IM, et al. 1999. Interpretation of the differences in the surface energetics of two optical forms of mannitol by inverse gas chromatography and molecular modelling. Int. J. Pharm. 191: 43–50.
36. Buckton G, Darcy P. 1999. Assessment of disorder in crystalline powders—a review of analytical techniques and their applications. Int. J. Pharm. 179: 141–158.
37. Ticehurst MD, Rowe RC, York P. 1994. Determination of the surface properties of two batches of salbutamol sulphate by inverse gas chromatography. Int. J. Pharm. 111: 241–249.
38. Ticehurst MD, et al. 1996. Characterisation of the surface properties of alpha-lactose monohydrate with inverse gas chromatography, used to detect batch variation. Int. J. Pharm. 141: 93–99.
39. York P, et al. 1998. Characterisation of the surface energetics of milled dl-propanol hydrochloride using inverse gas chromatography and molecular modeling. Int. J. Pharm. 174: 179–186.
40. Dove JW, Buckton G, Doherty C. 1996. A comparison of two contact angle measurement methods and inverse gas chromatography to asses the surface energies of theophylline and caffeine. Int. J. Pharm. 138.
41. Ahfat NM, et al. 2000. An exploration of inter-relationships between contact angle, inverse phase gas chromatography and triboelectric charging data. Eur. J. Pharm. Sci. 9: 271–276.
42. Thielmann F, Butler DA, Williams DR. 2001. Characterization of porous materials by finite concentration inverse gas chromatography. Colloids Surfaces A 187–188: 267–272.
43. Ohta M, Buckton G. 2004. The use of inverse gas chromatography to asess the acid–base contributions to surface energies of cefditoren pivoxil and methacrylate copolymers and possible links to instability. Int. J. Pharm. 272: 121–128.
44. Uhlmann P, Schneider S. 2002. Acid–base and eurface energy characterization of grafted polyethylene using inverse gas chromatography. J. Chromatogr. A 969: 73–80.
45. Hamieh T, Fadlallah MB, Schultz J. 2002. New Approach to characterise physicochemical properties of solid substrates by inverse gas chromatography at infinite dilution III.

Determination of the acid–base properties of some solid substrates (polymers, oxides and carbon fibres): A new model. J. Chromatogr. A 969: 37–47.

46. Hamieh T, Schultz J. 2002. New approach to characterise physicochemical properties of solid substrates by inverse gas chromatography at infinite dilution II. Study of the transition temperatures of poly (methyl methacrylate) at various tacticities and of poly (methyl methacrylate) adsorbed on alumina and silica. J. Chromatogr. A 969: 27–36.

CHAPTER 14

AN EXCIPIENT LIBRARY APPROACH TO ANALYTICAL DEVELOPMENT FOR LOW-DOSE, SOLID ORAL DOSAGE FORM DRUG PRODUCTS

QING CHANG, LISHENG KANG, KERI VARNER, JOYCE BRIDGES, NORMAN SESI, and MARGO PALMIERI

Analytical Sciences R&D, Lilly Research Laboratories, Eli Lilly and Company, Indianapolis, IN 40285

14.1 INTRODUCTION

In developing solid oral dosage form drug products at a dose less than 1 mg/dose unit, or low-dose, both formulation and analytical development may face extraordinary difficulties. Due to the high excipient-to-drug ratio, common development issues such as physical or chemical interactions between the API and the excipients, analytical interferences, and detection sensitivity are magnified. On one hand, drug product chemical stability, content uniformity, and drug release are among the top concerns in formulation development. On the other, because the drug and its process and/or degradation impurities need to be analyzed at ultra-trace levels (typically less than 1 μg/mL) in the presence of a large quantity of excipients, excipient background, peak separation, drug recovery, and detection sensitivity become big challenges to analytical development.

To illustrate, in complying with ICH guidelines[1] an impurity analysis for a low-dose drug product with a strength of 10 μg/dose unit may take place at an analyte concentration of about nanograms per milliliter. Performing analysis at such a low level requires a sensitive detection technique. Among a variety of common HPLC detection techniques,[2,3] mass spectrometry,[4,5] electrochemical detection,[6,7] chemiluminescence,[8] and fluorescence[9] are among the most sensitive and widely used. However, according to recent reviews on pharmaceutical and drug analysis,[10,11] HPLC with UV detection is found to be the technique of choice for routine HPLC

Formulation and Analytical Development for Low-Dose Oral Drug Products. Edited by Jack Zheng

analysis. This is understandable because in early-phase analytical development, the impurity profile is not yet well understood. Therefore, a universal or near-universal detection method such as UV is needed to ensure the capture of any new process- and/or degradation-related impurities. In late-phase drug development, UV detection proves to be one of the most rugged methods in quality control laboratories. Moreover, a method based on UV detection can be easily transferred and implemented due to the commonality of UV measurement among laboratories. The drawback to UV detection is its poor sensitivity at low analyte concentrations. One way to compensate is to inject larger volumes of sample onto the HPLC column (e.g., 1000–2000 μL) (see Hernández et al.[12] and Broquaire et al.[13]).

While the detection sensitivity issues may be solved through the application of advanced techniques, the excipient chromatographic background presents a tougher problem. Excipient background is not typically discussed in pharmaceutical analysis,[14] because, other than for excipient stability, it is seldom a major problem in typical-dose drug development. (It should be pointed out that, in liquid oral dosage form drug products, it is common to have excipient interference, especially resulting from colorants and flavorings. However, a discussion of this topic is beyond the scope of this chapter. Interested readers are referred to Niazi.[15]) In contrast, in situations where the drug is at a low dose, a sensitive detector capable of measuring small analyte signals will also pick up undesired excipient background interferences that would not normally pose a problem at typical dosage. This dramatically increases the complexity of low-dose method development.[16] Since there is no general approach to reducing excipient background, solutions are developed on a case-by-case basis. This is very costly in drug development.

To address the challenges in low-dose drug product development, we recently initiated an excipient library approach, which follows the philosophy, "an ounce of prevention is worth a pound of cure." The idea was to create a library of excipient-related information such as chromatographic background, stability, compatibility, and effect on drug recovery and release. This library serves as a general tool for low-dose drug development. Using the library, development teams are able to screen for the most appropriate excipients at the development planning/design phase on the basis of both formulation and analytical requirements. This approach aims to reduce analytical development difficulties where possible.

As the initial addition to the library, we collected excipient-chromatographic background information on 36 common excipients. In the following sections, we will discuss why we collect this information, what effect the excipient background has, how we control the background, and finally, how we utilize the library to facilitate drug development.

14.2 IMPORTANCE OF EXCIPIENT ABSORBANCE BACKGROUND TO LOW-DOSE IMPURITY ANALYSIS

For purity and/or impurity analysis using high-performance liquid chromatography, UV detection is still the method of choice for the reasons discussed earlier. In brief, for one reason it is the most popular detection method in use today,[11,17,18] thus facilitating method transfer between laboratories; and for another it is a near-universal detection method providing maximal opportunity for detecting unknown impurities. It is because of this second reason that UV detection is also subject to excipient background interferences, especially at low wavelengths. This interference is observed in typical dosage formulation, but is more pronounced in low-dose formulations.

14.2.1 Excipient Absorbance Background in Impurity Analysis for Typical Dosage Formulation

In this section, the term "typical dose" refers to dosage strengths of 1–100 mg API per dose unit. This corresponds to a sample concentration range from 20 μg API/mL to 20 mg API/mL, respectively. Though commonly not an issue, excipient absorbance background problems do exist and have been reported on a number of occasions,[19,20] particularly for API impurity-related assays. For example, in developing a method for analyzing clindamycin and six known impurities in a novel tablet formulation, Platzer and White[19] found the peak for triethyl citrate (an excipient in formulation) present at a size comparable to the impurity peaks. With the assistance of an HPLC method development software, DryLab®, the excipient interference peak was successfully separated from the analyte peaks. In this work, the concentration of clindamycin was at 3.5 mg/mL. In another work, Ciutaru et al.[20] developed and validated a method to analyze paclitaxel at a level of 0.6 mg/mL and its 11 known impurities in the presence of polyoxyl castor oil, a major excipient in the formulation. Paclitaxel is well known as a mitotic inhibitor, used in cancer chemotherapy and marketed as variety of commercial products.[21] However, according to Ciutaru et al.,[20] few methods were developed for quantitatively determining paclitaxel-related impurities and degradation products in finished pharmaceutical forms because the polyoxyl castor oil caused chromatographic interference, and therefore any analysis would required complex, time-consuming sample pretreatments. While Ciutaru and co-workers were able to distinguish 12 analyte peaks and six excipient-related interference peaks, complete chromatographic separation was unsuccessful. Quantitative analysis was only possible after subtracting excipient background from the sample chromatograms. In addition to the examples given above, excipient background is also found in other reports.[22–24]

It is clear that, although it is not a common issue for solid oral dosage forms, excipient background does need to be considered in method development for impurity analysis even in the typical-dose formulation.

14.2.2 Excipient Absorbance Background in Impurity Analysis for Low-Dose Formulation

In this chapter the term "low-dose" is defined as a dosage strength equal to or less than 1 mg API per dose unit, typically in the range of 0.001–1 mg/dose unit (or 1–1000 μg/dose unit). In contrast to typical dosage formulation, the excipient background in low dose becomes appreciable relative to analyte peaks and is a major consideration for impurity method development. For example, a typical sample preparation for low-dose analysis (i.e., 2 dose units/10 mL sample solvent) for a 10 μg/dose unit results in a sample solution of 2 μg API/mL. According to ICH guidelines for impurity analysis,[1] if the maximum daily dose of a new drug product is <1 g, any impurities greater than or equal to 0.1% must be quantified and reported. Therefore, the concentration of impurities at the 0.1% reporting threshold for the low-dose drug product is 2 ng/mL. To achieve this sensitivity using UV detection, the sample has to be either concentrated prior to injection[11] or injected at a larger volume (e.g., 1000–2000 μL vs the normal 10–100 μL). Because of the high excipient-to-drug ratio (e.g., 20,000 : 1 for a 10 μg API/200 mg unit dose) and low analyte concentration, chromatographic background peaks introduced by excipients, sample solvent, and mobile phase solutions can be quite significant and can interfere with the analyte measurement. As a precautionary step, it is recommended that trace amounts of environmental contaminants or impurities in the sample solvent and mobile phase be removed prior to use, using a method, such as that described by Ringo and co-workers.[25] It is our experience that the total organic carbon in double-distilled, de-ionized water should be controlled at less than 25 ppb. It should be realized, however, that controlling the background interference from excipients is much more difficult than controlling that from the sample solvent and mobile phase.

Figure 14.1a shows a chromatographic background of excipients generated by injecting 1800 μL of placebo sample solution extracted using a sample solvent containing a mixture of acetonitrile and water (20 : 80, v/v), 27 mM trifluoroacetic acid (TFA) and 20 mM sodium lauryl sulfate (SLS). The placebo formulation was designed for use with an API dosage-strength of 1–100 μg/dose unit. SLS, a surfactant, was added to the sample solvent to assist complete drug extraction, and the sample preparation followed the typical sample preparation procedure described above. Although the drug recovery was deemed acceptable as demonstrated using spiked placebo samples, the method was practically useless for impurity analysis due to the presence of excessive excipient background. In order to reduce the background, different surfactants, surfactant concentrations, mobile phase, sample solvents, and gradients were investigated. This led to a set of workable conditions and a tolerable background chromatogram as shown in Fig. 14.1b. While the resulting background was still not ideal, it was usable.

Significant background interference was also reported by Nygaard and co-workers.[11] In their work, they were trying to develop an improved method to determine process and degradation impurities in Vagifem® estradiol vaginal tablets at a dosage strength of 25 μg in an 80 mg tablet, representing an excipient-to-drug ratio of 3200 : 1. Using an existing method, the tablet was first extracted using ethanol, a solvent known to have good solubility for the drug and poor solubility for a major excipient in the formulation. The supernatant was then separated, dried, and redissolved to get a 16-fold more concentrated sample for subsequent HPLC injection. However, placebo samples prepared using this procedure showed tremendous background peaks, despite the discriminating solubility of ethanol to the drug and excipient. This makes the use of the method challenging and an improved method necessary. In the improved method, based on the understanding that most

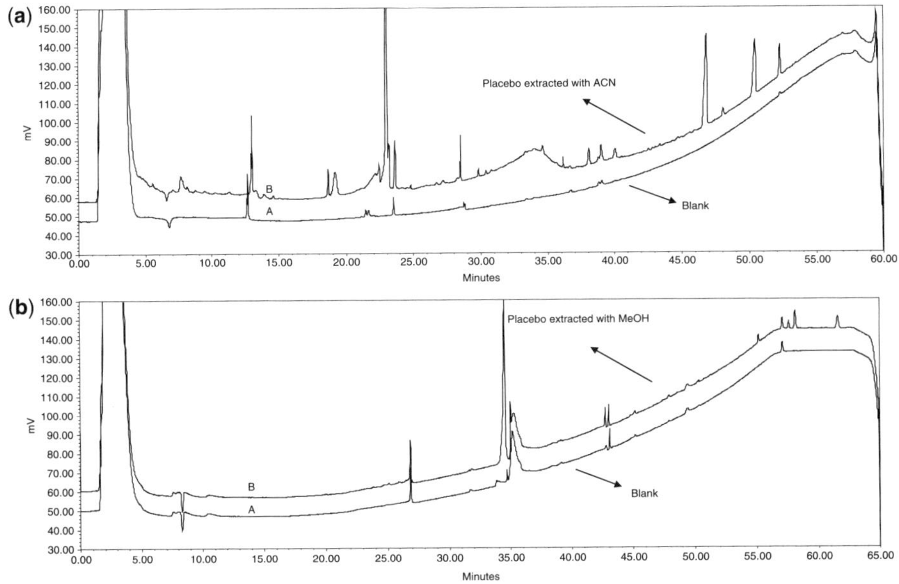

Figure 14.1 Chromatographic background of placebo containing HPC, lactose, MCC, MS and SLS, (a) extracted using a sample solvent of 20% ACN–80% H_2O–27 mM TFA–20 mM SDS and run under a gradient from 25% ACN–75% H_2O–7 mM TFA to 95% ACN–5% H_2O–7 mM TFA; and (b) extracted using a sample solvent of 30% MeOH–70% H_2O–27 mM TFA–20 mM SDS and run under a gradient from 35% MeOH–65% H2O–7 mM TFA to 90% MeOH–10% H_2O–7 mM TFA. In both cases, samples were injected at 1800 μL onto a Zorbax SB-C_8, 4.6 × 150 mm, 3.5 μm column at 30°C with a flow rate of 1 mL/min. The detection was at 226 nm.

of the excipients were water-soluble and the analytes were water-insoluble, a second extraction step was introduced to the dried supernatant obtained per the existing method procedure. The optimal extraction system contained water and toluene, determined after screening methylene chloride, chloroform, toluene, and hexane for effectiveness in reducing placebo interference. This additional extraction step dramatically reduced excipient background. The accuracy of the method with respect to API and its 10 possible impurities, spiked at three different levels, was within 80–140% with only one exception at 191.7%, and this was considered acceptable. Though not a simple approach, the improved method is practically more useful.

14.2.3 Excipient Library Approach for Low-Dose Impurity Analysis

As demonstrated above, tackling the excipient absorbance background problem is challenging in low-dose analytical development. Though approaches may be different, it is clear that none of the solutions come easily. They come at the expense of longer development times and more intensive manpower. Therefore, the question facing a development scientist is whether there are more effective approaches to low-dose analytical development that deal with the excipient absorbance background issue. The answer is yes!

In reviewing the difficulties, experiences, and lessons learned in low-dose, drug product development, a group of Lilly scientists proposed an excipient library approach. The idea was to set up a database of commonly used excipients, containing information such as excipient chromatographic background, excipient-to-drug compatibility, excipient-to-excipient interaction, and excipient effects on drug recovery and release. By having this database available, formulation and analytical scientists would be able to search and review the excipient information during the initial formulation design phase, and come out with an integrated approach taking into account both excipient functionality and potential analytical challenges. In return, analytical scientists would be able to develop high-quality methods to provide reliable feedback to formulation for further formulation optimization. Over time, new excipient information would be added to the library and available for future low-dose drug development. Through such a team effort and preventive approach, formulation and analytical scientists could help each other and make their low-dose development work more efficient and cost effective. Thus, the use of the library are two-fold: (1) to screen excipients whenever possible to meet formulation requirements and minimize potential analytical difficulties; and (2) to guide analytical method development when a formulation is selected. In order to take full advantage of this approach, we need to understand the factors that influence excipient absorbance background.

14.3 FACTORS AFFECTING EXCIPIENT ABSORBANCE BACKGROUND

Three primary factors contribute to chromatographic background, namely excipients, impurities in the excipients, and analytical method utilized in the analysis. Depending upon the chromophores in the molecules, excipients can exhibit quite different spectral characteristics from one to another. Obviously, the stronger the UV absorption at the detection wavelength, the greater the background the excipient generates. As will be demonstrated in following sections, excipient background typically shows up as a huge, prolonged solvent front and/or a broad hump in a portion of the chromatogram. Besides the excipients themselves, impurities in the excipients, which contain chromophores, can also impact the background. However, unlike excipients, the background generated by impurities typically appears as extra chromatographic peaks, causing complexity and difficulties in peak separation. As will be illustrated later, background interferences from excipients and their impurities are further dictated by quantity, type of excipient used, and the analytical method applied. The same excipient, when used as a binder, may display less background than when used as a film former, simply because 10 times less quantity is required. Nevertheless, it is possible to reduce the excipient background through optimization of the analytical method parameters, such as mobile phase system, pH control of the mobile phases, and detection wavelength. In the following sections, we shall first discuss the method parameters that affect the excipient background, followed by the contribution of excipients and their impurities to the background, and finally, excipient-control strategies. The excipients used in the discussion are listed in Table 14.1.

TABLE 14.1 Excipient Function Class, Unit Percentage Weight, Names and Nominal Individual-Excipient-to-Drug (or IE/D) Ratios by Assuming a Formulation Unit of 200 mg Total Weight, Containing 10 μg API

Class	Common Name	Abbreviation	Nominal IE/D Ratio (at Upper End of Range)
Binder (1–6%)	Hydroxyl propyl cellulose	HPC	1200 : 1
	Hydroxyl propyl methyl cellulose	HPMC	1200 : 1
	Maltodextrin lycatab DSH	MLDSH	1200 : 1
	Povidone	Povidone	1200 : 1
Disintegrant (1–6%)	Crospovidone XL	CXL	1200 : 1
	Sodium croscarmellose	SCC	1200 : 1
	Sodium starch glycolate	SSG	1200 : 1
Filler (50–99%)	Dibasic calcium phosphate	DCP	19800 : 1
	Lactose	Lactose	19800 : 1
	Mannitol	Mannitol	19800 : 1
	Microcrystalline cellulose	MCC	19800 : 1
	Starch with silicone	SWS	19800 : 1
Film former (10–40%)	Acacia	Acacia	8000 : 1
	Eudragit® EPO	Eudragit® EPO	8000 : 1
	Hydroxyl propyl cellulose	HPC	8000 : 1
	Hydroxyl propyl methyl cellulose	HPMC	8000 : 1
	Hydroxypropyl methylcellulose acetate succinate	HPMCAS	8000 : 1
	Sucrose NF (a coating binder)	Sucrose NF	8000 : 1
Lipids/PEG (50–99%)	Captex	Captex	19800 : 1
	Gelucire 44/14	Gelucire	19800 : 1
	Labrasol	Labrasol	19800 : 1
	Poly ethylene glycol 3350	PEG3350	19800 : 1
	Vitamin E TPGS	VE	19800 : 1
Lubricant/glidant (0.5–1%)	Colloidal silicon dioxide	CSD	200 : 1
	Magnesium stearate	MS	200 : 1
	Stearic acid	SA	200 : 1
	Talc	Talc	200 : 1
Pellet core (20–90%)	Cellets	Cellets	18000 : 1
	Non-pareil beads	NPB	18000 : 1
	Sugar spheres	SS	18000 : 1
Plasticizer (1–10%)	Glycerin	Glycerin	2000 : 1
	Poly ethylene glycol 400	PEG 400	2000 : 1
	Propylene glycol	PG	2000 : 1
Surfactant (0.5–1%)	Cremorphor 35	Cremorphor 35	200 : 1
	Sodium lauryl sulfate	SLS	200 : 1
	Tween 80	Tween 80	200 : 1

14.3.1 Effect of Mobile Phase System

Figure 14.2 shows the chromatograms of excipients commonly used as binders, obtained using mobile phase systems containing either phosphate buffer/acetonitrile (ACN) (Fig. 14.2a) or phosphate buffer/methanol (MeOH) (Fig. 14.2b). The pH of the phosphate buffer used in both mobile phase systems was maintained at pH 2.0, and data were collected at 210 nm which is the cut-off wavelength of a MeOH-containing mobile phase. The effect of mobile phase system on chromatographic background can be demonstrated by examining the chromatographic behavior of two excipients. The first one involves hydroxyl propyl cellulose (HPC) (see Table 14.1 for abbreviations). Using the phosphate buffer–ACN mobile phase system (Fig. 14.1a), HPC exhibits a significant hump in the chromatogram between

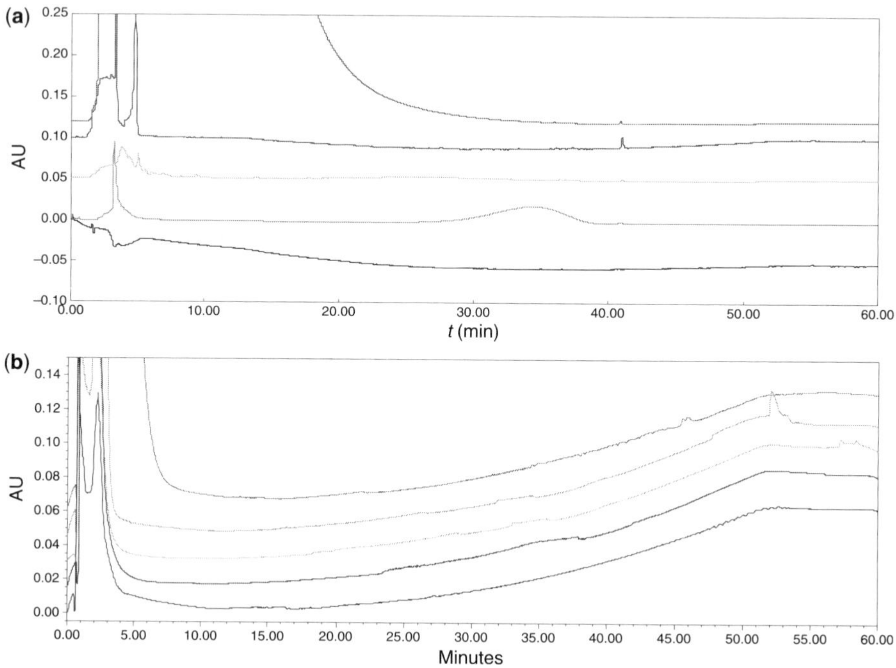

Figure 14.2 Chromatograms of excipients in binder class in different mobile phase systems. In both plots, the curves from the bottom are blank, HPC, HPMC, MLDSH and povidone, respectively. The sample solvent and mobile phase used are (a) 20% ACN–80% pH 2, 25 mM phosphate buffer and a gradient from 30% ACN–70% pH 2, 25 mM phosphate buffer to 80% ACN–20% pH 2, 25 mM phosphate buffer, respectively; and (b) 20% MeOH–80% pH 2, 25 mM phosphate buffer and a gradient from 30% MeOH–70% pH 2, 25 mM phosphate buffer to 80% MeOH–20% pH 2, 25 mM phosphate buffer, respectively. In both cases, samples were injected at 1800 μL onto a Zorbax SB-C_8, 4.6 × 150 mm, 3.5 μm column at 35°C with a flow rate of 1 mL/min. The detection was at 210 nm. An on-bench examination of the mixture of 80% ACN–20% pH 2, 25 mM phosphate buffer revealed no precipitation, so it was suitable as the mobile phase.

30 and 40 min, which is absent when a phosphate buffer–MeOH mobile phase is used (Fig. 14.2b). The other example is the excipient povidone. The large, broad solvent front for povidone in the phosphate buffer–ACN system becomes significantly smaller when the phosphate buffer–MeOH system is used. In both cases, the material used, that is, HPC or povidone, was from the same manufacturer and the same lot. While the cause for such mobile phase-dependent behavior of the excipients was not investigated (it is possibly attributed to a conformation change of the polymeric molecules in different solvent environment), these examples demonstrate that the choice of mobile phase influences the chromatographic background. Therefore, by properly selecting the mobile phase, excipient background can be minimized. Unlike for HPC and povidone, the chromatographic background for many excipients, such as maltodextrin lycatab DSH (MLDSH), is not affected by mobile phase system used.

14.3.2 Effect of Mobile Phase pH

Mobile phase pH can have significant impact on the chromatographic background as well. This is illustrated in Fig. 14.3. At low pH (Fig. 14.3a), numerous excipients display considerable disturbance in the chromatographic background, causing significant challenges to analytical method development. However, most of the disturbance either disappears or is remarkably reduced at high pH (Fig. 14.3b), making the use of these excipients possible. The pH-dependent excipient background is more or less expected, because most excipients possess polar groups in their structure,[26] which are subject to pH change. Consequently, pH change could potentially lead to a change in excipient's physical–chemical properties, such as solubility, protonation or hydrogen-bonding state, which could in turn lead to a change in UV absorption. For example, it is well known that Eudragit® Type E excipients, including Eudragit® E PO used in this study, are polymers of dimethylaminoethyl methacrylate, and the dimethylaminoethyl groups can be protonated under acidic condition, forming polycations.[27,28] A turbidity acid–base titration showed poly-[*n*-butyl methacrylate-(2-dimethylaminoethyl)-methacrylate-methyl methacrylate] copolymer with ratio 1 : 2 : 1 was water-soluble in acidic conditions up to pH 6.0.[27] This indicates that at pH 2 and pH 7, Eudragit® E PO might be present in two different protonation states, which could lead to the pH-dependent chromatographic behavior of Eudragit® E PO as shown in Fig. 14.3a, b. Nevertheless, like the mobile phase system, pH of the mobile phase can be an effective parameter in controlling excipient background.

14.3.3 Effect of Detection Wavelength

For most excipients, chromatographic background is more significant at lower detection wavelengths. At low wavelengths, for example, 210 nm, the significant background introduced by HPC, povidone, and EPO is obvious, making them undesirable excipients from an analytical perspective (data not shown). However, if the method can adopt a higher detection wavelength, for example, 280 nm, the background becomes negligible, and all the excipients can be used without concern. As a

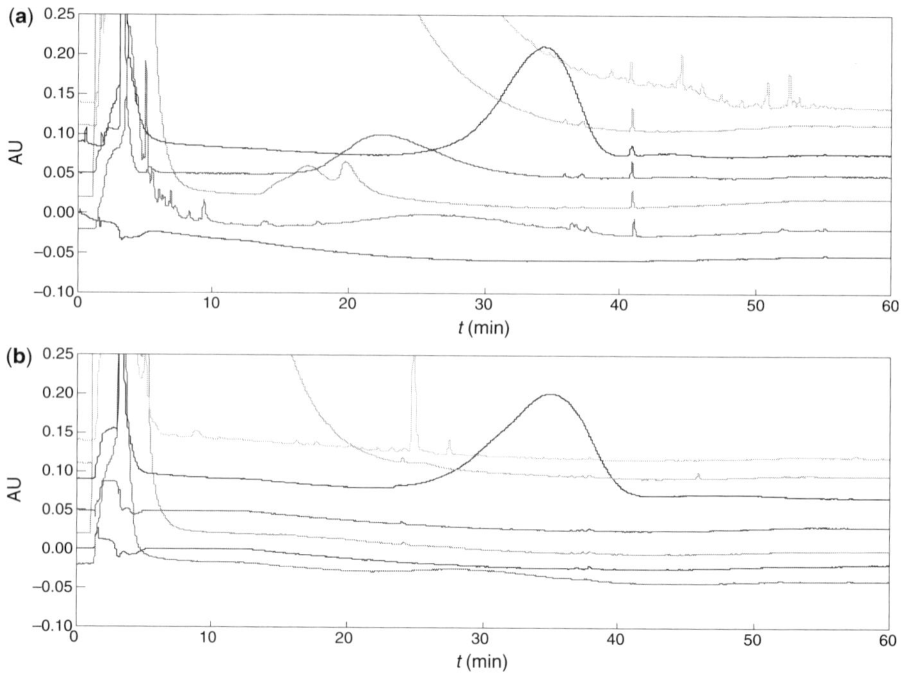

Figure 14.3 Chromatograms of excipients in film-former class under different mobile phase pH. In both plots, the curves from the bottom are blank, HPMC, acacia, sucrose NF, HPC, povidone and Eudragit® EPO, respectively. The sample solvent, mobile phase and column used are (a) 20% ACN–80% pH 2, 25 mM phosphate buffer, a gradient from 30% ACN–70% pH 2, 25 mM phosphate buffer to 80% ACN–20% pH 2, 25 mM phosphate buffer and a Zorbax SB-C8, 4.6 × 150 mm, 3.5 μm column at 35°C, respectively; and (b) 20% ACN–80% pH 7, 25 mM phosphate buffer, a gradient from 30% ACN–70% pH 7, 25 mM phosphate buffer to 80% ACN–20% pH 7, 25 mM phosphate buffer and a Zorbax XDB-C_8, 4.6 × 150 mm, 3.5 μm column at 35°C, respectively. In both cases, samples were injected at 1800 μL, the flow rate of mobile phase was 1 mL/min and the detection was at 210 nm. An on-bench examination of the mixture of either 80% ACN–20% pH 2, 25 mM phosphate buffer or 80% ACN–20% pH 7, 25 mM phosphate buffer revealed no precipitation, so they were suitable as the mobile phase.

general rule, high detection wavelength is preferable, provided that it is adequate for the intended use of the method.

The effect of HPLC method parameters on the excipient background has been described. It should be recognized that excipients themselves can also have an impact on the background, as will be illustrated in the next sections.

14.3.4 Excipient Types and Quantity Used

Depending on the class of excipients and quantity used in a formulation, the impact of an excipient on chromatographic background can be quite different. On one hand, binders, film formers, lipids, and surfactants display significant background absorbance, especially in a phosphate buffer–ACN system at low pH. In addition to what was illustrated in Figs. 14.2 and 14.3, Fig. 14.4a shows the chromatograms of excipients commonly used as surfactants. All of the surfactants generate background disturbance between 28–48 min in the chromatograms, which may cause concerns for impurity analyses at a low-dose. On the other hand, disintegration agents, fillers, lubricants, pellet core, and plasticizers generally exhibit negligible impact on the background. This is true in both phosphate buffer–ACN and phosphate buffer–MeOH systems at either low or high pH. Figure 14.4b shows the chromatograms of fillers displaying very limited background interference in comparison with those of surfactants due to the latter's greater UV absorption. It is interesting to note from Table 14.1 that the quantity of the fillers used in generating Fig. 14.4b is about 99 times greater than that of the surfactants shown in Fig. 14.4a. As expected, the background of an excipient is proportional to the quantity used (cf. HPC quantity used in generating Fig. 14.3a is six times more than that in Fig. 14.2a). Therefore,

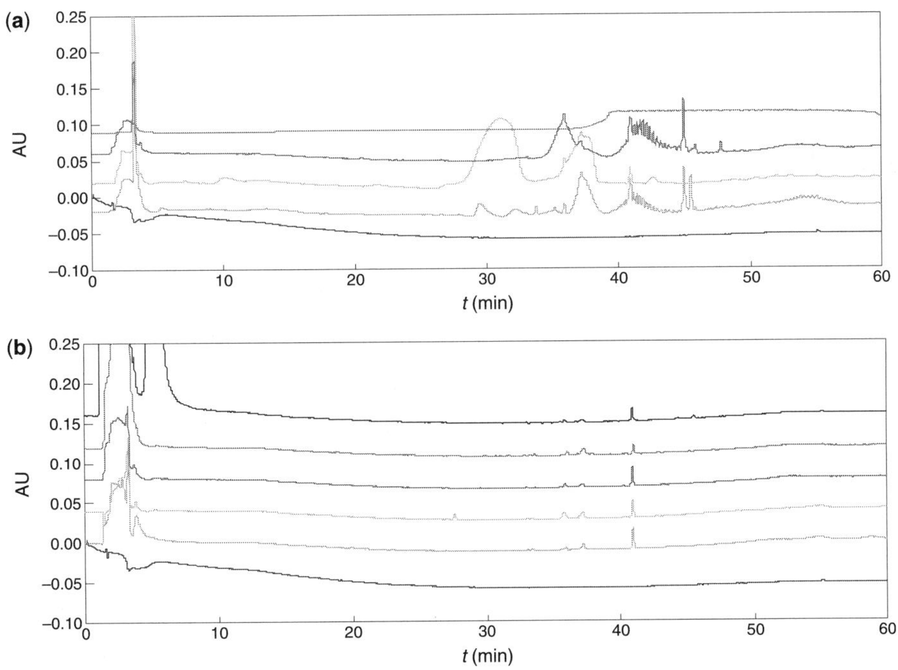

Figure 14.4 Chromatograms of excipients in different classes. Plot (a) represents excipients in surfactant class. The curves from the bottom are blank, cremorphor 35, SLS, Tween 80 and VE, respectively. Plot (b) represents excipients in the filler class. The curves from the bottom are blank, DCP, lactose, mannitol, MCC and SWS, respectively. In both plots, the sample solvent and mobile phase used are 20% ACN–80% pH 2, 25 mM phosphate buffer and a gradient from 30% ACN–70% pH 2, 25 mM phosphate buffer to 80% ACN–20% pH 2, 25 mM phosphate buffer, respectively. The samples were injected at 1800 μL onto a Zorbax SB-C_8, 4.6 × 150 mm, 3.5 μm column at 35°C with a flow rate of 1 mL/min. The detection was at 210 nm.

the least amount of an excipient should be used, providing a successful formulation is achievable.

14.3.5 Excipient Source and Lot-to-Lot Variability

A study was conducted to evaluate the chromatograms of microcrystalline cellulose (MCC) obtained from different suppliers and different lots from the same supplier using phosphate buffer–MeOH mobile phase at pH 2.0 and 7.0, respectively, and a detection wavelength of 210 nm. Based on this limited data, the background differences of MCC from different suppliers or different lots are quite negligible. The disruption in the chromatographic traces observed is likely instrument-related, since it is also seen in the blank. Variability between manufacturers and lots could be better seen for excipients with stronger background absorbance. Understanding the impact of excipient sources and lot-to-lot variability on the chromatographic background helps establish an effective excipient control strategy. Therefore, further collection of data on this subject needs to be continued.

14.3.6 Consideration in Excipient Control Strategies

To control excipient effect on chromatographic background, both the excipient itself and the impurities within the excipient need to be considered. As noted earlier, excipients typically appear chromatographically as a broad solvent front or hump. These characteristics are relatively well-defined, and therefore, the interference can be either eliminated or minimized through optimizing HPLC method parameters. In cases where the interference persists (e.g., the hump in HPC chromatogram traces in Fig. 14.2a), analyte peaks may still be quantifiable, because they are usually sharp enough to be reliably integrated using the broad hump as baseline.

In comparison, it is more difficult dealing with excipient impurities. These impurities may result from processing and/or degradation of the excipients, or even from degradation of the impurities themselves. A list of potential impurities in common excipients is provided in literature[29] and summarized in Table 14.2. For a given excipient, its process impurity profile can easily vary from manufacturer to manufacturer and even lot to lot. Such variations may be detected by a sensitive analytical method used for analyzing low-dose formulations and may show certain degree of interference with the analysis. An analytical method previously deemed adequate in separation may suddenly become inadequate due to a change in excipient source. Therefore, the method specificity should be re-evaluated every time a new lot or new source of excipients is involved. From a practical point of view, in early phase development, it is desirable to plan and source sufficient supply of excipients once a unit formula is finalized. However, in late phase product development when a development decision on a compound is made, due diligence should be performed in terms of excipient suppliers and lot-to-lot variability to ensure development of a robust analytical method. Regarding the degradation impurities, the best approach to minimize issues is through proper selection of excipients up front. From this

TABLE 14.2 Residual Impurities Carried Through Common Excipients

Excipient	Residuals
Poly vinyl propylene (PVP), Polysorbates, benzyl alcohol	Peroxides
Magnesium stearate, fixed oils, paraffins	Antioxidants
Lactose	Aldehydes, reducing sugars
Benzyl alcohol	Benzaldehyde
Polyethylene glycol	Aldehydes, peroxides, organic acids
Microcrystalline cellulose (MCC)	Lignin, hemicelluloses

standpoint, understanding chemical properties of the excipients and the impurities, as given in Table 14.2, can be beneficial.

Many interactions between active pharmaceutical ingredients and excipient impurities are well understood. For example, small-molecule drugs containing primary, secondary, or tertiary amino groups have a propensity to interact with formic acid, its esters, and/or formaldehyde, a common residual impurity present in excipients such as polysorbate, povidone, and polyethylene glycol 300.[30,31] Formaldehyde is susceptible to partial conversion to formic acid on contact with air. In addition, formic acid may be present as an ester in excipients that have hydroxyl groups or alcohol impurities. Therefore, these impurities may coexist in excipients. Also, low levels of nonsaccharide organic residues present in microcrystallince cellulose, originating from lignin, may degrade to form free radicals,[32] potentially interacting with the excipients. In summary, selecting appropriate excipients up front can be an effective way in controlling excipient impurities.

14.4 USE OF EXCIPIENT LIBRARY

14.4.1 Excipient Screening Using the Library

As mentioned earlier, the purpose of the excipient library is to minimize excipient-related analytical challenges in low-dose drug product development. Having this in mind, formulation and analytical scientists can work together during the formulation design stage to identify a formulation that not only satisfies the formulation requirements in drug-product processing and performance, but also helps address analytical challenges. For instance, if two or more excipients in the same formulation functional class are acceptable from the perspective of formulation processing and performance, priority in selection of the excipients should be given to those with minimal chromatographic background. Let us say in developing a high-shear wet granulation for capsule or tablet, both povidone and HPMC may be utilized as a binder. The preference should be given to HPMC because of its minimal excipient background in both water–ACN and water–MeOH mobile phase systems (Fig. 14.2). If povidone must be used, the analytical method would need to use a water–MeOH mobile phase

TABLE 14.3 Excipients, Quantity and Individual Excipient-to-Drug (IE/D) Ratios in a Hypothetical Unit of Formulation in Comparison to Nominal Excipient-to-Drug Ratios

Material	Quantity, mg	Hypo IE/D Ratio	Nominal IE/D Ratio	Hypo/Nominal
API	0.01	NA	NA	NA
Lactose	171.99	17,199 : 1	19800 : 1	0.87
HPC	6	600 : 1	1200 : 1	0.50
SLS	1	100 : 1	200 : 1	0.50
MCC	20	2000 : 1	19800 : 1	0.10
MS	1	100 : 1	200 : 1	0.50
Total	200	20000 : 1	NA	NA

system buffered at either low or neutral pH. Based on the information in the library, these selections allow minimal excipient background.

14.4.2 Prediction of Placebo Chromatographic Background

All excipient background information is collected and stored electronically. This allows a user to access the data, manipulate the background traces based on the individual-excipient-to-drug ratio in use, and make a prediction of the background to assess any potential issues for analytical development. For example, assume a formulation containing API and excipients at unit quantities as outlined in Table 14.3. Based on the quantity information, one can easily calculate the hypothetical individual excipient-to-drug ratio for each of the excipients. Nominal individual excipient-to-drug ratios are listed from Table 14.1. By comparing the ratios, multipliers are obtained. Then, the data for relevant excipient background traces stored

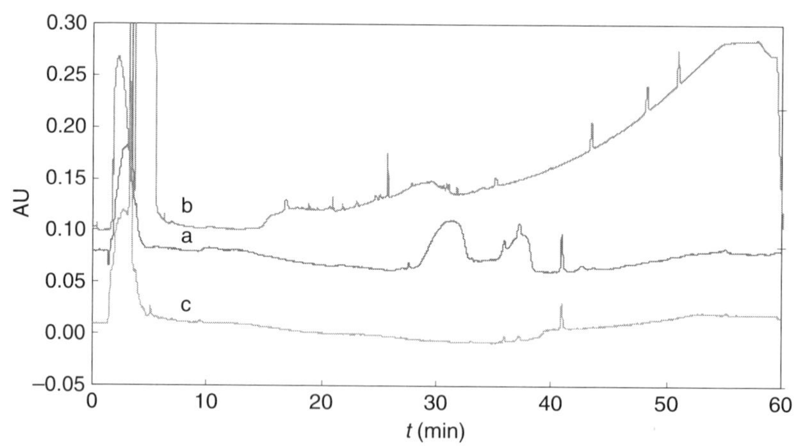

Figure 14.5 Chromatograms of either a placebo containing HPC, lactose, MCC, MS, and SLS, and predicted using the library and obtained from a historical run (curves a and b, respectively), or a placebo consisting of HPMC, mannitol, MCC, SA and VE, and predicted using the library (curve c).

TABLE 14.4 A Proposed, Optimal Formulation for Analytical Method Development

Material	Quantity, mg	Hypo IE/D Ratio	Nominal IE/D Ratio	Hypo/Nominal
API	0.01	NA	NA	NA
Mannitol	171.99	17199 : 1	19800 : 1	0.87
HPMC	6	600 : 1	1200 : 1	0.50
VE	1	100 : 1	200 : 1	0.50
MCC	20	2000 : 1	19800 : 1	0.10
SA	1	100 : 1	200 : 1	0.50
Total	200	20000 : 1	NA	NA

in the library can be multiplied to reflect the excipient background at this hypothetical excipient-to-drug ratio. Following this methodology, a simulated overall excipient background trace of a placebo containing the excipients specified in Table 14.3 is acquired [see Fig. 14.5, curve (a)]. Figure 14.5, curve (b) is a historically measured trace of a real placebo sample of the same formulation. Although the two traces are not quite identical, possibly due to the differences in HPLC conditions (see the figure caption for detailed conditions), or material source, the basic characteristics are similar. The double humps resulting from a combination of SLS and HPC, as shown in curve (b), are stretched in curve (a), and of comparable magnitude. Several sharp minor peaks in curve (a) are not seen in curve (b), indicating a possible difference in excipient impurity profile. Interestingly, by optimizing the excipient choice utilizing the library, a proposed, optimal formulation could be obtained that exhibits much clearer background [Fig. 14.5, curve (c)]. The excipient information of the proposed formulation is given in Table 14.4.

14.5 CONCLUSIONS

Analytical and formulation development for low-dose drug products can be very challenging, due to the high excipient-to-drug ratio and analyses at ultra-trace levels. The presence of significant excipient background interference often decreases the capability of analyzing drug-related impurities. Case-by-case resolution of such interference can be time-consuming and labor-intensive. To better address these difficulties, an excipient library approach is proposed and proves to be effective. Based on this approach, excipient background is minimized at the design/planning phase of formulation development, which helps reduce difficulties encountered during analytical development.

ACKNOWLEDGMENTS

The authors are grateful to a number of colleagues at Eli Lilly and Company, including Drs Bernard Olsen and Steven Maple for their encouragement and general discussion, Dr Jack Zheng for extensive discussion on the Excipient Library concept and approach, Ms Li Liu for discussion on drug–excipient interaction, Dr Duane Pierson and Jeanette Buckwalter for kindly reading the manuscript and providing grammatical corrections, and Drs Timothy Wozniak and Paul Wright for technically reviewing the manuscript.

REFERENCES

1. International Conference on the Harmonization of the Technical Requirements for Registration of Pharmaceuticals for Human Use (ICH). 2003. Q3B (R2) Impurities in New Drug Products; February.
2. LaCourse WR, Dasenbrock CO. 1998. Column liquid chromatography: equipment and instrumentation. Anal. Chem. 70: 37R–52R.
3. Baumann W. Practical aspects of modern high performance liquid chromatography. In: Molnar I, editor. New York: Walter de Gruyter.
4. Niessen WMA. 1999. State-of-the-art in liquid chromatography–mass spectrometry. J. Chromatogr. A 856: 477–501.
5. Reemtsma T. 2003. Liquid chromatography–mass spectrometry and strategies for trace-level analysis of polar organic pollutants. J. Chromatogr. A 1000: 477–501.
6. Hensley K, Williamson KS, Maidt ML, Gabbita SP, Grammas P, Floyd RA. 1999. Determination of biological oxidative stress using high performance liquid chromatography with electrochemical detection (HPLC-ECD). J. High Resol. Chromatogr. 22: 429–437.
7. Inoue K, Kato K, Yoshimura Y, Makino T, Nakazawa H. 2000. Determination of bisphenol A in human serum by high-performance liquid chromatography with multielectrode electrochemical detection. J. Chromatogr. B 746: 17–23.
8. Yamaguchi M, Yoshida H, Nohta H. 2002. Luminol-type chemiluminescence derivatization reagents for liquid chromatography and capillary electrophoresis. J. Chromatogr. A 950: 1–19.
9. Todoroki K, Hayama T, Ijiri S, Kazuta A, Yoshida H, Nohta H, Yamaguchi M. 2004. Rhodamine B amine as a highly sensitive fluorescence derivatization reagent for saccharides in reversed-phase liquid chromatography. J. Chromatogr. A 1038: 113–120.
10. Gilpin RK, Gilpin CS. 2007. Pharmaceuticals and related drugs. Anal. Chem. 79: 4275–4294.
11. Rao RN, Nagaraju V. 2003. An overview of the recent trends in development of HPLC methods for determination of impurities in drugs. Journal of Pharmaceutical and Biomedical Analysis 33: 335–377.
12. Hernández F, Hidalgo C, Sancho JV, López FJ. 1997. New method for the rapid determination of triazine herbicides and some of their main metabolites in water by using coupled-column liquid chromatography and large volume injection. J. Chromatogr. A 778: 171–181.
13. Broquaire M, Guinebault PR. 1981. Large-volume injection of biological samples dissolved in a noneluting solvent: a way to increase sensitivity and a means of automating drug determination using HPLC. J. Liq. Chromatogr. 4: 2039–2061.
14. Ahuja S, Scypinski S, editors. 2001. Handbook of modern pharmaceutical analysis. San Diego, CA: Academic Press.
15. Niazi SK, editor. 2004. Handbook of pharmaceutical manufacturing formulations. Volume 3: Liquid products. Boca Raton, FL: CRC Press.

16. Nygaard L, Kilde HD, Andersen SG, Henriksen L, Overby V. 2004. Development and validation of a reversed-phase liquid chromatographic method for analysis of degradation products of estradiol in Vagifem® tablets. J. Pharm. Biomed. Anal. 34: 265–276.
17. Dolan JW. 2007. How little can I see? LCGC North America 25: 142–152.
18. Forget R, Spagnoli S. 2006. Excipient quantitation and drug distribution during formulation optimization. J. Pharm. Biomed. Anal. 41: 1051–1055.
19. Platzer DJ, White BA. 2006. Development and validation of a gradient HPLC method for the determination of clindamycin and related compounds in a novel tablet formulation. J. Pharm. Biomed. Anal. 41: 84–88.
20. Ciutaru D, Badea I, Lazar L, Nicolescu D, Tudose A. 2004. A HPLC validated assay of paclitaxel's related impurities in pharmaceutical forms containing Cremophor® EL. J. Pharm. Biomed. Anal. 34: 493–499.
21. Wikipedia, The Free Encyclopedia: Paclitaxel. Wikimedia Foundation, Inc. Available at http://en.wikipedia.org/wiki/Taxol. Accessed on 11 August, 2007.
22. Erturk S, Aktas ES, Ersoy L, Fıcıcıoglu S. 2003. An HPLC method for the determination of atorvastatin and its impurities in bulk drug and tablets. J. Pharm. Biomed. Anal. 33: 1017–1023.
23. Jabera AMY, Sherifeb HAAl, Omarib MMAl, Badwanb AA. 2004. Determination of cetirizine dihydrochloride, related impurities and preservatives in oral solution and tablet dosage forms using HPLC. J. Pharm. Biomed. Anal. 36: 341–350.
24. Matysova L, Solich P, Marek P, Havlıkova L, Novakova L, Sıcha J. 2006. Separation and determination of terbinafine and its four impurities of similar structure using simple RP-HPLC method. Talanta 68: 713–720.
25. Ringo MC, Allen JR, Mattocks DM. 2003. Mobile-phase cleanup using solid-phase extraction disks. LCGC North America 21: 168–178.
26. Bugay DE, Findlay WP. 1999. Pharmaceutical excipients. Characterization by IR, Raman and NMR spectroscopy. New York: Marcel Dekker.
27. Moustafine RI, Zaharov IM, Kemenova VA. 2006. Physicochemical characterization and drug release properties of Eudragit® E PO/Eudragitw L 100-55 interpolyelectrolyte complexes. Eur. J. Pharm. Biopharm. 63: 26–36.
28. Specifications and test methods for EUDRAGIT® E 100, EUDRAGIT® E PO and EUDRAGIT® E 12,5. Specification 2004; Röhm GmbH & Co. KG, Pharma Polymers, Degussa.
29. Crowley PJ, Martini LG. 2002. Excipients for pharmaceutical dosage forms, encyclopedia of pharmaceutical technology. New York: Marcel Dekker.
30. del Barrio MA, Hu J, Zhou P, Cauchon N. 2006. Simultaneous determination of formic acid and formaldehyde in pharmaceutical excipients using headspace GC/MS. J. Pharm. Biomed. Anal. 41: 738–743.
31. Nassar MN, Nesarikar VN, Lozano R, Parker WL, Yande P, Palaniswamy V, Xu W, Khaselev N. 2004. Influence of formaldehyde impurity in polysorbate 80 and PEG-300 on the stability of a parenteral formulation of BMS-204352: identification and control of the degradation. Product Pharm. Dev. 9: 189–195.
32. Lewis NG, Davin LB, Sarkanen S. 1999. The nature and function of lignins: comprehensive natural products chemistry. In: Pinto BM, editor. Pergamon Press: Oxford; Chapter 18; 3.

CHAPTER 15

CLEANING VERIFICATION FOR HIGHLY POTENT COMPOUNDS

BRIAN W. PACK
Analytical Sciences R&D, Lilly Research Laboratories, Eli Lilly and Company, Indianapolis, IN 46285

15.1 INTRODUCTION

When considering cleaning verification activities for highly potent compounds, there is very little guidance provided as to the lower safety acceptance limit that should be considered. The Code of Federal Regulations PART 211—Current Good Manufacturing Practice for Finished Pharmaceuticals Subpart D—Equipment Section 211.67 on equipment cleaning and maintenance states that "Equipment and utensils shall be cleaned, maintained, and sanitized at appropriate intervals to prevent malfunctions or contamination that would alter the safety, identity, strength, quality, or purity of the drug product beyond the official or other established requirements." And that "written procedures shall be established and followed for cleaning and maintenance of equipment, including utensils, used in the manufacture, processing, packing, or holding of a drug product."[1] There is intentionally no mention of acceptance limits that should be considered; it is up to the manufacturer to document the cleaning rationale (process and acceptance limits) that maintains the quality and purity of the subsequent drug product being manufactured. In accordance with 21 CFR 211.67, the International Conference on Harmonization (ICH) has issued recommendations on Equipment Maintenance and Cleaning (Q7A, Sections 5.20–5.26) for compliance and safety that include very similar requirements with more elaboration on specific details.[2] Again, there is a reiteration that written procedures shall be established and that detailed cleaning agent selection and preparation, responsibilities, schedules, and cleaning acceptance limits be documented with rationale. All of which are outlined in order to prevent cross contamination between different manufactured lots. This cross-contamination concern applies not only to the active pharmaceutical ingredient; it also applies to residual cleaning

Formulation and Analytical Development for Low-Dose Oral Drug Products. Edited by Jack Zheng

solvents and detergents. The requirement again states that cleaning acceptance limits must be documented. The ICH Q7A, Good Manufacturing Practice Guide for Active Pharmaceutical Ingredients, goes on to say (Section 12.78 Cleaning Validation/ Section 12.81 Validation of Analytical Methods) that analytical methods should be validated in accordance with ICH, Q2 (R1) guideline on Analytical Methods[3] and that the methods should:

1. exhibit sensitivity to detect residues or contaminants;
2. establish sufficient detection limits to detect the acceptable level of the residue or contaminant;
3. establish the attainable recovery level;
4. have residue limits that are practical, achievable, verifiable and based on the most deleterious residue;
5. and have limits based on the minimum known pharmacological, toxicological, or physiological activity of the API or its most deleterious component.[2]

Point number 4 above states that residue limits should be "practical, achievable, and verifiable based on the most deleterious residue." In the case of potent compounds, it is generally the compound itself that would be the most deleterious residue. The philosophical argument around this requirement is focused on the word "practical." Analytical chemists would agree in principle that almost any amount can be detected, but the question is at what cost (time, extravagant sample preparation, or expensive instrumentation). Therefore, the word "practical" can come to mean something different depending upon perspective, phase of development, etc. To some it means, whatever is possible no matter the cost. To others, it may mean that as long as the method to determine residue limits is documented and the limits can be satisfied by the analytical method, then it is practical. The problem arises because there are several different ways to calculate an acceptable residue level that will provide drastically different acceptance values based upon known pharmacological activity and toxicological properties. These different methods to calculate acceptance limits will be presented in this chapter along with analytical methodologies that can meet the most stringent of the requirements. In addition, cleaning validation and cleaning verification will be discussed.

15.2 CLEANING VALIDATION VS CLEANING VERIFICATION

In the pharmaceutical manufacturing/packaging process, it is important to ensure the production equipment is properly cleaned in order to avoid cross-contamination of drug products.[4] The removal of drug residues is typically conducted by a series of cleaning procedures that can include acidic, basic, and detergent based cleaners. Two approaches can be utilized to demonstrate control and understanding of the cleaning process: (1) cleaning validation and (2) cleaning verification.

Cleaning validation is an extensive, multifunctional program where the entire manufacturing process is considered from the equipment that will be used to the analytical method that will be used to evaluate cleaning effectiveness.[5] Cleaning validation starts with the generation of a validation protocol. The validation protocol would include rationales in regards to cleaning agents and procedures,[6] equipment, equipment swabbing locations,[7] safety-based acceptance limits, selection of products used to demonstrate validation,[5,8] and validated analytical methodology.

When selecting representative products to validate a cleaning program, several approaches have been presented.[5,8] The most conservative approach would be to validate the cleaning procedure for all compounds manufactured. However, this approach is expensive, resource-consuming and is not typically practical. Therefore, manufacturing facilities may choose to validate on a subset of compounds and examine such parameters as solubility, potency (e.g., 1/1000 method), lot sizes (e.g., the 10 ppm method), toxicology (e.g., the Threshold of Toxicological Concern method), and cleanability.

Cleaning verification is confirmed at the completion of each manufacture (typically by submission of cleaning swabs or rinse solutions to the analytical laboratories) to demonstrate that the active pharmaceutical ingredient has been removed to a level below the preestablished acceptance limit. A cleaning verification program confirms the effectiveness of those cleaning procedures typically during phase I and phase II clinical trials; throughout these phases, analytical measurements provide a high degree of assurance that the target drug residue is below the safety acceptance criteria. In a manufacturing environment, cleaning validation is typically performed where verification is performed at predefined intervals.

For both cleaning verification and validation, the number of swabbing locations and swabbing sites are dictated by the product contact surface area (e.g., larger components may require a larger number of swabbing sites), energy dissipation (e.g., roller compaction or tablet pressing regions are more likely to accumulate product), composition of the product contact areas (i.e., polycarbonate vs stainless steel), and cleaning difficulty (tight corners, bends, and hard to reach places result in hard to clean locations that should be swabbed).[7] Again, a documented rationale is expected to exist in order to justify the swabbing strategy that included both the location and number of swabs to be taken.

15.3 ACCEPTANCE LIMIT CALCULATIONS

When determining the acceptance limit, a strong scientific rationale with relevant factors generally includes: (1) evaluation of the therapeutic dose of the actives; (2) toxicity of the potential contaminant; (3) solubility of the potential residue; (4) difficulty of cleaning; (5) visual examination; (6) the batch size of the subsequent products on the same equipment; and (7) how the product will be used.[9] Acceptance limit calculations take on the general form where two methods are typically used. Although some authors recommend adjusting the safety factor depending upon the dosage form,[9] it is most common to utilize the 1/1000th minimum dose and 10 ppm methods.[10–14] Recently, a third approach has been proposed based upon the application toxicological concern.[15] All approaches will be discussed in detail below.

The 1/1000th method assumes that pharmaceuticals are often considered to be nonactive at 0.1% of their normally prescribed dosages.[14] The following equation demonstrates how an acceptance limit is calculated utilizing the 1/1000th method:

$$\text{Acceptance limit}\left(\frac{\mu\text{g}}{\text{swab}}\right) = \frac{0.001\ \text{smallest strength product A (mg/day)}}{\text{Maximum daily no. of dosage units product B (units/day)}} \times \frac{\text{Lot size product B (no. of dosage units)}}{\text{Shared surface area (cm}^2\text{ or in}^2\text{)}} \times \frac{\text{Swab area (cm}^2\text{ or in}^2\text{)}}{1\ \text{swab}} \times \frac{1000\ \mu\text{g}}{1\ \text{mg}} \times RF \quad (15.1)$$

where RF represents the recovery factor established during analytical method validation. Typical ranges for RF are between 0.5 and 0.9; however a lower RF may be acceptable with justification. Utilization of the 1/1000th principle takes into account that in a multiproduct facility a typical dosage form (>10 mg/unit) may be manufactured after a potent compound (<0.1 mg/unit). This method of calculating an acceptable residue focuses on how much of lot A will end up in each subsequent dosage form and ultimately consumed by the patient taking clinical trial lot B. Depending upon the phase of development, the lot size may be small, there may be a small shared surface area in the manufacturing area, or the products may have an unoptimized formulation (multiple dosage forms taken/day). As with all methods of determining the acceptable residue that can remain after the manufacture of product A, it is assumed that the contaminant will be evenly distributed throughout the subsequent lot of material as opposed to the entire contamination going into one tablet or capsule.

The second method uses the 10 ppm limit historically used to calculate commercial manufacturing limits. This method allows the maximum carryover of product A to be calculated using lot sizes and shared equipment surface area, regardless of the potency of the prior lot. The formula below shows the method used to develop the 10 ppm acceptance limits:

$$\text{Acceptance limit}\left(\frac{\mu\text{g}}{\text{swab}}\right) = \frac{10\ \text{mg}}{1\ \text{kg}} \times \frac{\text{Lot size product B (kg)}}{\text{Shared surface area (cm}^2\text{ or in}^2\text{)}} \times \frac{\text{Swab area (cm}^2\text{ or in}^2\text{)}}{1\ \text{swab}} \times \frac{1000\ \mu\text{g}}{1\ \text{mg}} \times RF \quad (15.2)$$

The 10 ppm method delivers a somewhat conservative estimate in cases where the potency of product A is low and the lot size of product B is small. It is obvious from Eq. (15.2) that two variables drive the acceptance limit; the lot size of product B and the shared surface area. Of importance to note is that the potency of lot A is not considered in this calculation. For example, if the shared equipment surface area is constant between two drug product manufactures and the lot size for product B is 50 kg as opposed to 100 kg, the acceptance limit would be calculated to be half of that of the 100 kg lot size. An important aspect of the 10 ppm method is that it is independent of the potency or number of dosage units of either product A or product B. This calculation merely limits the absolute amount of product in A that can carry over to product B and be distributed evenly throughout all of the dosage forms in the second manufacture. Again, the acceptance limit in the ppm method is driven by lot size (kg) and shared surface area of the equipment.

A third approach utilizes the concept of threshold of toxicological concern (TTC); this approach is an extension of setting acceptable daily intake values (ADI) and establishing permitted daily exposures (PDE) values. This approach has been recently published by Forsyth at Merck and Company.[16] The concept of TTC has been proposed with regards to the control of genotoxic impurities in the active pharmaceutical ingredient.[17] The application of TTC to API control has been accepted by the EMEA (European Medicines Agency) where a TTC value of 1.5 μg/day intake of a genotoxic impurity is considered to be associated with an acceptable risk (i.e., an excess cancer risk of <1 in 100,000 over a lifetime) for most pharmaceuticals. From this threshold value, a permitted level in the active substance can be calculated based on the expected daily dose. The approach proposed by Dolan et al. is a three-tiered approach where compounds that are likely to be carcinogenic would have a limit of 1 μg/day ($<0.8\%$ of compounds known to pharmacologically active),[15,16] compounds that are likely to be potent or highly toxic would have a limit of 10 μg/day, and compounds that are not likely to be highly toxic, carcinogenic, or potent would have a limit of 100 μg/day. The TTC calculation is given in Eq. (15.3):

$$\text{ARL (mg/swab)} = \frac{\text{ADI } (\mu\text{g/day}) \times \text{SBS (kg)} \times \text{SA } (\text{cm}^2/\text{swab}) \times RF \times CF}{\text{MDD (mg/day)} \times \text{SSA } (\text{cm}^2)} \tag{15.3}$$

In this equation ARL is the acceptable residue limit, ADI is the acceptable daily intake, SBS is the smallest batch size, SA is the swab surface area, CF is the conversion factor (1000), MDD is the maximum daily dose of product B, and SSA is the shared surface area. At first glance, this calculation has desirable attributes of both the 10 ppm method and the 1/1000 method. For example, the 1/1000th method and the TTC method take into account the maximum daily dose of product B. Likewise the 10 ppm method and the TTC method take into account the lot size of product B. The main difference between the calculations is that the ADI is justified based upon the toxicological threshold classification in the TTC method; in the 10 ppm and 1/1000th methods it is based upon some general assumptions around potency and the assumed therapeutic potency of general pharmaceutical compounds. However, the TTC approach yields drastically different acceptance limits, driven primarily by a higher ADI based upon toxicologically accepted limits, which is one of the primary considerations outlined in ICH Q7A.[2] This approach would seemingly be much less conservative than the previously illustrated examples, but has single patient exposure built into the calculation.

The regulatory agencies have been very careful not to mandate to manufacturers how to calculate safety acceptance limits. As a result, a clinical trial material manufacturing area may choose any of the outlined approaches to calculate cleaning acceptance limits as long as a supporting rationale is provided. An example is provided where the acceptance limits are calculated by all three methods outlined above. The table below lists the product and equipment characteristics used to calculate the safety acceptance limits for a comparison utilizing the 1/1000th minimum dose, the 10 ppm, and the TTC methods. Example calculations are provided for each method of calculation. Although not realistic to expect 100% recovery from a swabbed surface, *RF* is assumed to be 1.0 for each calculation. All other parameters are outlined in Table 15.1.

1. The 1/1000th method:

$$\text{Acceptance limit}\left(\frac{\mu\text{g}}{\text{swab}}\right) = \frac{0.001 \times 0.01\ (\text{mg/day})}{5\ \text{units/day product B}} \times \frac{\text{Product B (10,000 dosage units)}}{\text{shared surface area } 25{,}000\ \text{cm}^2} \times \frac{\text{Swab area } 25\ \text{cm}^2}{1\ \text{swab}} \times \frac{1000\ \mu\text{g}}{1\ \text{mg}} \times RF$$

1/1000th safety acceptance limit $= 0.02\ \mu\text{g/swab}$.

TABLE 15.1 Lot Size and Dose Strength Assumptions Used for Safety Acceptance Limit Calculations

Product	Lowest Dose Strength (mg/tablet)	Lot Size (kg)	Lot Size (units)	Maximum Daily Dose (units)	Maximum Daily Dose (mg)	Shared Surface Area (cm^2)
A	0.01	20	10,000	1	0.01	NA
B	20	5	10,000	5	100	25,000

2. The 10 ppm method:

$$\text{Acceptance limit}\left(\frac{\mu g}{\text{swab}}\right) = \frac{10\,\text{mg}}{1\,\text{kg}} \times \frac{\text{Lot size product B } 5\,\text{kg}}{\text{Shared surface area } 25{,}000\ \text{cm}^2} \times \frac{\text{Swab area } 25\ \text{cm}^2}{1\ \text{swab}} \times \frac{1000\,\mu\text{g}}{1\,\text{mg}} \times RF$$

10 ppm safety acceptance limit = 0.05 μg/swab.

3. The TTC method:

$$\text{ARL (mg/swab)} = \frac{\text{ADI } (10\,\mu\text{g/day}) \times \text{SBS } (5\,\text{kg}) \times \text{SA } (25\,\text{cm}^2/\text{swab}) \times RF}{\text{MDD product B } (100\,\text{mg/day}) \times \text{SSA } (25{,}000\,\text{cm}^2)}$$

TTC safety acceptance limit = 0.5 μg/swab.

As can be seen from the above results, the acceptance limit will vary among the three methods. In this scenario, the 10 ppm method is 2.5 times higher than the 1/1000th method and the TTC method is an order of magnitude higher than both approaches. With a supporting rationale, all three acceptance limits can be perfectly valid. To further illustrate the differences among the three equations, Table 15.2 was generated to illustrate the impact of the potency of product A on the calculated acceptance limit. All parameters are the same as those outlined in Table 15.1; the strength of product A is varied between 100 and 0.01 mg/tablet. For example, as the potency of product A increases (i.e., active per tablet decreases), the cleaning acceptance limit goes from 200 μg/unit area (100 mg tablet), to 0.02 μg/swab for the 1/1000th method. The acceptance limit of 200 μg/unit area would not be used because it would not pass the standard requirement to be visually clean, which is generally accepted to be 100 μg/unit area, or less; the limit would therefore default to that

TABLE 15.2 Using the Assumptions in Table 15.1 to Calculate Acceptance Limits by the Three Approaches Outlined in the Text

	Product A			
	100 mg/Tablet	1.0 mg/Tablet	0.1 mg/Tablet	0.01 mg/Tablet
1/1000 method Acceptance limit	200 μg/swab	2.0 μg/swab	0.2 μg/swab	0.02 μg/swab
10 ppm method Acceptance limit	0.05 μg/swab	0.05 μg/swab	0.05 μg/swab	0.05 μg/swab
TTC method Acceptance limit (ADI = 10 μg/day)	0.5 μg/swab	0.5 μg/swab	0.5 μg/swab	0.5 μg/swab

value. Of importance to note is that the acceptance limits for both the 10 ppm method and the TTC method remain unchanged across the dose range of product A because the limits provided by those calculations are dictated solely by lot size and daily intake, respectively, with no dependence upon the potency of lot A. In this example, the 10 ppm and the TTC method would probably be considered too stringent for the 100 mg tablet example. For this reason, frequently more than one calculation is considered when establishing safety acceptance limits for a manufacturing facility. From the example in Table 15.2, the TTC approach would not typically require analytical techniques beyond HPLC-UV or TOC.

Table 15.2 outlines typical dosage ranges in a multiproduct manufacturing facility for clinical trial materials. Limits are evaluated annually based upon manufacturing sizes, equipment used, and potency of compounds. The acceptance limits are typically based upon the worse case between the 10 ppm, and the 1/1000th method. The TTC method has not gained widespread acceptance as of yet but deserves consideration based upon toxicology arguments and has been implemented elsewhere in the pharmaceutical industry (e.g., the control of mutagens in APIs).

After the limits are calculated for all products that are to be processed and all equipment used, the limits are compared. The smallest limit calculated for a product using all of the calculations becomes the acceptance limit for the cleaning verification for that product. If product B, the lot to be manufactured next, is unknown at the time of manufacture of Product A, the worse case should be assumed in the calculation. For example, if the smallest lot that has ever been manufactured in the facility is 5000 dosage units, or alternatively 1 kg, those values should be used in the equation to generate a maximum allowable carryover of product A. To reiterate some of the initial points, the rationale for which equation is utilized should be documented, and the limits that are established should be practical, achievable, and verifiable based on the most deleterious residue.

15.4 ANALYTICAL METHOD VALIDATION

ICH Q7A (12.74) recommends that the typical method validation parameters outlined in ICH Q2(R1) should be considered for cleaning verification assays.[2] Cleaning verification can be a challenging analytical problem in the pharmaceutical industry when, for example, a compound is considered to be extremely potent, possesses a poor chromophore, or has a combination of the two. Typically, the analytical method employed involves HPLC with UV detection.[18–20] As described previously, the acceptance criteria are established to ensure human safety and are based on toxicological and pharmacological data, dose strengths, equipment surface area, manufacturing batch size, number of dosage units per batch, smallest strength manufactured, and product contact surface area.[14,21] With all other considerations being equal (e.g., lot size and shared surface area), a lower cleaning acceptance limit is required for a smaller dose strength, as it is assumed to be more potent. Three different approaches have been outlined above where an adequate margin of safety is provided; one approach is to employ a risk factor of 1/1000th to the no-effect or low-effect dose levels used in the clinical trials. In cases where the therapeutic dose is projected to be in the low micrograms per day or per capsule range, the cleaning-verification acceptance limit can be driven into the ng/swab (or ng/cm^2) regime. For example, a dose of 10 μg API (active pharmaceutical ingredient)/capsule might require that the clinical trial manufacturing or clinical trial packaging equipment be cleaned to a level below 50 ng/25 cm^2 or 50 ng/100 cm^2, respectively. With a direct-sampling cleaning-verification strategy (i.e., swabbing), this acceptance limit of 50 ng/swab will result in analytical samples that are approximately 10 ng/mL with a 5 mL dilution in sample solvent. Although it is not impossible to reach this limit with conventional HPLC-UV when the compound of interest has a high molar absorptivity, it can be difficult for most compounds.

When dealing with low-level cleaning verification assays, several factors contribute to the complexity of the analysis. When considering that the allowable API residue may be 2 ng/cm^2 or less, the first difficulty arises during sampling of the surfaces with swabs. Such a low limit makes the sample extraction from a surface challenging during the swabbing process due to some level of affinity of the analyte to the surface. The small amount of analyte absorbed onto a surface, or unextracted from the swab, may account for only a small fraction of the total analyte at a relatively high acceptance limit. However, the same absolute amount of loss becomes a significant fraction of the total analyte when the acceptance limit is low. As a result, lower recovery from a surface may be expected as the dose is reduced and is dependent upon the material of construction that is swabbed (i.e., polymeric surface vs stainless steel vs hard anodized aluminum, etc.) and its affinity to an analyte. Therefore, the previously cited limit of 20 ng/25 cm^2 or 20 ng/100 cm^2 calculated in Table 15.2 could result in an analytical sample that is 2–5 ng/mL when corrected for the above-mentioned recovery challenges. The combination of low acceptance limits and potentially low recoveries can present a significant analytical challenge. At such a low level, the detection limit may not be easily achieved with HPLC-UV. Other detection techniques used in conjunction with HPLC, such as fluorescence and electrochemical detection, are effective and afford excellent sensitivity, but are compound-specific and may be somewhat limited as to the number of compounds where these techniques will be preferred. As a result, the advantages associated with these techniques are limited to a smaller subset of compounds, especially in the case of fluorescence where derivatization is required. Charged aerosol detection (CAD) is a relatively new detector on the analytical scene and offers excellent sensitivity; it has been demonstrated to have equivalent response factors for a large number of compounds and low nanogram sensitivity.[22] It is abundantly clear that the analytical chemist must understand the molecule of interest (e.g., Can it be ionized? Can it be oxidized or reduced? Does it fluoresce? Is it nonvolatile in the case of CAD?) and the safety acceptance limit when choosing the appropriate technique. Regardless of the analytical technique chosen for cleaning verification, there are certain components that are expected of any method validation activity and those expectations are outlined in the ICH guidelines on Analytical methods Q2 (R1).[3] For a quantitative impurity test, validation is required for specificity, limits of detection and quantitation, linearity, accuracy, precision (repeatability and intermediate precision, depending upon the phase of development), range, and robustness.[3] Each of these validation criteria are listed below in Table 15.3 with a brief explanation on the applicability to cleaning verification assays. A limit test for cleaning verification assays is often employed during clinical trials. With a limit test, a result of "pass" or "fail" is reported. The limit test significantly simplifies the validation of the cleaning verification assay. In order to validate a limit test, specificity, LOQ, accuracy, and stability must be evaluated at the acceptance limit. Linearity and range may be excluded. A drawback of the limit test is that the ability for trending the cleaning efficiency (except through failures) for a particular process, or compound, is eliminated because a quantitative result is not reported. Due to the fact that the formulation and the process are likely to evolve and the attrition of compounds during development is high, one

TABLE 15.3 Validation Requirements for Limit and Quantitative Swab Assays[3]

Requirement	Description	Limit Test	Quantitative Test
Specificity[a]	The ability to assess unequivocally the analyte in the presence of components which may be expected to be present. Interferences from swabs and surfaces should be considered	+	+
Accuracy/recovery	The amount of material recovered from surface, swab or rinse solution compared to accepted reference value. A correction factor should be established in the analytical method to represent incomplete recovery	+	+
Intermediate precision[b]	Intermediate precision expresses within-laboratories variations: different days, different analysts, different equipment, etc. This characteristic may be assessed on the worst-case surface(s) representing poor recovery and/or high variability	−	+
Repeatability/ precision	Precision under the same operating conditions over a short interval of time. Precision on standards and samples should be evaluated	+	+
Reproducibility	Reproducibility expresses the precision between laboratories (collaborative studies, usually applied to standardization of methodology). May be considered during method transfer. This characteristic may be assessed on the worst-case surface(s) representing poor recovery and/or high variability	−	+

(Continued)

TABLE 15.3 *Continued*

Requirement	Description	Limit Test	Quantitative Test
Quantitation limit	The lowest amount of analyte in a sample which can be quantitatively determined with suitable precision and accuracy. The QL must be sufficient to ensure that a response corrected for the lowest accuracy/recovery can be quantitated	+	+
Detection limit	The lowest amount of analyte in a sample which can be detected but not necessarily quantitated as an exact value	−	+
Linearity	Linearity is assessed to cover the full range of acceptance/reporting limits required by the method	−	+
Range	The interval between the upper and lower concentration of analyte in the sample (including these concentrations). Taken from the linearity assessment on standards or recovery from spikes to cover desired reporting range	−	+
Robustness	Capacity to remain unaffected by small, but deliberate variations in method parameters (e.g., extraction time of the swabs)	−	−
Standard stability	Stability of standard solutions should be established	+	+
Sample stability	Unextracted Swab (analyte on swab before solvent added), rinse solution, and swab extract stability should be assessed	+	+

− signifies that this characteristic is not required to be evaluated for cleaning verification; + signifies that this characteristic is required to be evaluated for cleaning verification.
[a]Not needed for nonspecific analytical methods (e.g., total organic carbon). All of the compound detected must be attributed to the target analyte unless rationale supporting an alternative has been documented.
[b]In cases where reproducibility has been performed, intermediate precision is not needed.

might argue that trending does not provide much value here. However, if the compound makes it to market, a quantitative assay is expected for commercial manufacturing before the cleaning process has been validated and to verify validation periodically.

15.4.1 Swab Selection

Although swab selection is not included as a requirement in Table 15.3, it is a parameter that should be considered at some point in the development of a swab assay. From a practical view point, it could be evaluated once for a facility and then replicated on all other compounds. Cleaning verification methods for swabs are typically validated by demonstrating recovery from a "test coupon." This coupon is made from a material that is representative of the manufacturing equipment in regards to material of construction (e.g., 316L stainless steel) and surface finish. A known amount of analyte will be spiked onto the coupon; the coupon will be swabbed in a methodical manner illustrated below in Fig. 15.1 (e.g., 10 swipes in the vertical, rotate the plate and 10 swipes in the horizontal directions for a 2×2 in. coupon). The number of swab strokes in each direction should be considered during the validation based upon the analyte recovery and the coupon size. For example, a 4×4 in. coupon may require 20 strokes in each direction or, alternatively, swipes in the diagonal direction could be utilized. Regardless, the method should be evaluated to replicate the swabbing practice that will be utilized in the manufacturing area. The swab will then be extracted in solvent, where the mobile phase is most convenient, and analyzed. Depending upon the swab, 5–20 mL is an appropriate extraction solvent to ensure a reproducible extraction without overdilution of the analyte, which could ultimately impact the analytical detection. When Texwipe® Large 714A Alpha swabs are utilized, an extraction volume of 5 mL is fairly common. Smaller volumes may be considered to improve the signal-noise ration (S/N) of the analyte, but it must be understood that the gains are not that substantial. For example, if an S/N of 20 was observed for the analyte when the swab was diluted into 5 mL, the analyst could expect that an S/N of 33 would be obtained by changing the extraction volume to 3 mL. Therefore, other avenues should be considered during method development before optimizing the swab extraction volume (i.e., different detection techniques that will be discussed later).

Although swab assays are different conceptually than both the impurity and the potency assay, the same scientific rationale governs the development of these assays. Many of the references listed in Table 15.4 outline different validation approaches. Seno outlined validation practices in the Japanese pharmaceutical industry for cleaning verification,[23] and Kirsch outlined an approach for swab method validation that is consistent with ICH guidelines for method development.[24] An important aspect of any cleaning-verification assay begins with swabbing the

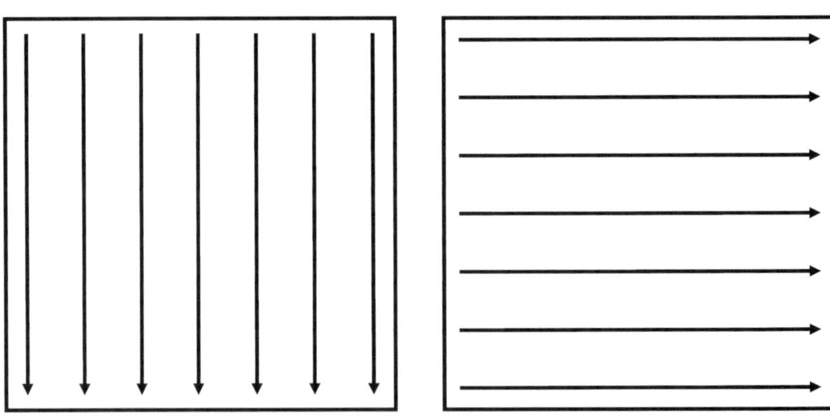

Figure 15.1 Illustration of typical swabbing practice.

TABLE 15.4 Selective Analytical Techniques for Cleaning Verification with Associated Analytes and Reported LOD, if Available

Selective Techniques				
Detection Technique	Analyte	Reported LOD	Estimated LOQ[a]	References
HPLC-UV	Amlodipine	0.02 μg/mL	0.7 μg/mL	37
	Ertapenem	0.0006 μg/mL	0.002 μg/mL	38
	Sulfadoxine	0.12 μg/mL	0.4 μg/mL	39
	Acetylsalicylic acid	0.04 μg/mL	0.1 μg/mL	40
	Sumatriptan succinate	0.003 μg/mL	0.01 μg/mL	41
	Losoxantrone	0.005 μg/mL	0.02 μg/mL	42
	Bisnafide	0.004 μg/mL	0.01 μg/mL	43
	Nonoxynol-9	0.06 μg/mL	0.2 μg/mL	44
UV	Any compound with chromophore	Typically higher than HPLC-UV	Typically higher than HPLC-UV	No references for cleaning verification
HPLC-MS	Proprietary	0.00002 μg/mL	0.00007 μg/mL	45
	Proprietary	0.0005 μg/mL	0.002 μg/mL	26
	Proprietary	<0.004 μg/mL	0.01 μg/mL	46
Ion mobility spectrometry (IMS)	Diphenylhydramine	0.0009 μg/mL	0.003 μg/mL	47
	Tamoxifen	0.05 μg/mL	0.2 μg/mL	48
	Proprietary	0.25 μg/mL	0.8 μg/mL	49
Gas chromatography	Methenamine hippurate	Not reported	Not reported	50
HPLC-ELSD	2-Amino-bicyclo[3,1,0]hexane-2,6dicarboxylic acid	0.26 μg/mL	0.9 μg/mL	51
TLC	Chloramphennicol	0.003 μg	0.01 μg	52
OPLC	Steroid hormones	0.03 μg	0.1 μg	53
CE	No reference to compounds	Typically higher than HPLC-UV	Typically higher than HPLC-UV	54
Atomic absoprtion	Cisplatin	0.0005 μg/mL	0.002	55
HPLC-electrochemical	Clarithromycin	0.3 μg/mL	1.0 μg/mL	56
	isoproterenol sulfate	0.1 ng/mL	0.2 ng/mL	57
Spectroscopy	Proprietary cleaning agent	4 μg/cm^2	13 μg/cm^2	58
		Not stated	Not stated	59
	Bovine serum albumin	low μg/cm^2	low μg/cm^2	60
HPLC-fluorescence	Norfloxacin	5 ng	20 ng	61
HP-TLC-fluorescence	Norfloxacin	5 ng	20 ng	61
Ion exchange conducitivity	Cleaning agent	0.1 μg/mL	0.3 μg/mL	62
Ion exchange–UV	Cleaning agent	1 μg/mL	3 μg/mL	63
Charged aerosol detection	Mometasone Furoate	0.6 ng	2 ng	
	Albuterol	1.5 ng	5 ng	22
	Loratadine	1.4 ng	5 ng	

[a]LOQ = 3.33 × LOD (assumes a S/N of 3 for LOD and a S/N of 10 for LOQ).

surface. Swabs are typically constructed of a polyester knit that will not leave behind fibers after swabbing and possess minimal extractable materials.[25] Extractables from the swabs are extremely important when considering assays for potent compounds. In a severe case the extractable peak itself may have a larger response than the analyte. This situation will drive a high level of specificity or selectivity in the analytical method. For example, in the work by Liu,[26] a large polymer peak (approximate size of the analyte peak at 10 ng/mL) from the swab was observed in the chromatogram when positive ionization mode electrospray was utilized; by switching to negative ionization mode electrospray ionization mass spectrometry, this peak was eliminated. Although switching ionization modes in electrospray mass spectrometry may not always be possible, it was presented here as an example of problems that arise for low-dose drug product swab analyses that do not present a problem at higher levels. Jenkins et al. did an extensive evaluation of swabbing materials as a function of the residual particles left on the surface after swabbing.[27] Quartz wool was found to give excellent recovery of analyte; however, it left an excessive amount of particles on the surface. Glass-fiber swabs and cotton swab also suffered from high levels of residual particles left behind on the surface. This point will be discussed further in regards to direct swab analysis for ion mobility spectrometry. Knitted polyester demonstrated the best balance between recovery, residual particle, and background levels. A guideline for swabbing technique that discusses swabbing procedures, solvent selection, and recovery as a function of the coupon tested is presented by Yang et al.[28]

15.4.2 Specificity

Specificity should be demonstrated from interferences (i.e., extractables) that arise from the cleaning swabs and/or blank surfaces. Specificity between the excipients utilized in the drug product manufacture is desirable, but not required. However, if the excipient is suspected to influence the response of the analyte via ion suppression in mass spectrometry or ion mobility spectrometry, for example, specificity would then be required. In most cases, if specificity is not achieved it must be assumed that the peak response is from the active pharmaceutical ingredient. If the interference is low enough, it may be acceptable as long as it does not unduly bias the recovery results and/or it can be accounted for appropriately through background subtraction. Significant interference from a surface may indicate compatibility issues for the selected sampling solvent and may vary (drop) over time as surfaces on equipment are repeatedly cleaned.

15.4.3 Detection and Quantitation Limits

The limit of quantitation, as opposed to the limit of detection, is the most important attribute of the swab method because it has been previously determined, from a safety and cross-contamination standpoint, that residual material above the cleaning acceptance limit is of serious concern. The LOQ is defined as a percentage relative standard deviation (percent RSD) of 10%, and the LOD is defined as a percentage RSD of 33%. These values are typically determined on low-level injections of the standard. The sensitivity of the method must be sufficient to ensure sample responses near the lowest acceptance limit are quantifiable. For typical swab assays, this requirement may necessitate an LOQ of 0.1 μg/mL (0.5 μg/swab limit, 1 swab extracted into 5 mL of solvent). As the compound becomes more potent, method LOQ requirements can be driven to the low ng/mL regime. Larger percentage RSD values may be acceptable (e.g., 20%) as the acceptance limit is reduced for a swab assay (including recovery from surfaces). However, the assay pass–fail limit should be lowered in such a way that this variability is accounted for. For example, if 80% recovery was obtained during validation with a 15% RSD for a 0.5 μg/swab limit, the assay pass–fail limit could be reasonably lowered to 68% to take into account the swabbing variability. The method assay pass fail limit would then be 0.34 μg/swab.

15.4.4 Linearity

Linearity is assessed to cover the full range of acceptance limits required by the method. Linearity has been performed in a couple of different manners. First, linearity has been performed through the preparation of standards that are equal to the resulting swab solution concentration after putting the swab into solvent. The second approach would involve spiking plates at many different levels and evaluating the recovery at each level. The second approach is problematic in that recovery is usually observed to decrease as the spiked level on the surface decreases. Thus, it may be unreasonable to expect linearity over a large range. However, if the range is kept narrow, either approach is suitable. Linearity is assessed to cover the full range of acceptance limits required by the method. If linearity is established, a quantitative result is typically expected across a range for tracking purposes so that the effectiveness of the cleaning process can be monitored. From a conservative standpoint, a recovery factory could be established at the low end of the reporting range and applied to all levels above that.

15.4.5 Accuracy and Recovery

When compared to a typical potency assay, this validation parameter is the most variable Eq. (15.4) represents the typical calculation that is used to determine the analytical recovery for the method. The spiked amount is based upon the predetermined acceptance limit (see Section 15.3 for different methods of calculating this value).

$$\text{Recovery}(\%) = \frac{\text{Spiked amount determined } (\mu\text{g})}{\text{Actual spiked amount } (\mu\text{g})} \times 100 \qquad (15.4)$$

In order to reproducibly add μg quantities to the surface, the analyte of interest is first dissolved in a solvent, usually methanol. Methanol is used because many analytes are soluble in this organic solvent and it dries rapidly. Thus method development can proceed without waiting and an additional drying step, as required with aqueous solvents, is not necessary. It is not uncommon to see relative standard deviations of recovery results for cleaning range from 2% to 20%, or higher, depending upon the surface investigated. In addition, the recovery of an analyte from the test surfaces is not expected to be complete. Depending upon the surfaces material of construction (e.g., a stainless steel vs cast iron), acceptance limit (e.g., 0.5 μg/swab vs 100 μg/swab), and the solubility of the compound, recoveries as low as 20%, or lower, may be acceptable and accounted for in the method calculations through the use of recovery factors. The minimum sample response (extract concentration) must be not less than the quantitation limit of the assay to ensure that analyte levels close to the lowest acceptance limit are quantifiable.

15.4.6 Intermediate Precision

With the above-mentioned variability that may be observed during accuracy/recovery determinations, it must be realized that acceptance criteria around intermediate precision must be set accordingly. Consider a cleaning verification of 50 ng/swab, for example; it is quite likely that if analyst A could obtain a recovery of 80% for a 50 ng/swab limit, analyst B could obtain a value of only 70% for the recovery. When looking at the residual surface analyte difference between the two analysts, analyst B would have left an additional 5 ng (0.8 ng/cm^2 for a 2.5 $\times$ 2.5 cm test coupon) across the tested surface area. Thus, those two results should be considered equivalent. It is easy to see that swabbing technique can play a crucial role in swabbing success when such small amounts are considered. As illustrated above, as the compound becomes more potent, the residual differences between analyst A and analyst B may be in the nanogram regime.

15.4.7 Range

The range of acceptable method performance is based upon the LOQ and the linearity assessment and is defined as the interval between the upper and lower concentration of analyte in the sample (including these concentrations). The estimate of range is typically taken from the linearity assessment on standards or recovery from spikes to cover desired reporting range.

15.4.8 Robustness

Robustness is the capacity to remain unaffected by small, but deliberate, variations in method parameters. In a typical HPLC validation this exercise would include minor variations in flow rate or pH of the buffer. When considering cleaning verification, this parameter may be extended to extraction time of the swabs, pH of extraction solvent, etc. However, it is fairly uncommon to evaluate such parameters due to the above-mentioned variability that may be found in swab methods.

15.4.9 Standard and Sample Stability

Stability of the unextracted swabs is determined in order to allow time for transport of the swabs between swabbing and analytical testing. Standard stability and swab extract stability (after the sample solvent has been added to the swab) are determined to facilitate analytical testing. Swab and extract stability must be assessed after contact with each of the representative product contact surface materials since sample stability can be affected by surface-specific contaminants. In addition, polymeric surfaces may contribute to the background in a low-level assay.

15.5 GENERAL ANALYTICAL TECHNIQUES

With the advances in analytical technology and detection schemes, it should be a rare exception for the toxicologically determined cleaning limit not to be attained. However, when selecting the appropriate analytical technique for cleaning verification, several parameters must be considered, such as the acceptance limit for the cleaning verification assay, the molar absorptivity of the molecule, solubility,[29] ionization or oxidation potential if alternative detection techniques are an option. In addition, the benefits of a selective assay required vs a nonselective assay should be considered. In a nonselective assay, the bulk properties of a rinse or swab solution are determined to ascertain if there is any deviation from the control (i.e., the blank in the same solution). The advantage of this approach includes that a variety of residues may be detected which include cleaning agents, excipients, previously manufactured products, degradation products, and active pharmaceutical ingredients. It should, however, be realized that the source of the contamination would remain unknown after this assay. The analyst would only know that the equipment had a detectable residue, which may or may not allow for the cleaning process to be improved on subsequent manufactures. Many nonselective analytical techniques are presented in the literature for cleaning verification assay. pH,[30] conductivity,[31] total organic carbon,[32–37] and visual inspection[30,35,37] have all been presented to verify removal of residual cleaning agent or API. The most prevalent of the nonselective assays is total organic carbon (TOC). This has the advantages of good sensitivity, rapid analysis time, and the ability to detect all residual carbon—independent of the source.[32] Difficulties could arise with nonspecific techniques due to the disparity of limits between the cleaning agents and the highly potent compounds. For example, a typical cleaning agent may have an acceptance limit of 100 μg/unit area. However, the calculation methods detailed above and the resulting limits outlined in Table 15.2 illustrate that, when the dose of product A is 1 mg, the acceptance limit is 2 μg/swab or less depending upon lot and equipment size. When using a nonspecific technique, all response must be assigned to the analyte. Therefore 2% of the allowable limit of cleaning agent would cause the swab assay to fail. In essence, the cleaning agent residual plus the residual API plus any soluble excipients must be less than the API acceptance limit. Based upon the above scenario, and the sensitivity of the methods, TOC is the only nonselective method that has the potential to be utilized for a low-dose compound if a stringent calculation drives the acceptance limit into the sub-microgram regime. In general, specific techniques are typically recommended for trace analysis as they will provide fewer false failures of the cleaning process.

For a selective technique, the target analyte is known before method validation. Table 15.4 outlines many of the feasible selective analytical techniques; the list is not all inclusive because of the multiple detection schemes that can be implemented with HPLC. HPLC is used exhaustively in the pharmaceutical industry. As a result, cleaning verification assays by this approach outnumber all others. Typically, at the time of manufacture, the potency assay has been developed and validated for the drug product. Therefore, the swab method is commonly very similar, if not identical, to the potency method. Characteristic swab assays would most often be isocratic methods with reduced run times. In addition to HPLC with UV detection, many other detection schemes are outlined in Table 15.4. The analytical chemist chooses these techniques based upon the chemical properties of the target molecule and the cleaning acceptance limit, which was previously established based upon dose and equipment surface-area considerations. For example, a molecule that does not possess a chromophore and is somewhat potent would pose an interesting analytical challenge. The analyst might consider evaporative light scattering detection, electrochemical detection, charged aerosol detection, or mass spectral detection to name a few possibilities. UV detection is listed in Table 15.4 where a specific example for a cleaning verification assay could not be located; however, depending upon the molecular properties of the compound, this technique would be a viable option for a cleaning verification assay. Of course, all techniques (and probably more) listed in Table 15.4 could be utilized depending upon the molecule of interest when the acceptance limit is routine. However the list of practical choices is greatly reduced when considering assays for potent compounds. When choosing the analytical technique to utilize, one must of course consider the acceptance limit. When more than one analytical technique will suffice, the phase of development should be considered. For example, if the method will be transferred to a QC laboratory and the acceptance limit is expected to stay extremely low, instrument availability could be the limitation and drive the ultimate decision on analytical technique. Therefore, if HPLC-MS, large-volume injection HPLC-UV, and HPLC-electrochemical will meet the requirements of the acceptance limits, the analyst should work closely with the receiving laboratory to ensure that it is comfortable with the technique and that they have the instrumentation that is to be validated. On the other hand, if the method is developed for a clinical phase I trial and speed is of the essence, it may be quickest to develop an LC-MS method and to reevaluate the practicality of transferring an LC-MS method to a QC laboratory if the molecule survives the high attrition rate of early clinical trials. Figure 15.2 illustrates preferred analytical methods as dictated by the acceptance limit of the cleaning assay. In each box a rank order is provided for that range of acceptance limits. For example, in the range of 10–100 mg/swab, it would be rare to consider analytical techniques other than HPLC-UV, UV, or TOC. Of course, the chemical properties of the compound could force you to consider other techniques (e.g., lack

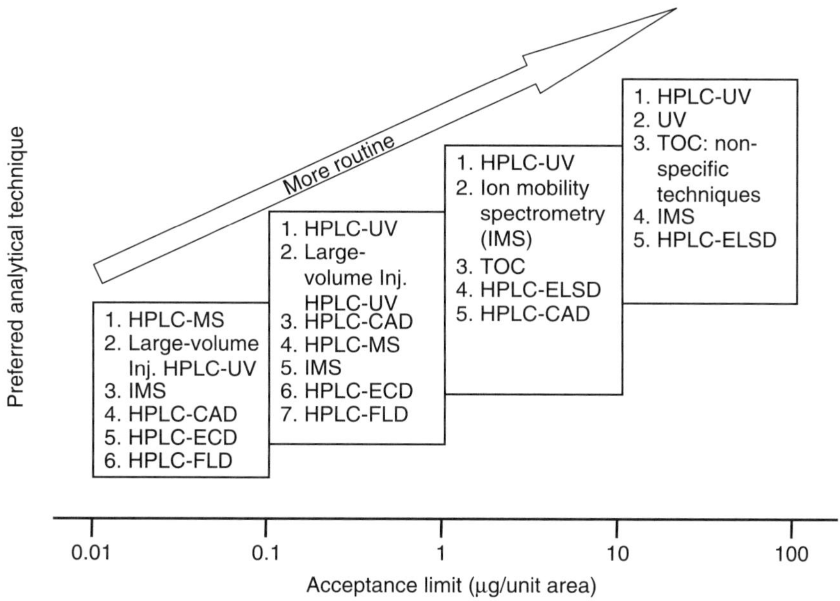

Figure 15.2 Preferred analytical technique for a given acceptance-limit range.

of chromophore would drive the decision to use HPLC with either CAD or ELSD). As with Table 15.4, the techniques indicated in Fig. 15.2 are not all inclusive, but are presented based upon availability and best practices. Figure 15.2 is divided on the x-axis by acceptance limits ranging from 0.01 to 100 μg/unit area. From Fig. 15.2, it is illustrated that HPLC-UV would be the preferred choice in most situations. This decision would be made regardless of clinical phase due the prevalence of HPLCs in the pharmaceutical industry, the ease of use and turnaround time of the analytical results. Many techniques are listed for multiple ranges of acceptance limits. For example, HPLC-MS is indicated as the top choice for the range of 0.01–0.1 μg/swab. As the acceptance limit increases, however, it moves down the list as to when you would consider this analytical technique due to the fact that it is more complicated to use and costlier to purchase and maintain. However, if the acceptance limit is greater than 10 μg/swab and the molecule does not have a chromophore, LCMS may be the first choice or alternatively the analyst may choose CAD or ELSD, or the nonspecific TOC. Alternatively, other factors may lead the analyst to choose techniques other than those indicated. For example, if at-line analysis of cleaning verification samples is desired, IMS may be the logical choice. If the reported limit of quantitation is examined in Table 15.4, it is apparent that many analytical techniques may reach the desired acceptance limit. It is clear that there is an abundance of decisions to make in regards to analytical techniques. The analyst should choose the technique that is easiest to execute routinely, implement, and ultimately transfer to a quality control laboratory.

15.6 ANALYTICAL TECHNIQUES FOR LOW-DOSE COMPOUNDS

As previously stated, there are many analytical approaches that have been successfully utilized for cleaning verification assays. All of these approaches will not be discussed here. A general rule of thumb would be if HPLC-UV will work, that should be the first choice due to its prevalence in the pharmaceutical industry. There have been several examples in the literature where extremely low-level cleaning verification assays have been validated with HPLC-UV. For example, Shea et al. developed a cleaning verification assay utilizing HPLC-UV for the determination of Losoxantrone, which is a cytotoxic compound for breast cancer.[41] In addition to illustrating a step-by-step approach for developing a cleaning verification assay, they demonstrated that the HPLC-UV method had a detection limit of 2 ng/mL. In another example, a HPLC-UV assay was developed for the compound Bisnafide, which is also a cytotoxic compound.[43] For this assay, the method was sensitive to 4 ng/mL of Bisnafide. In a separate work, an HPLC method was validated for fentanyl, alfentanil, and sufentanil in swab samples.[64] Efficient chromatography with moderate run times (<12 min) and high sensitivity were achieved for all compounds. Detection limits were reported to be from 2 to 10 ng/mL for this class of compounds by utilizing wavelengths that corresponded to the maximum absorbance of each compound.

An interesting approach presented by Raghavan and Mulligan involved the use of atomic absorption (AA) spectroscopy. The determination of cisplatin in cleaning validation rinse solutions was performed with a very sensitive AA method.[55] In this work, cisplatin was first derivatized with diethyldithiocarbamic acid to yield a platinum complex that was subsequently detected by AA. The sensitivity of this method was reported to be 0.5 ng/mL of cisplatin. Valvis and Champion presented a strategy for cleaning and decontamination of potent compounds by establishing meaningful criteria for acceptance criteria as a foundation for developing a sound analytical method.[65] They reported an analytical method that was capable of detecting two unspecified compounds at 0.05 μg/mL.

Again the point is that, for any given molecule, the choice of analytical technique may vary. The techniques outlined below may, in general, provide the highest probably of technical success for very stringent acceptance limits. In addition, the techniques are listed in the order of preference for cleaning verification assays that would have an acceptance limit of 50 ng/swab (most potent compounds in Table 15.2) or lower, and this will be the focus of the remainder of this chapter.

15.6.1 HPLC-Mass Spectral Detection

Advantages:

- sensitive;
- selective;
- specific;
- rapid method development.

Disadvantages:

- expensive to purchase and to maintain;
- typically requires additional training;
- more complex than UV;
- buffer selection limited to volatile mobile-phase additives.

For pharmaceutical compounds, LC-MS has found extremely wide acceptance due to the low-level detection that can be achieved, in addition to the selectivity and specificity that are attained by using HPLC in conjunction with MS detection. LC-MS is also convenient because of its compatibility with reversed-phase HPLC mobile phases. Volatile mobile phase additives such as trifluoroacetic acid, formic acid, and ammonium hydroxide are very common and can be utilized not only to aid in the chromatographic separation but also to influence the ionization state of the molecule (i.e., acid modifiers to protonate $[M + H]^{+1}$, and basic modifiers to deprotonate $[M - H]^{-}$). This requirement may require a modification of the potency method if phosphate was utilized; however, it is not viewed as a major drawback.

Simmonds et al. perfomed a comparison of LC-MS vs HPLC-UV for three propietary compounds.[46] In this work, the LOQ improved in going from HPLC-UV to LC-MS for all three compounds. For compound 1, the LOQ improved from 0.1 to 0.005 μg/mL; for compound 2 the LOQ improved from 0.015 to 0.004 μg/mL; and for compound 3 the LOQ improved from 0.02 to 0.005 μg/mL. This improvement in sensitivity is one of the primary drivers to choose LC-MS over competing techniques when low-level detection is required. In addition, extraction conditions were optimized, linearity of response, accuracy, and the impact of residual excipients were evaluated to support a single set of robust conditions, consistent with the requirement outlined in Table 15.3, which worked for all three compounds. On the use of LC-MS for cleaning verification, Forsyth and Van Nostrand reported that method development times and chromatographic run times are generally shorter.[66] In addition, the sensitivity can be the same as HPLC-UV, or better. However, they consider the LC-MS method to be less rugged and more costly than conventional HPLC with UV detection. Recently, Kolodsick et al. reported an excellent application of LC-MS/MS (utilizing a triple quadrupole mass analyzer) for enhanced sensitivity and specificity of drug residues for cleaning validation in manufacturing equipment.[45] The work by Kolodsick advocated the use of internal standards to correct for ion suppression effects. Two alternatives were illustrated: (1) isotopically labeled analytes; and (2) structural analogs. Data were presented on linearity and precision improvements achieved through the use of internal standards. Sensitivity requirements for method validation were satisfied with a low level solution at 10 ng/mL, which resulted in detection limits in the range of 0.02–0.2 ng/mL for all compounds investigated.

In a work by Liu et al.,[26] a cleaning-verification assay was validated for a highly potent family of compounds utilizing a swab-sampling procedure and LC-MS for separation and detection of the analytes. Due to the high potency of the compound, the LC-MS method was validated at a level of 50 ng/25 cm^2 and 50 ng/100 cm^2

because a slightly difference safety acceptance limit was calculated for the CT packaging area as opposed to the CT manufacturing area. These acceptance limits correlate to a 10 ng/mL solution after extraction in 5 mL of sample solvent, and to 3 ng/mL samples after correction for sampling losses. This validation exercise included recovery estimates from all drug product contact surfaces within the clinical trial manufacturing equipment, namely, stainless steel, anodized aluminum, Rilsan®-coated aluminum, bronze, polyvinylchloride, and Oilon®. The limit of detection for the LC-MS method was determined to be less than 0.5 ng/mL, or less than 0.1 ng/cm^2, of the analyte. This method did not employ an internal standard as did the work by Kolodsik.[45] Long-term performance of the validated method was also reported. The precision on replicate injections of the standard prepared in the range of 3-6 ng/mL was typically better than 8.0% relative standard deviation (RSD) over the course of one year, which resulted from 10 cleaning-verification submissions. The specific validation strategies and detection techniques pertinent to low-dose compounds were discussed. The method was validated for specificity, limit of detection, recovery, precision, and stability of standard and sample solutions which are consistent with the expectations for a limit test outlined in Table 15.3. In addition, the stability of the swab samples with analyte was evaluated to determine the allowable time interval between sampling CT equipment and extraction of the analyte with sample solvent. The assay pass–fail limit was determined to be 3 and 4 ng/mL for two new chemical entities (NCE). Figure 15.3 is an example chromatogram of

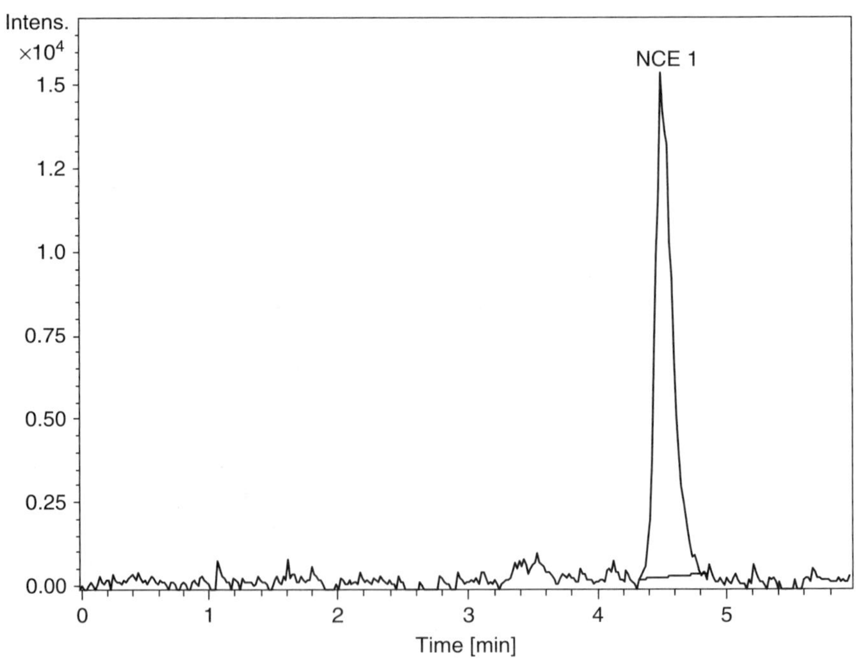

Figure 15.3 Chromatogram of an NCE at 3 g/mL which would represent a 50 ng/swab extracted into 5 mL and the limit corrected for a 30% recovery on representative coupons.

TABLE 15.5 Chromatographic Conditions Used to Obtain the Chromatogram in Fig. 15.3

	Chromatographic Conditions
Column	Zorbax RX C_{18}, 150 × 4.6 mm, 5 μm
Column temperature	30°C
Mobile phase	80% methanol/20% pH 4.5 ammonium acetate buffer
Flow rate	0.4 mL/min
Injection volume	100 μL

a 3 ng/mL system suitability injection on an NCE at Eli Lilly and company.[26] The conditions used to generate this selected ion chromatogram are outlined in Table 15.5. As can be seen from the figure adequate sensitivity was obtained even at a level of 3 ng/mL. This level accounted for a 30% RF on a 50 ng/swab limit where a 5 mL extraction volume in mobile phase was utilized.

In summary, LC-MS offers excellent sensitivity for many classes of pharmaceutical compounds. Due to the fact that MS is becoming more "routine" (i.e., it is essentially another detector), LC-MS should be the first consideration for all cleaning verification assays that are less than 0.1 μg/swab. In the citations outlined above, LC-MS has been shown to offer excellent sensitivity and specificity for the analytes of interest. The mass spectrometric conditions can be optimized in a flow injection mode to allow for rapid method development. All LC-MS analytical methods were validated in a way consistent with the requirements outlined in Table 15.3. The applications cited utilized LC-MS because of the sensitivity requirements of the safety acceptance limits; however, if the molecule of interest poses unique detection challenges such as a poor chromophore, LC-MS should be considered for assays at the level of 1.0 μg/unit area, or less. Above 1.0 μg/unit area there may be more attractive options for these swab determinations.

15.6.2 Large-Volume Injection HPLC-UV

Advantages:

- sensitive;
- selective;
- specific (wavelength selection);
- routine.

Disadvantages:

- large void volume;
- reproducibility of retention time may be a problem;
- peak identification (due to low signal level);
- other impurities in chromatogram.

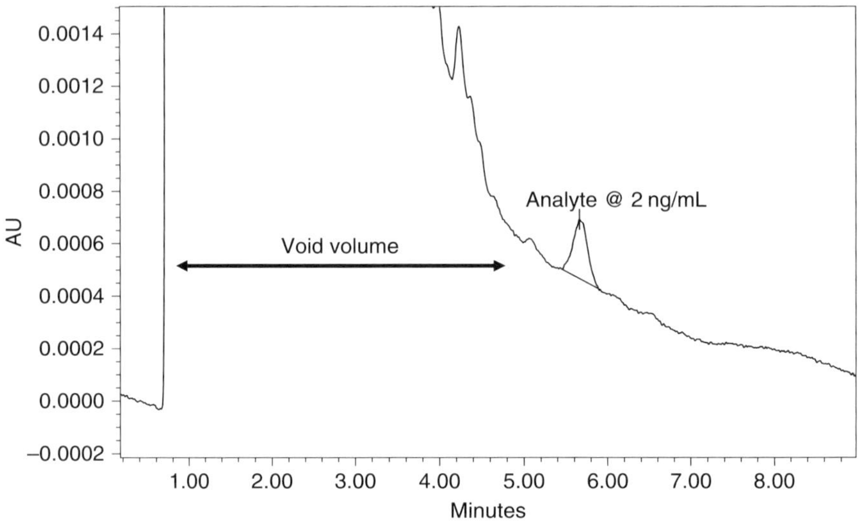

Figure 15.4 Chromatogram of compound A at concentration of 2 ng/mL utilizing an injection volume of 900 μL.

Typically, one of the first steps that is taken in method development to improve sensitivity is to increase the injection volume from a conventional injection of 10 μL to 100 μL, the maximum injection volume on many commercial instruments. Many HPLCs can be updated to include a large volume injection kit by utilizing an increased syringe size or larger metering valve, so that 900 μL to 2 mL may be injected onto an analytical column. In going from 10 to 100 μL, an order of magnitude in sensitivity is gained. By increasing the injection volume from 100 to 900 μL, nearly another order of magnitude in sensitivity is gained, and so on. Figure 15.4 illustrates a 2 ng/mL injection of compound A (a new chemical entity in phase I clinical trials). In Fig. 15.4, the peak of interest can clearly be distinguished from the baseline. The experimental conditions are outlined in Table 15.6. Of particular note in

TABLE 15.6 Experimental Condition Used to Generate the Large-Volume Injection HPLC Analysis in Fig. 15.4

Instrument	Agilent 1100 HPLC with large volume injection kit
Mobile phase composition	70/30% methanol/water + 0.1% trifluroacetic acid
Flow rate	1.3 mL/min
Column	HiChrom Ace-3 Phenyl, 75 × 4.6 mm, 3 μm particle size
Column temperature	40°C
Wavelength	220 nm
Sample solvent	Mobile phase
Injection volume	900 μL

Table 15.6 is that the HPLC column is a typical analytical column; however the injection volume is 900 μL, and the sample solvent is the mobile phase.

However, there is a price to pay for added sensitivity that is gained by utilizing large-volume injection. The disadvantage starts with the void volume; due to the 900 μL injection, the void lasts approximately 5 min and it may be argued that it does not return to baseline until approximately 8 min. Due to this long void volume time, turnaround time and method development time may be increased in comparison to LC-MS. In addition, sample solvent matching to the mobile phase is of the utmost importance. The solvent strength of the sample solvent must be less than or equal to that of the mobile phase to ensure that acceptable peak shape is obtained. Also, a stronger sample solvent may cause the analyte peak to elute in the void volume due to the size of the injection volume. Special care should be take to purchase high-purity solvents; impurities present in the solvents and acid modifiers may be detected and interfere with the analyte of interest, and without the specificity of mass spectrometry may become problematic. While this technique is not elegant, even with the caveats mentioned above, it is fairly straight forward to develop a low-level swab assay using a large volume injection. Due to the simplicity of this technique, the method can be simply transferred to a QC laboratory with minimal capital expenditures (large volume upgrade kit). In addition, there will be no additional training required since it is simply an HPLC assay with a larger injection volume. If there is a need to develop a more sensitive assay than large volume injection HPLC-UV or LC-MS, a large volume injection LC-MS method could be developed to provide a straightforward mechanism to improve the LC-MS sensitivity by a factor of 9, by increasing the injection volume from 100 to 900 μL. This combination may not suffer from the void volume effect observed in Fig. 15.4, due to the fact that an m/z is detected.

The choice between large volume injection HPLC-UV and LC-MS as the preferred analytical technique is not clear cut. The decision of one technique over the other may simply come down to a matter of preference and availability of instrumentation.

15.6.3 Charged Aerosol Detection

Advantages:

- sensitivity;
- dynamic range;
- uniformity of response;
- ease of use.

Disadvantages:

- cannot be used on semivolatile components;
- buffer selection limited to volatile additives;
- response can change based upon mobile-phase composition.

Charged aerosol detection (CAD™) is a rather new analytical technology on the scene. It was first introduced in 2002 by Dixon and Peterson.[67] Since that time, there have been several publications on the application of CAD™ as an HPLC detector.[22,68–70] CAD is a unique technology, in which the HPLC column eluent is first nebulized with nitrogen, the large droplets are removed via an impactor in the spray chamber and the resulting small droplets are dried to remove mobile phase, producing analyte particles; at this point CAD™ is very similar to the nebulization and drying steps involved in evaporative light scattering detection.[51] After particles are formed, a secondary stream of nitrogen becomes positively charged as it passes a high-voltage, platinum corona wire (see Fig. 15.5); the charge is then transferred to the opposing stream of analyte in a small mixing chamber. The charged analyte particles are then transferred to a collector where a signal is generated that is directly proportional to the quantity of analyte present.

In the work by Forsatz and Snow, three APIs and one excipient were determined by HPLC-UV and HPLC-CAD™.[22] The APIs were mometasone furorate, a moderately potent glucocorticoid steroid used in the treatment of inflammatory skin disorders, albuterol, a short-acting β2-adrenergic receptor agonist used for the relief of bronchospasm in conditions such as asthma, and Loratadine, a drug used to treat allergies. The excipient evaluated was lactose. In this work, the signal-to-noise ratio was compared at 10 ng for each of the APIs. Sensitivity was comparable for both albuterol and loratadine when compared to HPLC-UV, while CAD™ offered

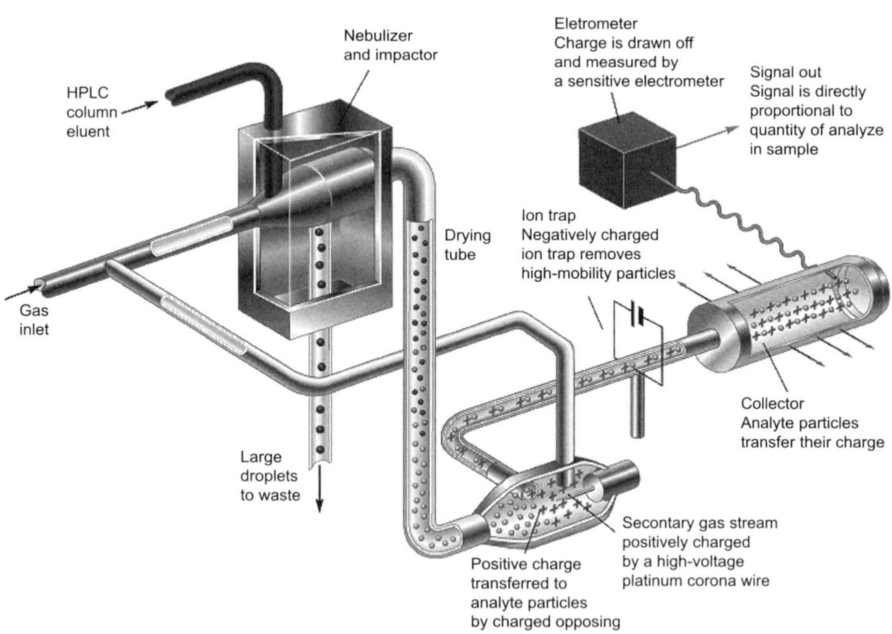

Figure 15.5 Instrument schematic of the CAD™ (charged aerosol detection). (Reproduced with permission from ESA Bioscience.) (See color insert.)

an improvement in sensitivity by a factor of approximately 3 for mometasone furorate. In addition, to sensitivity, this work also evaluated the response factors for the analytes. When comparing the responses at 205 nm, mometasone furorate had a response that was approximately 47% of that of loratadine, whereas for the CAD™, the responses for mometasone furorate and albuterol were equal across the investigated range and the loratadine response was within approximately 30%. Lactose was investigated and of course did not invoke a UV response; however, it responded very similarly to the APIs. Equal response across a wide range of compounds is seen as a distinct advantage to this detector.[68] This work also presented a linear response whereas a nonlinear response had been presented previously, but explained that it was a fairly narrow range investigated. The CAD™ response had been previously reported to be nonlinear and represented by Eq. (15.5):

$$y = ax^b \tag{15.2}$$

where y = peak response, x = analyte mass, and b = the exponential response factor (sensitivity).[69]

One aspect of CAD detection to be aware of is that analyte response is directly proportional to percentage of organic; however, the magnitude of this effect is very similar for all compounds.[69] Therefore, a shift in retention time will cause a difference in response. Because of the uniformity of response characteristics outlined above, CAD™ is a very interesting option as a universal detection system for HPLC. From the author's experience, it is a very simple detector to utilize and can be integrated with laboratory data collection system quite easily with the analog output.

15.6.4 Ion Mobility Spectrometry

Advantages:

- minimal sample preparation (no sample preparation with direct swab analysis);
- simple to operate;
- rapid analysis;
- sub-ng absolute detection limits;
- no solvent waste.

Disadvantages:

- limited number of swab types that can be utilized;
- compounds must be amenable to thermal desorption;
- ion suppression a concern.

There are currently two vendors of ion mobility spectrometers: Smith's detection offers the Ionscan® and GE Sensing offers the Ion Trap Mobility Spectrometer®. A description will be provided with an emphasis on their applicability to analyzing swabs with nanogram amounts of residue with no preference to either vendor. For reference, Fig. 15.6 is a schematic of the GE ITMS system.

The theory of operation of ion mobility spectrometry is that the velocity (V) of an ion down the drift tube is directly proportional to the applied electric field (E).[47–49] K is commonly referred to as the mobility constant and can be used to correct for temperature and pressure.

$$V = K \times E \tag{15.3}$$

A solid or liquid sample can be introduced to the analyzer by thermal desorption. The resultant vapors are swept through the inlet by the carrier gas and ionized by a radioactive ^{63}Ni source. Discreet packets of ions are then pulsed down the flight tube under a controlled potential. The arrival of the ions at the detector is inversely proportional to the mass of the molecule. Thus, the smaller ions arrive at the detector first, and the larger ions arrive later. At that point the signal is amplified and read out via an appropriate computer interface. Both commercially available instruments are capable of generation and detection of both positive and negative ions.

Since the theory of operation is similar, with some subtle difference, for both instruments the absolute sensitivity (mass detected) for both instruments should be similar. The critical attribute where the two instruments vary, which drives the utility for swab determinations at extremely low levels is in sample introduction. To reach the submicrogram/swab regime, direct swab analysis may be required. Recall the acceptance limits calculated in Table 15.2. Using the assumptions in Table 15.1, a 1 mg tablet will drive the acceptance limit to 2.0 μg/swab, a 0.1 mg tablet will drive the acceptance limit to 0.2 μg/swab and a 0.01 μg tablet will drive the acceptance limit to 0.02 μg/swab. With direct swab analysis, ion mobility should be able to attain the required sensitivity for most compounds with this limit as the absolute amount on the swab would be 20 ng. However, if a typical dilution is required and deposition of a small aliquot

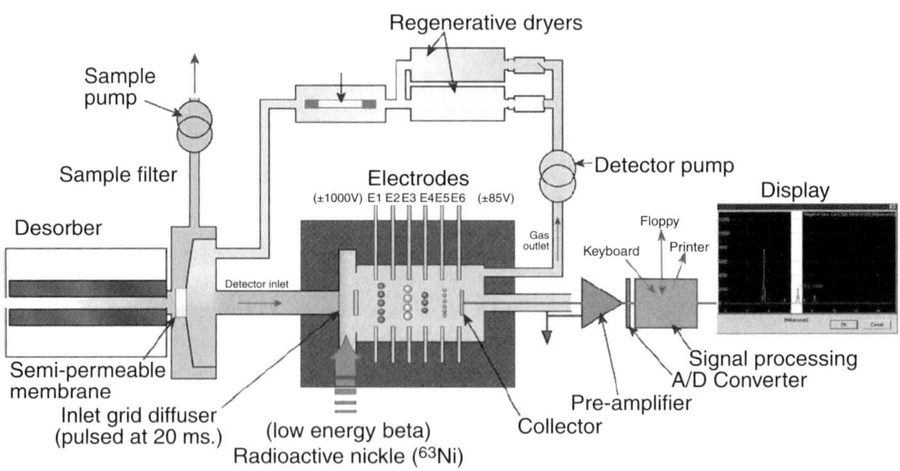

Figure 15.6 Instrument schematic of GE ITMS. (Reproduced with permission from GE Sensing.) (See color insert.)

before desorption into the IMS, the absolute amount introduced into the IMS is much smaller. For example, assume that a standard Texwipe® swab is utilized for cleaning verification and reconstituted into 5 mL of sample solvent; 20 ng/swab is now converted to 4 ng/mL. Typically, 1 μL is introduced into the desorber, although injections can be stacked and allowed to dry in order to preconcentrate the analyte (although, this procedure would sacrifice one of the primary benefits of speed). Therefore the absolute amount introduced into the IMS becomes 4 pg, which is quite challenging to detect for most compounds. However, if the acceptance limit is 1–5 μg/swab, this mode of sample introduction will become feasible to detect most compounds that can be ionized. In the latter scenario, sample preparation of the swabs would become the limiting factor for turnaround time, whereas direct swab sampling allows for more real time analysis. However, if the acceptance limit is in the 5–100 μg/swab regime, direct swab analysis may prove to be too sensitive for the application. Both instruments offer advantages and disadvantages and should thoroughly evaluated for the particular application, analyte, and range of reporting limits.

In Table 15.3, are outlined the requirements for method validation. One requirement is that specificity should be considered in the presence of substances that may be present during sample analysis. In the case of cleaning verification, these substances would include residual API, excipients, and cleaning agents. Typically a visual clean has to be established before a swab can be submitted to the laboratory. Commonly that limit is 100 μg/unit area. If there were 100 μg of an excipient or cleaning agent in the presence of the analyte, ion suppression of the analyte and interference with the mobility time of the analyte would need to be considered during the analytical method validation. Many excipients and components of cleaning agents can serve as ionization scavengers (depending upon positive and negative ionization mode). Therefore, it is possible in the presence of cleaning agents to not get an equivalent response for the analyte of choice when other components are present. The severity of the ion suppression should be carefully evaluated during the method validation so that it can be clearly integrated into the method. This problem could me more prevalent with direct swab analysis because the swab would be simply swiped on the manufacturing equipment and then inserted into the IMS instrument. With indirect swab analysis, a very small injection volume should reduce the risk of ion suppression. Regardless, the control strategy should be carefully outlined so as to never pass a swab that should otherwise fail, which would ultimately impact the integrity of the subsequent lot. Another factor to consider with IMS technology is the swabs that can be used. As mentioned previously swab composition should be considered for such factors as analytical recovery and shedding of particles. Polyamide (glass fiber) swabs have been shown to leave fibers behind after swabbing[25] and should be removed from the manufacturing equipment, before the next manufacture.

15.6.5 HPLC-Electrochemical Detection

Advantages:

- sensitivity;
- selective (voltage selection can discriminate against background).

Disadvantages:

- ruggedness;
- compounds must be capable of being oxidized or reduced.

Electrochemical detection (ECD) in conjunction with HPLC is a well-established technique in pharmaceutical analysis. Typical applications allow for background signals to be reduced in complicated matrices because of the lack of response of electro-inactive species. A good example is in a recent work where the excellent sensitivity of ECD is demonstrated for the determination of olanzapine in brain tissue.[71] The utility of this technique is structure dependent and hinges on the ability to oxidize or reduce the compound of interest. As a result, unique specificity can be obtained. Olanzapine, is a member of the benzodiazepine class of drugs, and is a potent postsynaptic dopamine receptor antagonist. The clinical indication for Olanzapine is for the treatment of schizophrenia. In this work,[71] an oxidation voltage of 0.31 was utilized. A linear range was observed from 0.2 to 10 ng/mL. This range would correspond to a range of 1–50 ng/swab (assuming a 5 mL dilution volume and 100% *RF*).

In addition to complicated biological matrices, HPLC-ECD has been successfully applied to impurity determinations in both active pharmaceutical ingredients[72] and pharmaceutical formulations.[73] In the work by Blazewicz et al.,[72] rocuronium and its associated impurities were determined at a level 45 ng/mL (LOQ) and the impurities were determined in the range from 25 to 750 ng/mL. This study utilized amperometric detection at a potential of 0.9 V vs an Ag–AgCl reference electrode. While these levels would not meet the most stringent requirements outlined in Table 15.2 for a dose of 0.01 mg/tablet (0.02 μg/swab into 5 mL dilution = 4 ng/mL), this sensitivity would suffice for the limit calculated for the 0.1 mg/tablet (0.2 μg/swab into 5 mL dilution = 40 ng/mL). The work by Marszall[73] illustrated the use of HPLC-ECD for a formulated product. The analytes of interest were thiamine hydrochloride, pyridoxine hydrochloride, and cyanocobalamin. In this study coulometric detection was utilized. The detection limits were calculated to be 9.2, 2.7, and 0.08 ng/mL for thiamine, pyroxidine, and cyanocobalamin, respectively. Assuming that the LOQ would be 3.33 times the reported LOD, this sensitivity would suffice for the most challenging limit in Table 15.2 for cyanocobalamin, and would suffice for the other two compounds at the next highest dose range.

In regards to cleaning verification assays, Elrod et al. published a manuscript on the determination of isoproterenol sulfate.[57] Detection was achieved using a glassy carbon electrode operated at 0.65 V vs an Ag–AgCl reference electrode. It was demonstrated in the work that isoproterenol sulfate was detectable at 0.1 ng/mL and could be quantitated at 0.2 ng/mL. Recovery was evaluated at 40, 80, and 120 ng spiked onto a swab, stainless steel and glass. Excellent recovery (>82%) and precision (<12.8%) were demonstrated for both surfaces. Although not applied to acceptance limits in the ng/swab regime, Rotsch et al. demonstrated the use of HPLC-ECD for the cleaning verification of clarithromycin.[56] The need for ECD was driven in the work by the fact that clarithromycin does not have a chromophore;

however, it does contain an electroactive tertiary amine. The recovery of clarithromycin was demonstrated on glass, plexiglass, and stainless steel from 9 to 103 μg. The recovery ranged from 70% at the lowest spike levels to 100% at the higher levels. Recovery of clarithromycin was demonstrated in the range of 0.97–20.67 μg and was found to be greater than 89% in all cases.

Based upon the advantages of the other techniques presented prior to LC-MS, large volume injection HPLC-UV, and HPLC-CAD, the decision to use electrochemical detection would be driven primarily by a unique analytical need, equipment availability and previous experience of the analytical chemist. A complex chemical matrix should not be of concern; at most there could be some residual cleaning agent and residual excipients in addition to the active pharmaceutical ingredient. Since the matrix in cleaning verification is typically simple, electrochemical detection would not be the primary detection technique. However, the sensitivity afforded by ECD is excellent and can meet the most stringent of the acceptance limits outlined in Table 15.2.

15.6.6 HPLC-Fluorescence

Advantages:

- extremely sensitive (pg/mL);
- selective;
- routine;
- linear range similar to UV.

Disadvantages:

- most compounds do not naturally fluoresce;
- derivitization is typically required.

There are several examples where fluorescence detection has been utilized within the pharmaceutical industry.[74–76] However, very few publications exist where fluorescence was required for cleaning verification assays.[61] Presumably, acceptance limits have not typically required the sensitivity that is afforded by fluorescence detection; thus alternative techniques were utilized. A typical fluorescent detector is arranged such that the fluorescent light is viewed at an angle to the exciting incident light beam. The spectrometer can either be grating- or filter-based. Due to the fact that the resulting emission wavelength is at a longer wavelength than the incoming excitation wavelength and the signal is measured off-axis of the emission wavelentgh, the resulting background signal is very low. Thus, the signal-to-noise of this measurement is very high. This instrumental setup accounts for the enhanced sensitivity and selectivity of utilizing fluorescence in conjunction with HPLC. The disadvantages outlined above are inherently linked together in that, if the compound does not naturally fluoresce, it must be derivatized in order to utilize fluorescent detection.

If derivitazation is required, the functional groups on the molecule must be considered. For example, for fluorescent derivativizayion of phenols, primary amines, and secondary amines, dansyl chloride (5-dimethyl aminonaphthalene-1-sulfonyl chloride) and 4-chloro-7-nitrobenz-2,1,3-oxadiazole (NBD chloride) are options;[77] 1-anthroylnitrile for hydroxy compounds,[75] 4,7,-phenanthroline-5,6-dione (phanquinone), fluorescein isothyocyanate, fluorescamine, and ninhydrin work well for amino acids.[76] If the compound does fluoresce, the advantages outlined above can immediately be realized. For example, in the work by El-Gindy et al., fluorescent detection was utilized for the determination of trazodone HCl.[78] In this work, an excitation wavelength of 320 nm was utilized in accordance with an emission wavelength of 435 nm. It is this function of fluorescence that affords it the selectivity (i.e., molecule dependent excitation and emission wavelengths) and sensitivity that is sought after with this technique. Although this work demonstrated the application of spectrofluorimetric detection for a potency assay, the susbsequent quatitation limit was calculated to be 0.05 μg/mL. This quantitation limit would be equivalent to a 0.25 μg/swab limit (when the swab is diluted into 5 mL extraction solvent), which would be appropriate for many cleaning verification limits.

An excellent example of utilizing fluorescent detection for cleaning verification is presented by Simonovska et al.[61] In this work norfloxacin was the analyte. Norfloxacin is a quinolone/fluoroquinolone broad spectrum antibacterial agent. In this work, the method was validated for removal of resides at the allowable limit of $10\ mg/m^2$. In comparison to how the limits have been expressed in this chapter, that limit would be equivalent to 25 μg/swab (based upon a 5×5 cm surface coupon). This paper describes high-performance thin-layer chromatography for the direct fluorescent detection of norfloxacin. The excitation wavelength was 280 nm and the emission wavelength was 446 nm. This work illustrated the excellent sensitivity (5 ng norfloxacin) that can be obtained. In addition, the authors were advocating the use of imaging detectors (CCD in this case) for the quantitative evaluation of many samples (spots) and rapid turnaround time as compared to classical densitometry. Linearity was demonstrated from 10 to 90 ng of norfloxacin.

As with electrochemical detection, the decision to use fluorescent detection would be driven primarily by the analytical need to investigate this technique as opposed to other options (e.g., LCMS). Equipment availability and previous experience of the analytical chemist would be secondary considerations, but would contribute to the decision. The strength of fluorescence detection is in the specificity that can be achieved through the selection of excitation and emission wavelengths in order to discriminate against a complicated background. As with ECD, FD exhibits excellent sensitivity in many cases and can meet the most stringent of the acceptance limits outlined in Table 15.2.

15.7 CONCLUSIONS

This chapter presented the challenges associated with cleaning verification assays for very potent compounds. Three different approaches to calculating acceptance limits for a manufacturing facility were presented. The 10 ppm, 1/1000th, and TTC methods were illustrated to produce significantly different acceptance limits that could ultimately drive that acceptance limit into the low nanogram regime depending upon the calculation utilized. Discussion around the variables that influence this acceptance limit calculation and analytical techniques that have been utilized for cleaning verification experiments were presented. These techniques were broken into two categories: (1) nonselective, and (2) selective. Five different analytical detection methodologies were presented as preferable options when validating a cleaning verification assay. The techniques listed are not the only options, but the ones that will provide the highest probability of technical success for the largest subset of pharmaceutical compounds. Applications of LC-MS, large volume injection HPLC-UV, HPLC-CAD, electrochemical and fluorescence detection were presented as attractive options for low-dose cleaning verification applications.

ACKNOWLEDGMENTS

I would like to thank Dr Tim Wozniak for his helpful comments and Jamie Veltri for her contributions to the large-volume injection HPLC-UV section.

REFERENCES

1. 21 CFR 211.67, Code of Federal Regulations PART 211—Current Good Manufacturing Practice for Finished Pharmaceuticals—Equipment cleaning and maintenance, Subpart D—Equipment.
2. ICH Guidelines, Q7A, Good Manufacturing Practice Guide for Active Pharmaceutical Ingredients.
3. ICH Guidelines, Q2(R1), Validation of Analytical Procedures: Text and Methodology.
4. FDA. 1993. Guide to inspections of validation of cleaning processes.Washington, DC: Food and Drug Administration.
5. Garvey CR, Levy S, McLoughlin T. 1998. Pharm. Engng 18(4): 20–26.
6. Hwang RC. 2002. Am. Pharm. Rev. 5(3): 42–46.
7. Gerber M, Perona D, Ray L. 2005. Pharm. Engng 25(3): 46–54.
8. Agalloco J. 1992. PDA J. Parenteral Sci. Technol. 46 (5) 163–168.
9. Hall WE. 1999. Drug Manuf. Technol. Ser. 3: 269–298.
10. Valvis II, Champion WL Jr. 1999. Organic Process Res. Dev. 3: 44–52.
11. Alloco JP, Brame W, Ferenc B, Hall WE, Jenkins K, LaMagna JT, Madsen RE, Mullen MV, Wagen Knecht D, Wagner CM. 1998. PDA J. Pharm. Sci. Technol. 52: 1–23.
12. LeBlanc DA. 1998. Pharm. Technol. 22(10): 136–148.
13. Zeller AO. 1993. Pharm. Technol. Eur. 5: 18, 20, 22, 24–27.
14. Fourman GL, Mullen MV. 1993. Pharm. Technol. 17: 54–60.
15. Dolan DG, Naumann BD, Sargent EV, Maier A, Dourson M. 2005. Regul. Toxicol. Pharmac. RTP 43(1): 1–9.

16. Forsyth RJ, LeBlanc A, Voaden M. 2007. Pharm. Technol. 31(1): 74–83.
17. European Medicines Agency, Evaluation of Medicines for Human Use. Guideline on the Limits of Genotoxic Impurities, EMEA/CHMP/QWP/251344/2006.
18. Klinkenberg R, Stee RB, Ceccata A. 2003. J. Pharm. Biomed. Anal. 32: 345–352.
19. Mirza T, Lunn MJ, Keeley FJ, George RC, Bodenmiller JR. 1999. J. Pharm. Biomed. Anal. 19: 747–756.
20. Nozal MJ, Bernal JL, Toribio L, Martin MT, Diez FJ. 2002. J. Pharm. Biomed. Anal. 20: 285–291.
21. Boca MB, Apostolides Z, Pretorius E. 2005. J. Pharm. Biomed. Anal. 37: 461–468.
22. Forsatz B, Snow NH. 2007. LCGC 25(9): 960–968.
23. Seno S, Ohtake S, Kohno H. 1997. Accred. Qual. Assur. 2(3): 140–145.
24. Kirsch RB. 1998. Pharm. Technnol. 22(2, suppl.): 40–46.
25. Miscioscio K, Cooper DW. 2000. J. IEST 43(1): 31–37.
26. Liu L, Pack BW. 2006. J. Pharm. Biomed. Anal. 43(4): 1206–1212.
27. Jenkins KM, Vanderwielen AJ, Armstrong JA, Leonard LM, Murphy GP, Piros NA. 1996. PDA J. Pharm. Sci. Technol. 50(1): 6–15.
28. Yang P, Burson K, Feder D, Macdonald F. 2005. Pharm. Technol. 29(1): 84–94.
29. Max L. 1997. Pharm. Technol. 21: 56–73.
30. Westman L, Karlsson G. 2000. PDA J. Pharm. Sci. Technol. 54(5): 365–372.
31. Bristol P. 2004. Manuf. Chem. (Engl.) 75: 37–38.
32. Wallace B, Stevens R, Purcell M. 2004. Pharm. Technol. Aseptic Process. 28: 40–43.
33. Guazzaroni M, Yiin B, Yu JL. 1998. Am. Biotechnol. Lab. 16(10): 66–67.
34. Biwald CE, Gavlick WK. 1997. J. AOAC Int. 80(5): 1078–1083.
35. Holmes AJ, Vanderwielen AJ. 1997. PDA J. Pharm. Sci. Technol. 51(4): 149–52.
36. Mirza T, Lunn MJ, Keeley FJ, George RC, Bodenmiller JR. 1999. J. Pharm. Biomed Anal. (Engl.) 19: 747–756.
37. Klinkenberg R, Streel B, Ceccato A. 2003. J. Pharm. Biomed. Anal. 32(2): 345–352.
38. Sajonz P, Natishan TK, Wu Y, McGachy NT, DeTora D. 2005. J. Liquid Chromatogr. Relat. Technol. 28(5): 713–725.
39. Brindusa BM, Zeno A, Etheresia P. 2005. J. Pharm. Biomed. Anal. 37(3): 461–468.
40. Nozal MJ, Bernal JL, Toribio L, Jimenez JJ, Martin MT. 2000. J. Chromatogr. A 870(1–2): 69–75.
41. Nozal MJ, Bernal JL, Toribio L, Martin MT, Diez FJ. 2002. J. Pharm. Biomed. Anal. 30(2): 285–291.
42. Shea JA, Shamrock WF, Abboud CA, Woodeshick RW, Nguyen LQ, Rubino JT, Segretario J. 1996. Pharm. Dev. Technol. 1(1): 69–75.
43. Segretario J, Cook SC, Umbles CL, Walker JT, Woodeshick RW, Rubino JT, Shea JA. 1998. Pharm. Dev. Technol. 3(4): 471–476.
44. Shifflet MJ, Shapiro M, Levin C, DeNisco R. 2001. LC-GC 19(3): 312, 314–317.
45. Kolodsick KJ, Phillips H, Feng J, Molski M, Kingsmill CA. 2006. Pharm. Technol. 30(2): 56–71.

46. Simmonds EL, Lough WJ, Gray MR. 2006. J. Pharm. Biomed. Anal. 40: 531–638.
47. Kent P, Jose F, DeBono BJ, Azhar M. 2005. The Role of Spectroscopy in Process Analytical Technology. www.spectroscopyonline.com, January. Access date Nov 2007.
48. Debono R, Stefanou S, Davis M, Gaurav W. 2002. Pharm. Technol. 26(4); 72–78.
49. Munden R, Everitt R, Sandor R, Carroll J, DeBono R. 2002. Pharm. Technol. Eur. 14(10): 66–72.
50. Mirza T, George RC, Bodenmiller JR, Belanich SA. 1998. J. Pharm. Biomed. Anal. 16(6): 939–950.
51. Risley DS, Hostettler KF, Peterson JA. 1998. LC-GC 16(6): 562–568.
52. Vovk I, Simonovska B. 2005. J. AOAC Int. 88(5): 1555–1561.
53. Katona Z, Vincze L, Vegh Z, Trompler A, Ferenczi-Fodor K. 2000. J. Pharm. Biomed. Anal. 22(2): 349–353.
54. Fabre H, Altria KD. 2001. LC-GC Eur. 14(5): 302, 304, 306, 308–310.
55. Raghavan R, Mulligan JA. 2000. Drug Dev. Ind. Pharm. 26(4): 423–428.
56. Rotsch TD, Spanton M, Cugier P, Plasz AC. 1991. Pharm. Res. 8: 989–991.
57. Elrod L Jr, Schmit JL, Morley JA. 1996. J. Chromatogr. A 723: 235–241.
58. Mehta NK, Goenaga-Polo J, Hernandez-Rivera S, Hernandez D, Thomson MA, Melling PJ. 2003. Spectroscopy 18(4): 14–16, 18–19.
59. Smith JM. 1993. Pharm. Technol. 17: 88, 90–92, 94, 96, 98.
60. Urbas AA, Lodder RA. 2003. NIR News 14(2): 8–10.
61. Simonovska B, Andrensek S, Vovk I, Prosek M. 1999. J. Chromotogr. A 862: 209–215.
62. Weston A. 1998. Am. Biotech. Lab. 16(3): 30–33.
63. Shifflet MJ, Shapiro M. 2000. Int. BioPharm. 13(1): 51–54, 64.
64. Lambropoulos J, Spanos GA, Lazarides NV. 2000. J. Pharm. Biomed. Anal. 23: 421–428.
65. Valvis II, Champion WL Jr. 1999. Org. Process Res. Dev. 3: 44–52.
66. Forsyth RJ, Van Nostrand V. 2005. Pharm. Tech. 29(4): 134–140.
67. Dixon RW, Peterson DS. 2002. Anal. Chem. 74: 2930–2937.
68. Gamache PH, McCarthy RS, Freeto SM, Asa DJ, Woodcock MJ, Laws K, Cole RO. 2005. LC–GC 23: 150, 152, 154, 156, 158, 160–161.
69. Tadeusz G, Frederic L, Roman S, Pat S. 2006. Universal response in liquid chromatography using charged aerosol detection. Anal. Chem. 78: 3186–3192.
70. Inagaki S, Min JZ, Toyo'oka T. 2007. Biomed. Chromatgr. 21: 338–342.
71. Saracino MA, Gandolfib O, Dall'Olio R, Albers L, Kenndler E, Raggi MA. 2006. J. Chromatogr A 1122: 21–27.
72. Blazewicz A, Fijalek Z, Warowna-Grzeskiewicz M, Boruta M. 2007. J. Chromatogr A 1149: 66–72.
73. Marszall ML, Lebiedzinska A, Czarnowski W, Szefer P. 2005. J. Chromatogr. A 1094: 91–98.
74. Vienneau DS, Kindberg CG. 1997. J. Pharm. Biomed. Anal. 16: 111–117.
75. Takashi M, Nagashima M, Shigeoka S, Nishijima M, Kamata K. 1997. J. Chromatogr. A 775: 137–141.

76. Gatti R, Gioia MG, Andreatta P, Pentassuglia G. 2004. J. Pharm. Biomed. Anal. 35: 339–348.
77. Scott RPW. 1994. Liquid Chromatography for the Analyst, Chromatographic Science Series Vol. 67. Boca Raton, FL: CRC Press.
78. El-Gindy A, El-Zeany B, Awad T, Shabana MM. 2001. J. Pharm. Biomed. Anal. 26: 211–217.

PART III

CONTAINMENT TECHNIQUES FOR HIGHLY POTENT PHARMACEUTICAL COMPOUNDS

CHAPTER 16

CONTAINMENT CHALLENGES AND STRATEGIES FOR POTENT COMPOUNDS IN THE PHARMACEUTICAL INDUSTRY

VICTORIA CATHCART, SARAH JONES, and BEVERLY NICKERSON
Pfizer Global Research & Development, Groton and New London Laboratories, Pfizer, Inc., Groton, CT 06340

16.1 INTRODUCTION

During the drug discovery and development process, many of the chemical entities handled by scientists are considered to be "highly potent" or "very active," meaning that they have a pharmacological effect at very low concentrations. Novel drug compounds are designed to have pharmacological activity at the organ, tissue and cellular level. Activity considered to have a beneficial therapeutic effect in the clinic is often considered hazardous in an occupational environment. In addition to the compound under development, associated intermediates of the chemical synthesis, as well as impurities, may have toxic effects at low concentrations. Even in the analytical laboratory where the typical scale of sample handling may be of the order of several milligrams at most, health effects resulting from exposure may be seen. Some compounds may be biologically active at concentrations as low as nanograms per cubic meter; to put this into perspective, this is at a level that is a thousand times lower than the eye can see.

Laboratory and manufacturing operations can be conducted safely if the potential hazards of the compound are recognized and appropriate precautions are identified, evaluated, communicated and used correctly. By adopting good working practices, which include understanding the risks and determining the best containment strategy to control the risks for that situation, personnel will be protected from

Formulation and Analytical Development for Low-Dose Oral Drug Products. Edited by Jack Zheng

health risks associated with the chemicals with which they work. The principle stakeholders, or "drivers," for containment are health and safety, quality, environmental, and operational/financial. This chapter focuses on one of these areas: health and safety.

16.2 SAFE EXPOSURE CONTROL LEVELS—BANDS, LIMITS, AND HANDLING GUIDANCE

Before guidance on safe handling of potent compounds can be developed, it is helpful to try to understand as much as possible the potential hazards of the compound so that appropriate controls are selected. Selection of workplace controls should be made to target exposure points to these hazards, thus minimizing the risk of becoming inadvertently exposed to the compound. At the same time, it is desirable to make the controls as minimally burdensome as possible.

Characterizing the hazards of new chemical entities is as much of an art as it is a science. As they are new, there is usually no information available on the specific compound, and it can be several months to years after the discovery of the new chemical entity before it can be well-characterized from a health and safety perspective. This is due to a number of reasons. First, enough of the compound needs to be synthesized so that there is a sufficient quantity available for testing and analysis. As the yields early on are quite small, it may take several syntheses before there is sufficient material for testing. Secondly, complete hazard characterization is expensive; it is cost prohibitive to conduct extensive testing on every newly discovered compound. In addition, a vast percentage of new compounds will never become approved drugs.

Although an extensive data set is not generated for early drug candidates, there are some studies that are typically conducted when a compound is still in the preclinical (pre-Phase I) stage of development. In addition, other information can be reasonably speculated based on chemical structure, mechanism of action, and projection of dosage.

Given the limitations on conducting extensive testing, many pharmaceutical companies have developed a hazard characterization strategy, often referred to as "banding," "control banding," or "occupational exposure banding" (OEB). Banding is a system of categorizing substances according to a set of criteria, and managing the risk of exposure to the substances by handling the materials with a control methodology that corresponds to each category or band.[1] For example, if a substance meets the criteria to be categorized into "band 2," then the substance is handled using a set of preestablished handling guidelines developed to control risks of band 2 substances.

There is no one "official" set of banding criteria for pharmaceutical compounds, nor is banding standardized between pharmaceutical companies. Some companies have a three-band system, while others have a five-band system—one company's most potent compounds may be classified as a "band 3," while a "band 3" compound in another company may be slightly more hazardous than household dust. Therefore, when exchanging hazard information with a company, it is important to have an understanding of the banding system at that particular company.

16.2.1 Development of a Banding System

The starting point in the development of a banding system begins with the answer to these two questions:

1. At what point in time do I wish to be able to characterize materials into discrete bands?
2. What type of information is available at that point of time?

The answers to these questions are iterative—that is, it may be desirable to be able to characterize materials as soon as possible after discovery, however, if there is not sufficient data available to characterize the compound with reasonable certainty, the point at which the compound is characterized may need to be pushed back in time. Examples of information that could be available "early" (i.e., weeks to months after initial discovery) of the compound include:

- chemical structure;
- relative degree of activity;
- early genetic toxicology results (e.g., Ames test results);
- early estimates of projected dose in humans;
- mechanism of action;
- an estimate of half-life.

As the compound moves closer to entering Phase I clinical trials, more data are generated that can be used to develop classification criteria, such as acute oral toxicology data, greater understanding about the potential for reversibility of effects from exposure, as well as what effects of exposure were observed during studies and the seriousness of the effects.

Once it is determined what data are available, the next step is to establish the bands and assign data ranges within the appropriate bands. This step requires input from a multidisciplinary team of professionals with expertise in engineering, industrial hygiene, toxicology, and pharmacology. As the compound moves further along in development, more data are generated from toxicological studies as well as clinical trials. At some point, enough data are available to establish an occupational exposure limit (OEL). An OEL is the time-weighted concentration of a substance in air for a conventional 8 h work shift within a 40 h work week, to which it is believed that nearly all workers can be exposed to for their working life without adverse health effects. Table 16.1 summarizes some differences between an OEB and an OEL.

Similar to the OEB setting, there is not a specific method to setting OELs that is used by everyone. However, there are some recognized and peer-reviewed models[2] that many organizations use or modify. Although the type of data that is used in

TABLE 16.1 Comparison of OEB and OEL

	OEB	OEL
General description	Covers a range (band) of values	Expressed as a specific number
Method of determination	Set by comparing available data to preestablished list of criteria	Derived from an equation that considers toxicological endpoints, workplace factors, and safety factors
When it is set	Often set early in the drug development process when there is less information about the compound	Set later in the drug development process when the characteristics of the compound are better understood

the calculation of an OEL varies with the model used, some of the typical variables and constants used are:

- NOEL (no observable effect level) or NOAEL (no observable adverse effect level);
- LOEL (lowest observable effect level);
- human body weight (e.g., 70 kg);
- human breathing rate (e.g., 10 m^3 for an 8 h work shift);
- therapeutic dose;
- safety factors used to compensate for species differences, severity, unknowns, etc.

At this point, the OEB or OEL becomes a guide in the development of a compound handling guidance. By using knowledge of expected exposure levels for worker activities in combination with knowledge about protection factors expected from controls, one can develop procedures for handling the compound in such a manner that the worker's exposure is below the set exposure limits.

16.2.2 Safe Handling Guidelines for Potent Compounds

Safe handling of highly potent or low-dose compounds requires control of all worker exposures. What this means in practical terms is that several planning activities need to occur. The scale of this process depends upon the experience of staff who are planning the work and the maturity of the potent compound exposure control management system. In some cases this process can be a long-term project, involving a multidisciplinary review team comprised of users (e.g., scientists, technicians, support staff), containment engineers, industrial hygienists, ergonomists, and facility/space planners. In other cases the scope is significantly smaller, such as when a new compound is introduced into an experienced project team within an existing containment facility. Table 16.2 shows a recommended outline to follow in

TABLE 16.2 Steps in Developing a Handling Guideline for a Low-Dose Compound

Planning/Implementation Aspect	Responsibility
Make an *assessment of the risk* to workers' health in handling this material in the workplace	Cross functional team (e.g., users such as scientists, technicians, support staff, containment engineers, industrial hygienists, toxicologists)
Decide what precautions are needed. These precautions may include building or retrofitting a facility, investing in engineering solutions, developing specific training, or providing medical surveillance for employees involved in the work, etc.	Cross functional team (e.g., users such as scientists, technicians, support staff, containment engineers, industrial hygienists, ergonomists, facility/space planners)
Follow the *hierarchy of control* to ensure that exposures are prevented or adequately controlled	Industrial hygiene, engineering, facility management approval
Once implemented, *maintain controls* and ensure they are used correctly	Facility management, supervision
Monitor employee exposures where possible	Facility management through audit and inspection; industrial hygiene, occupational health support
Ensure employees are informed, trained and supervised to use the controls properly	Facility management, supervision, safety, industrial hygiene

developing a plan for handling a low-dose compound. Each of these steps is discussed in more detail in the section below and in the case studies in Section 4.

Assessment of the Risk to People. The first step in risk assessment defines the physical, chemical and pharmacological nature of the hazard. Considerations to be made may include:

- toxicological aspects often captured in an exposure standard such as an OEL or OEB;
- physical form (e.g., liquid or solid);
- whether the substance is concentrated or dilute;
- if it is a solid, the physical characteristics:[3]
    - powder mass and bulk density,
    - moisture content,
    - particle size and particle size distribution,
    - true density,
    - flowability/powder cohesion,
    - powder shape;

- whether it is a sensitizer (a sensitizer is a chemical that causes a substantial proportion of exposed people or animals to develop an allergic reaction in normal tissue after repeated exposure to the chemical[4]).

In addition, the route of exposure must be considered. There are five main ways that compounds can get into the body. These routes are:

- inhalation;
- direct skin contact;
- ingestion;
- inadvertent contact of the mucus membranes and skin by touching the eyes, nose or mouth after being in contact with the compound;
- inadvertent exposure by injection or breaking of the skin is also possible when handling needles or equipment with glass components.

Inhalation and direct skin contact are the most common routes of exposure. Since potent compounds tend to be handled in solid/powder or liquid form, control measures need to be used to prevent dust or liquid aerosols from becoming airborne, and subsequently being inhaled or coming into contact with the skin. In addition to inhalation, direct skin contact and inadvertent contact with powders or liquids are routes of exposure that need to be identified and minimized.

The next step of the risk assessment, led by an industrial hygiene professional, evaluates the likelihood that a person exposed to the identified hazards would experience an effect. It is important to note that even a positive therapeutic effect (e.g., cholesterol-lowering) is considered to be adverse in terms of occupational exposure. The goal is to return the person home in the same condition he/she arrived in. Questions addressed in this part of the risk assessment include:

- What are the likely routes of exposure to the worker? Typical incidents should also be considered here, for example, needle stick-related exposure when injecting the material into a chromatograph, inhalation when charging a tablet press, etc.
- What is the duration of exposure?
- Where could accidental contamination occur?

Decide What Precautions are Needed. When deciding on what precautions are needed to control worker exposure to a low-dose compound, the following key aspects have been found to comprise a successful planning strategy:

- Efforts should be focused at controlling the identified exposures at their sources. Taking this approach limits potential exposure for workers handling the compound and limits the amount of contamination that will migrate from the work area to other areas of the facility. All process equipment, analytical equipment and activity must be contained by some sort of engineering control when in use. Examples include reducing the number of manual interactions required by the scientist, use of contained formulation equipment, controlling dust emissions during transfers between equipment, enclosing point sources by enclosure or isolation.

- Provide appropriate local exhaust ventilation (LEV) plant (e.g., heating, ventilation, and air conditioning (HVAC) duct, fans, motors, filters, exhaust) and plan for maintenance and repair requirements of these systems. Use air pressure differentials and cascades to prevent migration of contamination into clean areas. Recirculation of general room air should be based on a risk assessment of the operation to ensure that airborne concentrations of the pharmaceutical compounds do not increase over time. Use high-efficiency filtration for exhausts and segregate the workspace from clean space, reducing to the greatest extent feasible the risk for environmental release (e.g., to air or water).
- Design the facility as an envelope around the exposure activity and adopt the following concepts:
  - general room design (i.e., flooring, ceilings, lighting, bench-tops, walls, general utility services, environmental control/ventilation);
  - use impervious smooth finishes of all walls, ceilings and floors within process/laboratory areas to prevent surface contamination build up and facilitate cleaning requirements, ensure smooth sealed transitions between surface finishes;
- Plan carefully with the users and understand how they will do their work, taking into consideration the following logistics:
  - personnel logistics (e.g., work flow, traffic, personal protective equipment (PPE) use, handling practices);
  - material logistics (e.g., material flow, material handling, process flow).

The above aspects are covered in more detail in Table 16.3.[1] It should be kept in mind that Table 16.3 discusses *general* facility designs to consider when developing a containment strategy for highly potent compounds. However, each consideration is subject to rigorous risk assessment. Practically, this means a determination of whether the consideration or practice is required or is a nice extra to control exposures to an appropriate level.

16.3 THE HIERARCHY OF WORKPLACE CONTROLS

Once the precautions that are needed to control exposures are determined, the next step is to compare the level of controls needed against what controls are already in place. There frequently are multiple control strategies that will minimize the potential for exposure. The determination of which control strategy is the best to use is determined by the hierarchy of control principle. Our particular approach to managing risk is to use this hierarchy to evaluate possible risk management approaches for a specific project in conjunction with a modified layer of protection analysis (LOPA) approach.[5]

TABLE 16.3 General Considerations to Make in Determining What Precautions are Needed for Handling a High-Potency, Low-Dose Compound

General Considerations	
1. General handling philosophy	Open handling of product not permitted. Keep containers closed. Avoid open handling on the bench. Use fume hoods, biological safety cabinet (BSC), or other ventilated control device for all aerosol generating activities
2. Access	Restricted access to work area required to authorized, properly trained personnel with medical clearance as applicable
3. Notices/signposting	Signs posted indicating compound and associated hazards
4. Other controls	Containment technology must be used to prevent emissions to the work area or egress of materials to surrounding "clean areas"
5. Rooms – entrances and exits	Isolated through airlocks for production and pilot plant scale (e.g., greater than 5 kg for powders or 100 L liquids). Production area negative to airlock; airlock negative to nonproduction areas Separate personnel and materials airlocks (same airflow design as production) are recommended (case-by-case) for kilo scale (i.e., less than production/pilot plant scale and greater than 1 kg powder or 22 L liquid). Air locks are not required for small-scale (e.g., less than kilo scale) operations
6. Changing facilities	Change/locker rooms and showers contiguous with work area for production, maintenance, service and personnel decontamination for production and pilot plant-scale operation (e.g., greater than 5 kg powder or 100 L liquid). Access to change/locker space and showers required for kilo and small-scale operations (e.g., less than production and pilot plant scale)
7. PPE decontamination	Decontamination of person (i.e., PPE is rendered safe to remove) required prior to entry to change/degowning room or other "clean areas"
Construction	
1. Materials of construction	Highly cleanable, moisture/chemical resistant, nonporous materials
2. Piping	Minimize exposed piping and mechanisms to facilitate cleaning. Consider separate mechanical room for pipe routes
3. Floors	Floors should be seamless and chemical resistant.
4. Ceilings	Ceilings designed to enable ventilation control and cleaning
5. Lights	Gasketted, recessed light fixtures
6. Surfaces	Surfaces should be nonporous, chemical resistant and easily cleanable and designed to limit dust settling

(*Continued*)

TABLE 16.3 *Continued*

Ventilation—Containment Strategy	
1. HVAC systems (exhaust air, recirculation)	Single-pass systems strongly recommended. Recirculation to production area not recommended. Arrangement of ventilation systems should provide for air flow direction away from breathing zone
2. Exhaust emission points	Designed to ensure that re-entrainment to supply does not occur
3. Exhaust to nonproduction areas	Recirculation of production/laboratory air into nonproduction ("clean") areas prohibited. Dedicated HVAC systems are required. Air flow away from breathing zone
4. Ductwork within building	All exhaust ductwork inside the building should be under negative pressure
5. Air cleaning devices	Where possible, air-cleaning devices should be located close to the process to avoid contamination of exhaust ductwork. Bag in/bag out (safe-change) filters or comparable required for all filtration systems
6. HVAC maintenance and Inspection	HVAC systems need to be properly maintained and periodically inspected. Isolated access recommended Standard operating procedures (SOP) should be developed to ensure this transpires
Air Flows	
1. Airflows	Prevent migration of contaminants into uncontrolled areas through use of directional airflows. Separate/dedicated work areas required
2. Airflow direction	All production/laboratory areas negative in pressure to all outer areas
3. Air pressure differentials	Air pressure differentials required to limit dust movement to outside areas. For large scale operations (greater than 1 kg powder or 22 L liquid), pressure differentials are to be monitored and alarmed. Design target of 15 Pa
4. Change out areas in airlocks	Change/locker rooms and showers contiguous with work area for production, maintenance, service and personnel decontamination for production- and pilot plant-scale operation (e.g., greater than 5 kg powder or 100 L liquid) Access to change/locker rooms and showers required for kilo- and small-scale operations (e.g., less than production- and pilot plant-scale)
5. Airlocks for maintenance service	Airlocks or technical spaces required for directional air flow for maintenance service and decontamination
HVAC Systems—General Ventilation	
1. General ventilation distribution/exhaust	General ventilation distributed at ceiling level; exhaust located at floor level behind process equipment or through LEV

(*Continued*)

TABLE 16.3 *Continued*

2. General exhaust filtration	Terminal high efficiency particulate air (HEPA) filtration at exhaust/return required for large scale operations (e.g., greater than 1 kg powder or 22 L liquid). Appropriate terminal filtration provided at exhaust/return for small-scale operations
3. Air exchange rates	Minimum of 15 air changes per hour
4. Air cleaning devices	Where possible, air-cleaning devices should be located close to the process to avoid contamination of exhaust ductwork
	Bag in/bag out (safe-change) filters or comparable required for all filtration systems
5. HVAC maintenance and inspection	HVAC systems need to be properly maintained and periodically inspected. Isolated access recommended. SOPs should be developed
HVAC Systems—Local Exhaust Ventilation (Applies to Open Handling and Transfer Operations)	
1. Local exhaust ventilation systems	LEV required at all dust- or vapor-generating operations and exhausted to the outside through HEPA filters. Full enclosure (containment) ventilation systems recommended
2. Exhaust point connections	Solid connect exhaust at all points where equipment must be opened for service; provide extra exhaust for unusual conditions
3. Capture devices	Fume hoods and other open-face containment devices are not permitted for production and pilot plant scale (e.g., greater than 5 kg powder or 100 L liquid)
	Fume hoods and other open-face containment devices are to be considered for kilo-scale (e.g., less than production/pilot plant-scale and greater than 1 kg powder or 22 L liquid)
	Fume hoods are acceptable with a face velocities of 80–120 fpm (0.4–0.5 m/s), or other containment measures (e.g., snorkel). Weighing hoods should maintain manufacturer-recommended face velocity for small scale (e.g., less than kilo-scale)
4. LEV exhaust recirculation	Recirculation of LEV exhaust air not permitted. LEV should be interlocked to processes
5. LEV exhaust filtration	Exhaust air must be HEPA-filtered after passing through dust collector, prior to discharge to outside for large-scale operations (e.g., greater than 1 kg powder or 22 L liquid)
	Consider filtering exhaust air with HEPA filters after passing through dust collector, prior to discharge to outside for small-scale operations (e.g., less than large-scale)
6. Equipment testing	Ventilation testing to ensure proper function and operation required. For containment devices, factory acceptance testing and site acceptance testing should be completed

(*Continued*)

TABLE 16.3 *Continued*

7. Safe change filters	Bag in/bag out (safe-change) filters or comparable required for all filtration systems
Room/Equipment Cleaning	
1. Dry sweeping	Dry sweeping prohibited
2. Vacuum	Use HEPA vacuum system before wet cleaning. Vacuum system should be dedicated for operating area
3. Vacuum filter change	Bag in/bag out (safe-change) filters or comparable required for all filtration systems
4. Cleaning	High-pressure hose or compressed air cleaning not permitted; use water mist for sufficient wetting period before washing
5. Equipment cleaning	Clean-in-place (CIP) systems strongly recommended for equipment for large scale operations (e.g., greater than 1 kg powder or 22 L liquid) Wash in place systems recommended for equipment for small-scale operations (e.g., less than large-scale)
6. Equipment access	Recommended that equipment be accessed for maintenance from outside containment area for large-scale operations (e.g. greater than 1 kg powder or 22 L liquid) Consider all equipment be accessed for maintenance from outside containment area for small-scale operation (e.g., less than large-scale)
7. Cleaning verification	For large-scale operations, equipment and workplace should be verified, as applicable, as clean by wipe sampling, for GMP areas
8. Renovations	Prior to removal, equipment should be thoroughly cleaned. Laboratories and productions areas should be handed over to contractors in a clean state. Equipment and area should be verified as clean using wipe sampling techniques (when compound specific analytical methods are available)
Maintenance	
1. Equipment design	Equipment should be designed for easy maintenance and cleaning
2. Preventative maintenance	All critical instruments/systems, alarms and performance indicators must be maintained in accordance with established preventative maintenance procedures. Consider specialized preventative procedures for activities within this band
3. Maintenance procedures	Specific procedures should be developed and implemented for equipment and facility maintenance. Where feasible, tools should be dedicated for the area. Follow equipment cleaning and decontamination procedures prior to performing maintenance work

We developed a simplified spreadsheet based tool that enables us to evaluate:

- How many layers of protection are needed for a project?
- How safe is the operation when all the layers are in place—or when one of them fails or is not used?
- What level of reliance are we placing on each layer? And is this acceptable?

The tool was developed using about five years of industrial hygiene data to support the logarithmic scales assigned to each control strategy. The layers of protection can be represented by the diagram shown in Fig. 16.1 and translate to levels of the traditional control hierarchy.

At the laboratory scale we have developed a strategy for handling highly potent pharmaceutical compounds by designing and building a number of laboratories with high-level containment equipment such as isolators to provide the facility to safely handle solids on scales of operation that range from analytical to kilolab. By putting samples into solution at the earliest stage possible and handling solutions of various concentrations, we have been able to demonstrate that exposures are controlled through industrial hygiene monitoring and measurement. For more details on this approach refer to Chapter 17.

Although use of isolators or other effective engineering controls is the preferred method of handling highly potent compounds in solid form, this is not the only possible approach. We have found that use of traditional laboratory controls and a combination of high level of PPE in conjunction with rigorous administrative controls can provide adequate protection. Before considering the use of any of these solutions in a workplace, make sure workers are fully informed about hazard identification, risk assessment and control options.

In combination, all three types of controls (e.g., engineering, administrative and PPE) are extremely effective. Use of only one approach may provide a range of protection from highly effective to not appropriate or adequate, depending upon the

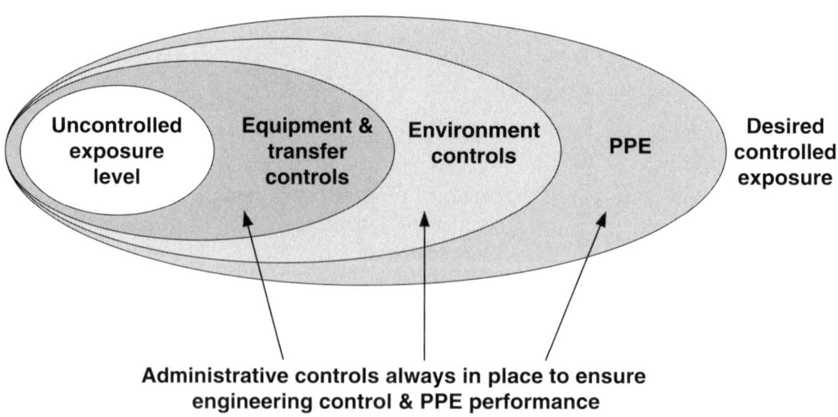

Figure 16.1 Layers of protection.

TABLE 16.4 Example of Risk Based Planning for Handling a Low-Dose Pharmaceutical Compound within a Research Laboratory

Unit Operation/Task	Step	Potential Route of Exposure	Duration	Qualitative Exposure Assessment (Person Handling the Material)	Precautions Required
Weighing low-dose material on a laboratory analytical scale	Subdividing material in powder form	Inhalation/skin absorption	<10 min	Low	*Engineering Controls* Work must be conducted in bench mounted weighing enclosure or isolator *General Controls Required* Only those specifically working on substance in laboratory Laboratory signed with hazard information on compound Name of Chemical Hazard: OEL ____ DO NOT ENTER Contact ____ for Entry Sticky mats, outside laboratory and immediately below subdividing area Ventilated weighing enclosure, • Double nitrile gloves • Disposable Tyvek® suit *or* disposable laboratory coat, shoe covers, disposable sleeves • PAPR (personal air powered respirator) *Isolator* • Normal laboratory attire *Waste* • Plastic lined drums with label on outside with name of compound and OEB level • Arrange waste collection
Serial dilutions of low-dose compound	Transfer compound in solution to flask via pipette in hood	Absorption (skin)	<5 min/transfer	Low	Nitrile double gloves, Tyvek® sleeves, disposable laboratory coat
		Inhalation	<5 min	Negligible	Laboratory hood
	Dilute with solvent or oil in hood	Absorption (skin)	<5 min	Low	Nitrile double gloves, Tyvek® sleeves, disposable laboratory coat
		Inhalation	<5 min	Negligible	Laboratory hood

(*Continued*)

TABLE 16.4 *Continued*

Unit Operation/Task	Step	Potential Route of Exposure	Duration	Qualitative Exposure Assessment (Person Handling the Material)	Precautions Required
HPLC	Transfer solution from flask to HPLC vials via pipette and cap vials in hood	Absorption (skin)	<5 min	Low	Nitrile double gloves, Tyvek® sleeves (see previous statement), disposable laboratory coat
		Inhalation	<5 min	Negligible	Laboratory hood
	Load HPLC vials into tray in hood	Absorption (skin) (from outside of vial)	<5 min	Negligible	Nitrile gloves, disposable laboratory coat
	Load Tray into HPLC	none	<5 min	N/A	N/A
	Unload Trays	Absorption (skin) (from outside of vials)	<5 min	Negligible	Nitrile gloves, disposable laboratory coat
	HPLC Waste Collection	Absorption (skin)		Low	Nitrile double gloves, Tyvek® sleeves (see previous statement), disposable laboratory coat Technique (use precautions when removing tubing to prevent drips)
		Inhalation	Several hours	Low	Top of bottle is capped Compound in very dilute concentrations compound in a liquid Distance (bottle on floor)
NMR	Load NMR tubes that have been prepared in containment area and are in a closed tube	Skin absorption		Negligible	Nitrile gloves Auto loader

situation. For this reason, many companies require that the hierarchy of control is followed to assure best protective measures are used, even when extremely small amounts of chemical are being handled. The selection process for any control combination is the outcome of a risk assessment where exposure variables are evaluated. When planning work with a high potent compound the following general aspects should be considered to reduce exposure potential:

- facility designs requirements that have been proven to control exposure to potent compounds;
- location where the work will be conducted;
- type of work that will be conducted;
- duration and frequency of the activities planned;
- exposure potential.

The example shown in Table 16.4 illustrates an assessment conducted when planning work in the laboratory environment; the controls are determined by employing the risk-based assessment process in conjunction with an understanding of the control measures that could be put into place.

16.4 CASE STUDIES

Two case studies have been developed based on a couple of activities that are performed on a regular basis within the pharmaceutical industry. These studies are intended:

- to illustrate how controls should be maintained;
- to demonstrate the type of performance evaluations that can be made to assess the effectiveness of engineering controls and workplace exposures (monitor employee exposures);
- to define the talking points to inform, train and supervise employees.

16.4.1 Case Study 1: Weighing Within a Ventilated Weighing Safety Enclosure

Many operations within the laboratory start with weighing. It is difficult to undertake precise weighing in conventional laboratory fume hoods, as the airflow and vibration inside an operating fume hood often disturb the balance. In order to accommodate the need for an engineered control at this scale of operation, dust control systems have evolved known as ventilated weighing safety enclosures or powder weighing hoods. Key characteristics of a ventilated weighing safety enclosure include:

- it accommodates a balance and/or microbalance with electrical ports integrated;
- hinged front openings for the placement of large items inside the units;

- low volume laminar airflow and airfoils which effectively minimizes turbulence;
- low vibration;
- constructed from transparent scratch resistant resin (acrylic) with stain-resistant recessed work surfaces (phenolic resin) to contain spills;
- removable air plenums or slot panels for ease of cleaning and decontamination;
- option for controlling wastes generated with "hazardous waste chute";
- face velocity alarm to indicate low flow.

Maintenance of Controls. These types of enclosures should be maintained in accordance with guidance from the manufacturer. As a minimum these units are tested on an annual basis to ensure that adequate face velocity is maintained and components (including terminal filtration units where requisite) are inspected. Prior to use, users inspect the unit to ensure that it is functioning correctly.

Employee Exposure Monitoring. Industrial hygiene assessments using surrogate monitoring techniques (with lactose) have been conducted during various subdivision operations on the open bench-top, within a ventilated weighing safety enclosure such as a Flow Sciences Hoods®, shown in Fig. 16.2, and chemical laboratory hoods. Initial studies were conducted to assess the need for ventilated weighing safety enclosures and included assessment of airborne exposure only, while later studies evaluated airborne exposure, as well as surface contamination. These studies looked at critical variables, such as face velocity, scale of subdivision

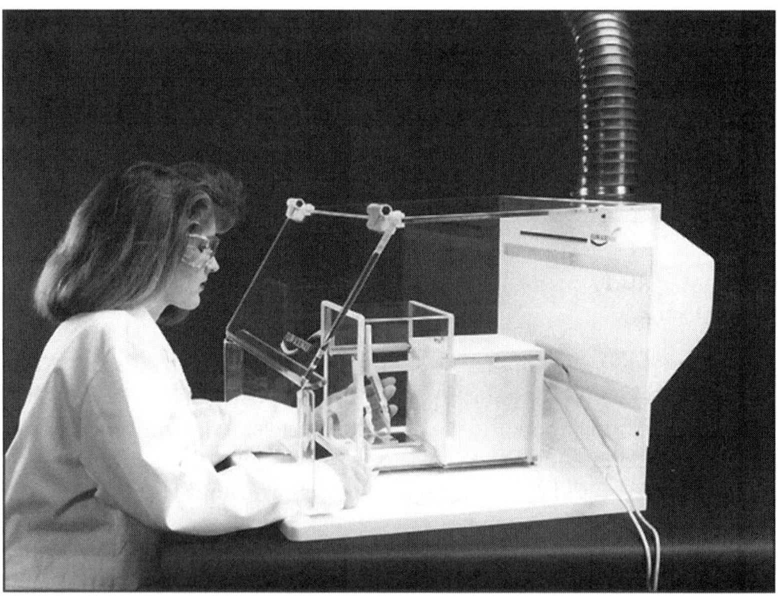

Figure 16.2 An example of a ventilated weighing enclosure.

work, sash position for chemical laboratory hoods and operator work practice. Area air sample concentrations for open bench-top applications ranged from 0.1 to 3 $\mu g/m^3$. It was found that various hoods reduced airborne concentrations by up to 90%. Surrogate monitoring conducted for various ventilated weighing safety enclosures at different face velocities during small-scale laboratory operations (up to 10 g) indicated that operator breathing zone concentrations were $<1.0\ \mu g/m^3$ at several different face velocities tested. Sampling conducted within ducted and ductless versions of these enclosures indicated that performance is not affected by terminal filtration arrangements.

Information and Training. The following personal work practices have been found to be important factors in minimizing potential exposure when weighing samples.

- Care should be taken to ensure that protective equipment is worn correctly, and that no exposed skin is visible; gloves and laboratory coats are worn to ensure that dermal contact is minimized and to provide a continuous protective barrier to the skin from powder contact. Disposable sleeve covers are also suggested if arms are inserted far enough that laboratory coats could be covered with hazard.
- All PPE should be removed and disposed of in the hazardous waste chute or disposal bag when removing hands from the enclosure to prevent dragging powders out of the unit. Users should be trained in aseptic glove removal technique to minimize aerosolization of material during a process where skin could become exposed.
- Weighing should be carried out carefully in order to minimize spillage and thus reduce exposure potential
- To minimize contamination, the powder should be carefully placed into the weigh boat. Dropping the material from a height should be avoided.
- All contaminated tools, particularly the spatulas used, should be placed into a beaker or another vessel. Any powder in the beaker can then be dissolved in a suitable solvent and be properly disposed of.
- For larger scale weighing, care must be taken when scooping material into flasks and beakers. The best technique would be to place the compound carefully into the base of the beaker (positioned at an angle), minimizing the generation of airborne dust. Consideration must be made of the design of the vessels; the use of a wide neck vessel and small scoop which can be inserted into the base of the vessel is recommended.
- Dropping the powder from a height leads to the creation of airborne dust, which will eventually settle onto the surrounding surfaces. In this case the contamination is gross and can be clearly seen.
- Unsealed containers such as weigh boats and conical beakers which contain compounds should not be removed from the powder weigh hood because the powder could become airborne during this process.

- If it is not possible to weigh directly into a sealable vessel within the weighing hood, then the powder should be transferred into a suitable sealable container prior to removal from the weighing hood. The use of a powder funnel will ensure that the compound is appropriately transferred. A surface wipe-down of any vessel leaving the enclosure should be done.
- Any contaminated equipment should be cleaned using wet cleaning methods, such as a wet cloth prior to removal from the weigh hood.
- Any contaminated cloth should be placed inside a bag within the weigh hood without obstructing the back baffle. This bag should be sealed, double bagged and disposed of, as a minimum, at the end of each working day (e.g., via a hazardous waste chute).
- Small amounts of powder spillage are inevitable; surfaces within containment units such as powder weigh hoods should be cleaned, as a minimum, at the end of each working day.
- Keep the vented enclosure on at all times, especially during the tare process. The balance should be tarred while under ventilation as this is the same atmosphere the actual weighing will occur in. Keeping the unit on, even when not in use, also helps prevent exposure due to previous users not cleaning the station correctly.

Note Regarding Chemical Laboratory Hoods. Industrial hygiene assessment for powder subdivision within chemical laboratory hoods indicates that face velocities should not exceed 100 feet per minute (fpm) with the sash in the lowered position. Personnel exposures at or below 1.0 $\mu g/m^3$ are achievable for both large-scale and small-scale subdivisions, provided that good work practices are adhered to. When face velocities are maintained between 80 and 100 fpm and the sash is in a lowered position, work practices affect personnel exposure concentration by greater than one order of magnitude. Face velocities above 150 fpm result in excessive turbulence and an inability to weigh accurately, due to air movement, vibration and product loss to exhaust.

"Visibly clean" is not an acceptable cleaning criterion. A detailed, sequential cleaning procedure is advisable, for surfaces inside and outside laboratory chemical hoods and ventilated weighing enclosures. If settling of powder occurs on the floor, this indicates that material is escaping and that additional administrative and personal protective controls are warranted when using chemical fume hoods for subdivision applications.

16.4.2 Case Study 2: Liquid Handling

While less hazardous than powders, potent compounds in solution may also become airborne and therefore lead to worker exposure. Operations that have the potential to create aerosols, such as sampling, sample preparation, sample transfers and purifications, should only be performed with appropriate engineering controls in place. It is important to clean surfaces that may have become contaminated during the handling of liquids or from the spill of droplets by these materials. These aerosol droplets, if left to dry, can result in powder deposits. If these powder deposits are agitated they can become airborne and potentially lead to exposure. For such operations it is particularly important to select the most appropriate chemically protective gloves, which afford protection to the solvents being used. The potential for exposure also exists when handling relatively small quantities of compounds, for example, when preparing analytical test samples.

Employee Exposure Monitoring. Industrial hygiene assessment of surface concentrations associated with a potent compound handled solely in liquid form within a chemical laboratory hood was conducted to assess the potential for downstream contamination potential. Handling operations assessed included dilutions of sample solutions and HPLC analysis. Wipe samples were collected from the following surfaces within and outside of the laboratory:

- bench-top within chemical fume hood—center;
- bench-top within chemical fume hood—left side near HPLC waste jar;
- center of chemical fume hood on air foil;
- floor below chemical fume hood;
- center island bench-top left side of sink;
- door knob on laboratory side of door leading to donning/doffing room;
- floor of donning/doffing room at door to laboratory.

Samples were collected using Texwipe 714A Alpha Swabs and a 100 cm^2 stainless steel template. Two swabs were used to wipe each location. The first swab was premoistened with methanol and used to wipe the surface. The swab was then placed in an amber glass vial and a second "dry" swab was used to re-wipe the same surface and was also placed in a vial. Following collection, each vial was sealed and sent with a blank to an accredited industrial hygiene laboratory for analysis. The analytical results indicated that the concentration of the potent compound was approximately equal to the company set cleaning guidance level of 1.0 $\mu g/100\ cm^2$ at the center of the chemical fume hood. All remaining surfaces were approaching or at the analytical reporting limit of 0.05 μg. The results of the wipe sampling are provided in Table 16.5.

It is common for numerical guidance limits to be developed to aid the evaluation of whether a surface is clean. Development of such guidance is tied to the development of hazard data and safe airborne exposure limits. When a compound is at the early stage of development it is likely that some sort of generic surface limit may be set (similar to an exposure band previously discussed). The use of these surface concentrations limits may be used to require additional cleaning and re-sampling if the limit is exceeded. In the case study examined here it is strongly suggested that additional cleaning is necessary for surfaces within the center of the chemical laboratory hood.

TABLE 16.5 Wipe Sampling Results

Location	Concentration (μg/100 cm^2)
Bench-top within chemical fume hood—center	0.96
Bench-top within chemical fume hood—left side near HPLC waste jar	0.06
Center of chemical fume hood on air foil	0.11
Floor below chemical fume hood	0.11
Center island bench-top left side of sink	0.12
Door knob on laboratory side of door leading to donning/doffing room	0.15
Floor of donning/doffing room at door to laboratory	0.13
Blank	<0.05 μg

<, Less than indicated reporting limit μg/100 cm^2. Bold indicates concentration equal to or exceeding the 1.0 μg/100 cm^2 guideline.

It is important to note that air sampling conducted during this study consistently demonstrated airborne concentrations below the analytical detection limit during activities conducted within the chemical laboratory hood.

Information and Training. General recommendations for handling potent compounds in liquid form include:

- Maintain vigilance over the use and disposal of PPE (e.g., safety glasses, disposable Tyvek® laboratory coat, disposable booties) during occupancy within the laboratory. In addition, it is recommended that disposable Tyvek® sleeves are used when transferring liquids, for example during dilution preparation.
- Ensure the waste drum is located at the at the exit door within the laboratory, so that removal of PPE is performed with the occupant on the "sticky mat" to prevent contamination of shoes.
- Perform thorough cleaning of bench-top within the chemical fume hood after each unit operation using a 3× cleaning technique. This technique is involves an initial surface cleaning with a deactivating agent, followed by a water and/or solvent rinse, and a third surface cleaning with a standard cleaning solvent such as isopropanol or methanol.
- It is recommended that periodic surface wipe sampling is conducted to monitor surface contamination within and outside of the laboratory and to maintain employee and supervision attention to good working practices.

Note About Cleaning Methods. A number of cleaning techniques can be used. For example, a balance brush could be used to sweep residual powder off the balance and onto a filter paper. However, this method is not ideal because the powder tends to be distributed over the base of the unit. Wet cleaning methods tend to be more effective and are therefore preferable. The powder must be soluble in the agent used, otherwise smearing occurs. Touching contaminated surfaces could also occur as a result of inadvertent contact and exposure. Be sure, during cleaning operations, to solubilize and remove the compound. Carefully consider the cleaning techniques and materials to be utilized before beginning the cleaning operation.

16.5 SUMMARY

The very same characteristics that make a pharmaceutical compound a "good medicine" also make it a challenge to develop and manufacture in a safe manner. Pharmaceutical compounds are intended to have a physiological effect on the patient. It is also desirable to have a drug that is efficacious with an easily managed dosing regimen, such as a once a day dosage. This translates into compounds that cause effects in very small quantities. This chapter has described a system of control methods that is used by many pharmaceutical companies to prevent their workforce from becoming exposed and experiencing effects from working with these compounds.

The system consists of two parts. The first part involves using either available information from the drug development process or making reasonable speculations to characterize the potential hazards to the workforce from exposure to the compounds. The second step involves using that information to assess the risk of exposure and recommend controls that prevent exposure. There is more than one suitable control method that can control most exposure points, and several examples have been provided. Finally, case studies have been provided to demonstrate the effectiveness of some of these control methods.

ACKNOWLEDGMENTS

The information included in this chapter is based on contributions over several years from many professionals in Pfizer's Occupational Hygiene Community of Practice, as well as from the professionals in Occupational Toxicology. In addition, we would like to acknowledge the contributions of Jorge Marzari, PhD, CSP in the application of the Layer of Protection Analysis approach to our risk assessment process. Much of the data used for the case studies was generated by Mike Burns and Jeff Kaminski of OccuHealth, Inc. Thanks to Flow Sciences Inc. for the photograph (Fig. 16.2) used in this chapter to illustrate experiences.

REFERENCES

1. Neuman BD, Sargent EV. 1996. Performance based exposure control limits for pharmaceutical active ingredients. Am. Ind. Hyg. Assoc. J. 57: 33–42.
2. Ku RH. 2000. An overview of setting occupational exposure limits (OELs) for pharmaceuticals. Chem. Hlth Safety 7(1): 34–37.

3. Pujara CP, Kildsig DO. 2001. Effect of individual particle characteristics on airborne emissions. In: Wood JP, editor. Containment in the pharmaceutical industry. New York: Marcel Dekker.
4. 29 C.F.R. § 1910. 1200, 2006.
5. Center for Chemical Process Safety. 2001. Layer of protection analysis—Simplified process risk assessment. New York: American Institute of Chemical Engineers.

CHAPTER 17

SAMPLE HANDLING AND CONTAINMENT IN ANALYTICAL TESTING LABORATORIES

S. DAVID PATTAVINA, NANCY SAGE, and BEVERLY NICKERSON
Pfizer Global Research & Development, Groton and New London Laboratories, Pfizer, Inc., Groton, CT 06340

17.1 INTRODUCTION

Active pharmaceutical ingredients (APIs) are designed to have pharmacological activity. While this activity may be of benefit to the patient, it can be hazardous to individuals who need to handle the material during analytical characterization and testing of the API and its dosage forms. The number of high potency pharmaceutical compounds is increasing. Reportedly, by the year 2010 approximately 90% of all pharmaceutical compounds will be potent compounds.[1] Sample handling practices and containment in the analytical testing laboratory are key considerations when managing potent APIs and low-dose drug products.

Pharmaceutical companies typically have several options regarding analytical testing of potent compounds: retrofit a standard analytical laboratory handle potent compounds, design and build an analytical containment laboratory or outsource the testing. Based on extensive experience using both standard analytical laboratories and containment laboratories for handling and testing potent compounds, some considerations and recommendations for handling and testing these compounds are discussed in this chapter. More emphasis is given to the option of using a containment laboratory since the industry trend is toward using more containment technology for handling these materials. This trend is due to the increase in the number of potent compounds under development as well as a heightened awareness of the hazards associated with these types of compounds. While outsourcing this type of work is a viable option, it is not discussed within this chapter.

Formulation and Analytical Development for Low-Dose Oral Drug Products. Edited by Jack Zheng

17.2 SAMPLE HANDLING CONSIDERATIONS

There should be written guidelines (e.g., handling guidelines) in place detailing how potent compounds are to be handled during analytical testing. These handling guidelines should include the specific hazard(s) of the compound, the minimum level of personal protective equipment (PPE) required, as well as any specified engineering and administrative controls that need to be in place and used.

Inhalation and direct skin contact are the most common routes of chemical exposure. The greatest exposure risk in handling potent compounds in an analytical laboratory therefore occurs when handling solid materials due to the potential to generate and inhale airborne dust particles of the compound. Once the potent material has been placed into solution, the airborne exposure risk is reduced and solutions of potent compounds may be handled in a manner similar to other nonpotent pharmaceutical compounds, assuming good laboratory practices are followed. Caution should be taken not to aerosolize the solutions since this could create an inhalation hazard. In addition, any sample solution spills should be adequately cleaned to prevent powder deposits of the compound from forming, which could potentially become airborne after the liquid has dried.

The solid form of the drug includes the API, tablet blends and granulations, tablet cores and film-coated tablets. The API, as well as blends and granulations, may pose the greatest concern for inhalation of drug particles, but it is important to recognize that tablet cores may also be a source of dust and potential inhalation exposure. Film-coated tablets generally do not have dust concerns; in most cases film-coated tablets, as long as they remain intact, can be handled in the same manner as nonpotent tablets.

Since the greatest exposure risk occurs in handling the potent compound in a solid or powder form, efforts should be made to minimize the need to handle this form of the drug. For example, the common practice of using a mortar and pestle to grind several tablets to make a composite sample for potency and purity testing should be avoided if possible. An alternative procedure would be to place intact tablets into a flask, add diluent, then disperse the tablets and extract the active ingredient by shaking, sonicating or homogenizing the sample solution. In some cases handling of the powder form of the drug cannot be avoided, such as when preparing API standard solutions for use in sample analysis. In this case, it would be desirable to prepare the standard or a stock standard solution using a diluent in which the compound is stable. One should then establish solution stability for the longest duration possible (e.g., 30 days) to minimize how often standard solutions need to be prepared. If necessary, one can prepare a stock solution in organic solvent or aqueous buffer to maximize stability, then prepare a working standard solution by diluting the stock solution to match the analysis buffer (e.g., HPLC buffer) prior to the analysis.

These general strategies can be used whether sample handling is performed in a standard analytical laboratory or in a containment laboratory. Considerations for these two different types of laboratories are discussed below. Furthermore, the use of automation to prepare samples for analytical testing in a contained environment is another option to reduce potential worker exposure to potent compounds. This option, however, can be cost-prohibitive and therefore is not discussed in this chapter.

17.3 HANDLING POTENT COMPOUNDS IN STANDARD ANALYTICAL LABORATORIES

Adapting a standard analytical laboratory (i.e., an analytical laboratory that contains no gloveboxes or isolators and has not previously been used for potent compounds) for handling and testing potent APIs and low-dose drug products has several advantages. The laboratory can be set up relatively quickly and requires minimal investment to implement, use and maintain. It is much less costly than designing and building a dedicated containment laboratory. Ensuring worker safety when handling potent compounds in such a laboratory relies extensively on the use of administrative controls, chemical fume hoods, ventilated weighing enclosures and PPE. This approach can provide protection for workers by minimizing exposure to the compounds being handled and tested. There are limits, however, to how effective this approach is for extremely potent and hazardous compounds. Several factors that need to be considered in ensuring safe handling of potent compounds in a standard analytical laboratory are discussed below. The shipping, receipt and transportation of potent samples are discussed in Section 17.5.

17.3.1 Laboratory Access

Access to the laboratory should be limited to personnel directly involved with the testing of the high potency material. Access should be regulated using a key card, as shown in Fig. 17.1, or other type of lock system to prevent persons who do not

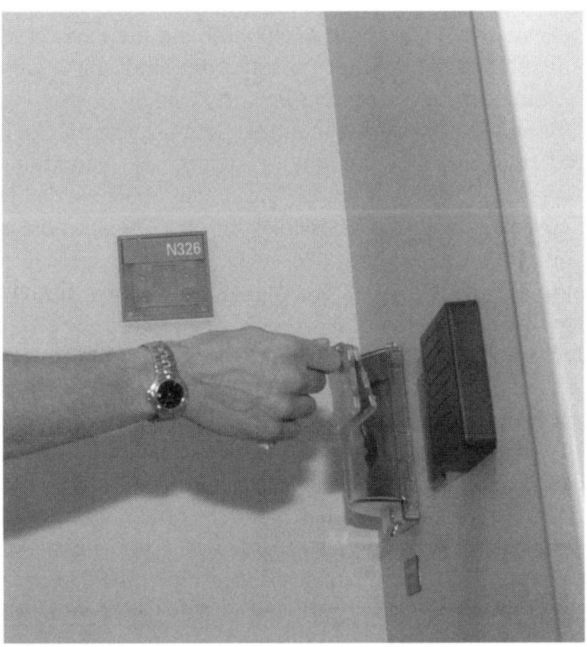

Figure 17.1 Accessing the laboratory by key card.

have proper authorization from entering the laboratory. There should be a single point of contact for persons needing access to the laboratory. This will ensure that personnel entering the area have been properly trained in potent compound handling and are aware of any risks associated with entering the laboratory. Personnel not trained in potent compound handling, such as maintenance staff, should be escorted by trained laboratory personnel at all times.

In addition to restricting access to the laboratory, signs should be posted at the entrance of the laboratory detailing the name of the compound being worked on as well as the hazards associated with that specific compound. A list of key contacts with intimate knowledge of the operations being performed in the laboratory should be placed outside the door. This is especially important in case the laboratory has to be entered during off peak hours by facilities personnel or an emergency response team. Individuals should not work in the laboratory alone; a buddy system should be utilized to ensure worker safety. An alternative to the buddy system would be to utilize closed circuit cameras to monitor activities in the laboratory from a remote location. The person responsible for monitoring an individual working in the laboratory must be vigilant and aware of activities in the laboratory at all times; there should be no extended periods of time where an individual is unsupervised.

17.3.2 Personal Protective Equipment

Proper PPE must be identified and utilized. The selection of PPE should be based upon the hazard(s) associated with the compound and the method of handling. The level of PPE required when handling potent compounds in a standard laboratory setting is more stringent than that required in a containment laboratory that is heavily dependent upon engineering controls (e.g., isolators). When handling a potent compound in a standard laboratory setting, the minimum PPE required should be appropriate gloves and safety glasses as well as dedicated laboratory shoes with shoe covers, a dedicated laboratory uniform (e.g., scrubs) and a disposable laboratory coat or coverall. Double gloves with sleeve covers can also be used as added protection to minimize the risk of exposure, especially during weighing operations in ventilated weighing enclosures.

Particular attention should be paid to the gloves worn in the laboratory. Gloves must not only protect the workers from the potent compounds, but they must also provide an acceptable level of protection from any reagents that are being used in the handling and testing of these compounds. If there is a possibility of inhalation of potent compounds, a suitable respirator containing a high efficiency particulate air (HEPA) filtration system or supplied breathing grade air should be employed. Additional respiratory protection may be needed if any reagents, such as solvents, posing an inhalation risk are being utilized in the laboratory. The site's Environmental Health and Safety department should be consulted to determine if medical monitoring of individuals working with potent compounds should be considered. This judgment should be made on a case-by-case basis, taking into account the specific hazards of the individual compounds being tested. After use, all PPE should be treated as hazardous waste and be disposed of accordingly.

17.3.3 Additional Controls

Every effort must be made to ensure that any potential contamination remains inside the laboratory and is not tracked into corridors or common areas. The airflow in the laboratory should be rebalanced such that the pressure inside of the laboratory is negative to that of the hallways or common areas. This negative pressure can prevent airborne materials from migrating outside the laboratory into common areas through doorways and other openings. Qualified personnel should check airflow in the laboratory, as well as in any chemical fume hoods or ventilated weighing enclosures, on a regular basis. This will ensure that the laboratory is kept at negative pressure and that these engineering controls (e.g., chemical fume hoods, ventilated weighing enclosures) are functioning properly.

A double door system with a gowning and degowning area is recommended since this can minimize the disruption of airflow into and out of the laboratory and provide a defined area for PPE disposal and storage. Sticky mats, also known as tack mats or adhesive mats, should be placed at all doorways to eliminate the possibility that material will be tracked outside of the laboratory on the soles of shoes. These mats should be changed on a regular basis to ensure their functionality; caution should be used when changing the mats.

An additional consideration is the use of absorbent, plastic-backed paper on laboratory benches or work surfaces. These papers can absorb any spills, minimizing the risk of forming powder deposits of the potent compound after the spill has dried.

17.3.4 Sample Handling

Proper sample handling and housekeeping procedures must be stressed. In general, there are several activities that by their very nature pose a higher risk for worker exposure. With respect to analytical testing, these high-risk exposure operations include weighing of dry solids, transfer of solids between containers, grinding operations, particle size measurements, and any operation that has potential to create an aerosol. All of these operations must be performed in a properly functioning hood or ventilated weighing enclosure; there should be no open bench-top handling of any materials when performing operations which result in the potential for creation of dust or aerosolized particles. In addition, traffic flow inside the laboratory should be restricted when handling potent compounds in the hoods to ensure that there is no disruption of air currents, such as can happen when walking by an open hood. Such disruptions could potentially compromise worker safety.

As previously discussed, once the solid or powder sample is in solution, the risk of worker exposure is greatly reduced. Handling precautions for the solution containing the potent compound may therefore be less stringent than for handling solids or powders of the same compound. Transportation of high potency materials to and from the laboratory is discussed in Section 17.4.

17.3.5 Removal of Hazardous Wastes

The level of treatment that waste generated in the laboratory is subject to should be evaluated on a case-by-case basis. Decisions regarding the level of waste treatment should take into account the medium that the potent compound is in. Solvent waste, by default, is more stringently regulated and undergoes different disposal protocols than an aqueous waste. Solvent waste contaminated with potent compounds would normally be treated in the same manner as solvent waste containing nonpotent compounds, but it should be noted on all containers that the waste contains a potent compound. Proper labeling of the waste containers will help to assure that personnel responding to an incident involving the waste will handle the situation in an appropriate manner.

Any aqueous waste, such as dissolution media, that is generated should also be evaluated on a case-by-case basis. Potent compounds are normally dosed in formulations containing milligram or lower levels of active compound. Dissolution or other aqueous wastes are therefore normally very dilute solutions. As long as there are no ecological toxicity issues, dissolution media and aqueous wastes containing potent compounds can normally be incorporated into the standard aqueous waste stream. If there are any toxicity issues associated with the wastes, the aqueous wastes and dissolution media should be segregated from the normal waste stream and treated in an appropriate manner.

In the case of nonsolvent contaminated solid laboratory waste, depending upon the potent compound being handled, it may be necessary to handle and dispose of the waste using a higher level of treatment than one would of a standard pharmaceutical waste solid, which would normally be considered a nonhazardous waste.

Glassware that has potentially been contaminated with a potent compound should be thoroughly rinsed and any active compounds neutralized, if possible, prior to removal from the laboratory for cleaning. All rinses and any materials used to wipe the container during the decontamination process should be handled as hazardous waste. All personnel involved with cleaning glassware should be trained on proper handling techniques to lessen the likelihood of accidental exposure. Procedures for removal of hazardous wastes from the laboratory should take into account not only the environmental or biohazard level of the waste but also the pharmacological effects of the potent compound.

17.3.6 Limitations

Ensuring worker safety when handling potent compounds in a standard analytical laboratory relies heavily on the use of chemical fume hoods, ventilated weighing enclosures, administrative controls and PPE to ensure worker safety. One of the drawbacks of this type of setup is that it can be extremely uncomfortable to work in the required level of PPE for long periods of time. In addition, the donning and doffing of PPE can take quite a bit of time and needs to be repeated every time an individual enters and exits the laboratory. Another drawback is the cost associated with purchasing and disposing of large amounts of PPE, which must be treated as hazardous waste due to potential contamination.

Equipment in the laboratory that comes into direct contact with a potent compound requires thorough decontamination before it can be removed from the laboratory. Some equipment cannot be adequately cleaned and must be disposed of as hazardous waste. For example, it was found that cooling fans on pieces of equipment (e.g., Endeavor Hydrogenator, HPLC systems) had spread trace levels of contamination throughout the equipment. This equipment could not be cleaned to an acceptable level and therefore had to be disposed of as hazardous waste. The use of isolators or containment laboratories, which is discussed in the next section, is an alternative approach that addresses these issues.

17.4 HANDLING POTENT COMPOUNDS IN A CONTAINMENT LABORATORY

A containment laboratory is a laboratory that has a high level of engineering controls, such as isolators or glove boxes, in place to ensure worker safety. When using a containment laboratory, the handling guidelines and procedures developed must address the operations of the containment laboratory, the containment equipment in the laboratory, as well as the handling of the potent compounds. In addition, the handling guidelines and procedures should cover how to deal with emergencies such as breach of containment. Specific areas that should be addressed in the handling guidelines or procedures are discussed below.

17.4.1 Containment Laboratory Access

Only personnel with an immediate need to enter the containment laboratory should be given access. Laboratory access should only be given after an individual has been trained not only on potent compound handling, but also on the operation of the containment laboratory itself and any isolators or glove boxes within the laboratory. If isolators are to be utilized, training should as a minimum include the operation and use of the isolators, leak detection in the isolators, visual and mechanical inspection of the isolator gloves, isolator glove change procedures and steps to be taken in the event of an emergency, such as a breach of an isolator glove.

17.4.2 Personal Protective Equipment

Unlike the standard analytical laboratory previously discussed, where worker safety is heavily reliant on PPE, chemical fume hoods, ventilated weighing enclosures, and administrative controls, a containment laboratory is heavily reliant on engineering controls such as isolators to ensure worker safety. In a situation where an isolator is being used to contain a potent compound, the requirements for PPE may be less stringent. Laboratory attire for handling potent compounds in an isolator laboratory includes disposable laboratory coats, dedicated laboratory shoes and appropriate gloves and safety glasses. In general, there is no need to wear a respirator in a containment laboratory as the isolator will contain any dust particles or aerosols that are generated. There are instances, however, where more or less PPE is warranted depending upon the specific hazards of the compound. Hazard data for the individual compound must therefore be taken into account when choosing the appropriate level of PPE. In addition, there should be a specific area set aside for the donning and doffing of PPE in the laboratory. All PPE, whether believed to have been contaminated with a potent compound or not, should be treated as hazardous waste and be disposed of accordingly.

17.4.3 Containment Laboratory Room Design or "Thinking Inside the Box"

As previously mentioned, a containment laboratory is heavily reliant on engineering controls (e.g., isolators) to ensure worker safety and comfort. In designing such a laboratory, every aspect of the laboratory is important and must be considered. An example of the design considerations for a containment laboratory is detailed below. This example also highlights what can happen when a key detail is not considered.

Our first containment laboratory was designed with little thought as to how the room itself should be built. The laboratory was essentially a regular chemistry laboratory with isolators placed inside the room, with an ante-room added on for donning and doffing PPE. When trying to balance the airflow for the laboratory (e.g., positive pressure in the hallway; slightly negative pressure in the ante-room, and more negative pressure in the laboratory), it was found that the proper airflow could not be attained. This was when the importance of room design was realized. It was found that the ceiling tiles installed in the laboratory were so permeable to air that it was impossible to maintain the proper air balance in the laboratory. This problem required a redesign of the laboratory to correct the defect.

The design of the new containment laboratory utilized essentially the same principles as a clean room but, for opposite reasons. The purpose of a clean room is to protect the product from contamination from the environment. In the containment laboratory, the goal is to protect the environment and personnel from the product. The way to accomplish both of these goals is essentially the same. The room needs to be sealed off from the rest of the building and airflow needs to be tightly controlled. The ceiling in the laboratory should be a "hard" ceiling and made as impervious to airflow as possible. In this case, a standard dry wall ceiling which was radiused (i.e., corners were curved not squared) to the walls and coated with an epoxy paint was installed. Using epoxy paint on the walls and ceiling not only made them impervious to air, but also made them water resistant. This had the effect of making the laboratory easier to clean in the event of any accidental contamination of the laboratory. The floor of the laboratory was also sealed and the material was extended up onto the walls with radiused corners. This not only prevented contamination from being trapped in the joints where the floors and walls meet, but also prevented damage to the walls when cleaning and, in the event of a flood, water would be less likely to exit the laboratory and contaminate other areas of the building. Airflow for the laboratory was balanced for positive pressure in the hallway, slightly

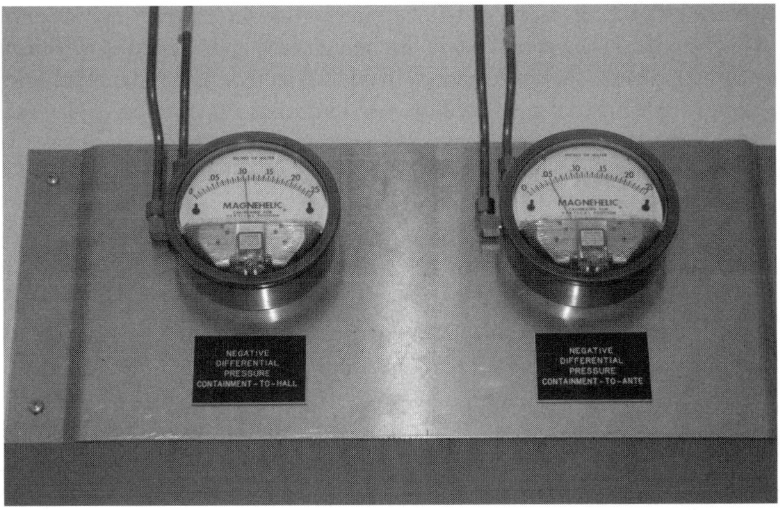

Figure 17.2 Magnahelic gages measuring pressure differentials between rooms in a containment facility.

negative pressure in the ante-room, and more negative pressure in the laboratory. Room pressures were constantly monitored using magnahelic gages as shown in Fig. 17.2.

All electrical outlets and light fixtures were fitted with gaskets and sealed to ensure that they were impervious to air and water. The room exhaust was filtered with redundant HEPA filters; this was the key consideration to prevent contamination of the ductwork. The exhaust system had redundant fans installed that were connected to emergency power to minimize the risk of failure. In the case of an ecologically toxic compound or reagent, the isolator drains had the ability to retain water or solvent discharge. The retained discharge could then be treated and neutralized prior to releasing it to a municipal wastewater treatment facility or sending it out as hazardous waste. In addition, the anteroom to the laboratory has a decontamination shower to allow employees to wash down with water in the event of a containment breach.

17.4.4 Isolator Design

For analytical testing purposes, there are two key considerations in designing an isolator. The first consideration is that the design of the isolator should be such that the individual utilizing the isolator is sufficiently protected from exposure to the material being tested. The second consideration is that the isolator construction must be such that the analytical equipment placed inside the isolator can function properly. These key design considerations are discussed in detail below.

Vibrations and Isolator Construction. When building an isolator to contain analytical equipment that is sensitive to vibrations, such as a balance, care must be taken to ensure that the equipment will be protected from excess vibration. Efforts to isolate vibrations from the analytical equipment can be approached in different ways. In general, the isolators should be placed in an area as free from vibration as possible. Site selection for the isolator is therefore of the utmost importance. Isolators, out of necessity, must to be placed in locations where there are sufficient utilities to support their operation, but every attempt should be made to locate them as far as possible from high traffic areas.

The isolator construction itself also plays a major role in the vibration dampening process. Isolators should be constructed on heavy, rigid steel stands. Although adjustable height isolators are beneficial for accommodating the height requirements of different users, the legs should be pinned securely in place before use. Isolator stands should be placed upon solid foundations to impart as much rigidity to the structures as possible. The outer shell of the isolators is typically made of 7-16 gage sheet metal. Although sheet metal is sufficiently strong for the sides and back of the isolator, it tends to have too much flex to be utilized for floor material in the isolator, especially in larger units. Half-inch plate stainless steel isolator floors offer superior strength and rigidity to the isolator and are worth the additional expense. Motors, fans, and blowers should be mounted on vibration dampening mounts to isolate them as much as possible from the isolator structure. Vibration sensitive equipment in the isolators should be placed on vibration dampening platforms.

Power Outlets. Isolators must be built with a sufficient number of power outlets. Service ports are any penetrations of the isolator shell that are made for utilities. The location of service ports containing power outlets is critical for the placement of analytical instrumentation inside of the isolators. The power outlets should be water-resistant to allow for cleaning of the unit after use. A disadvantage of the service port and power outlet penetrations is that each penetration of the isolator shell has the potential to become a point for an air leak or containment breach. This potential can be minimized by utilizing degradation resistant seals on the service ports. Cables and wiring that penetrate the isolator shells can be placed through self-sealing rubber grommets. Although grommets seal the outside of the cable, they still allow for air leakage through the cable. An alternate design involves stripping the outer casing and insulation from the individual wires. The wires are then encased in epoxy resin and sealed into the service port, creating a leak tight seal. These encased wires do pose a maintenance disadvantage, in that the cables are difficult to replace.

The number of penetrations made to the isolator shell should be kept to a minimum. Whenever possible, service port penetrations of the isolator floor should be avoided. Not only is it more difficult to make penetrations to the heavy plate floor, but these penetrations also take up valuable floor space in the isolator and thereby limit the placement of equipment and the amount work that can be performed in the isolator. Making the penetrations to the top or upper portions of the sides or back of the isolator is preferable whenever possible.

Isolator Gloves and Glove Ports. The glove port size and design are important considerations for the design of the isolator. The ports that were used in the isolators for the containment laboratory previously described were 12 inches in diameter, which made movement within the isolator easier than the more standard 8-inch size. A drawback is that the large size of the ports can affect the ability to view inside the isolator. The use of oval glove ports should be considered as they seem to improve both dexterity and visibility when compared to the use of smaller circular ports, which can adversely impact one's range of motion.

Figure 17.3 shows an isolator with different sized glove ports. The use of larger glove port openings, such as 12-inch openings, also allows the glove box or isolator to be operated at a lower negative pressure. The standard isolator with 8-inch glove ports operates at approximately −0.5 to −0.7 inches of water gage. This is sufficient negative pressure to supply approximately 125 feet per minute air velocity across the glove port opening should a glove become detached from the glove port. When utilizing a 12-inch glove port, the same 125 fpm air velocity can be obtained using −0.2 to −0.3 inches of water gage. By operating at lower negative pressure, the operator experiences less fatigue as there is less resistance to movement in the gloves.

Glove material of construction and size should also be considered when designing an isolator. There is a variety of gloves available for isolator use. Be sure to install gloves that are compatible with the materials handled in the isolator. Glove manufacturers (e.g., North Safety Products, Cranston, RI; Renco Corp., Manchester, MA) can provide chemical compatibility charts to help in glove selection. A popular glove on the market for analytical use is the 15 mil Hypalon® (DuPont Performance

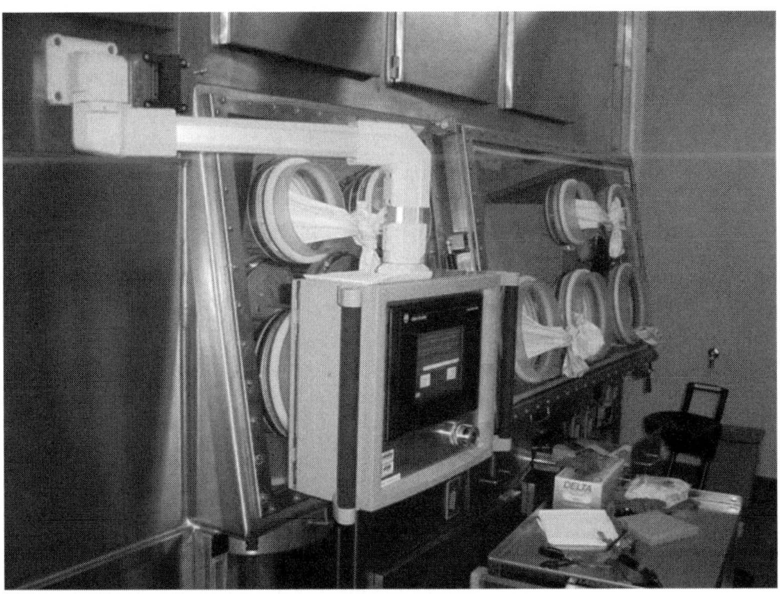

Figure 17.3 Isolator with multiple glove ports in different sizes.

Elastomers, Wilmington, DE), which has good chemical resistance to a wide variety of chemicals.

Gloves are available in both ambidextrous and hand-specific types. In general, hand-specific configurations should be utilized wherever possible, as they tend to be more comfortable and easier to use. The smallest hand size glove that can be utilized is preferable as it increases dexterity. A second set of disposable gloves should always be worn inside the isolator gloves to decrease the likelihood of the user's hand being exposed to hazardous material should a puncture or rip of the primary glove occur. The addition of a disposable cotton glove liner over the secondary disposable gloves aids in the insertion and removal of hands into and out of the isolator gloves.

An alternative type of glove is the two-piece glove. The sleeve part of the glove has an accordion appearance that makes range of motion for different size people much easier. The gloves that connect into the sleeve are available in different thicknesses and materials of construction. When making glove selections, base the selection of the glove material on the variety of chemicals used and the permeation data available for these compounds. Two-piece gloves are generally available only in smaller port sizes. If the isolator does not have the required glove port size, there is the possibility of purchasing a mold designed for the specified size port. These molds tend to be expensive and a cost–benefit analysis may need to be performed to determine if this is a viable option.

Equipment Accessibility. When designing an isolator, care must be taken to not make the isolators so deep that the back of the isolator cannot be reached from the glove ports. If there is an oversized piece of instrumentation that needs to be placed inside of the isolator, consider designing an isolator that has glove ports on both the front and back sides. This will not only aid in retrieving materials that are dropped in the isolator and end up in the back corners, but will also aid in servicing and repairing any malfunctioning equipment by allowing for easier access to the back and sides of the instrument. This is important because, although it is easy to clean and decontaminate the outside surfaces of the equipment, cleaning the inside (especially if cooling fans are present on the instrument) is difficult if not impossible.

Isolator Cleaning. Isolators should be built with cleanability in mind. All stainless steel should be buffed to a number 4 finish. All corners and joints should be radiused (i.e., curved, not squared). Buffing to a smooth finish and having radiused corners prevents scratches, cracks and crevices where material can accumulate and become trapped. Spray bulbs and wands built into the isolator facilitate the cleaning of the interior of the isolator. These spray bulbs and wands can utilize either water or a water/detergent mix. Most analytical equipment, being electric, is not cleanable using water. In order to clean the isolator itself, the analytical instrumentation must be unplugged and protected with some sort of cover.

An alternative to using spray bulbs and wands to clean an isolator is utilizing disposable wipes soaked in an appropriate solvent to clean all areas that had potential to become contaminated with high-potency material. This allows the material to be solublized and removed from the surface. This wipedown can then be followed with another disposable wipe that has been wetted with a sodium hypochlorite solution. This procedure degrades and neutralizes a wide variety of APIs. A final rinse is then made with a disposable wipe wet with deionized water. All cleaning materials should be treated as waste that has been contaminated with high-potency compound and with solvents.

Glove boxes and isolators have been used extensively in the nuclear industry and only more recently in pharmaceutical research. The one advantage that the nuclear industry has over the pharmaceutical industry when it comes to handling hazardous materials in glove boxes and isolators is that the detection of trace amounts of radioactive material on items removed from the isolator is relatively easy using a hand-held detector. Dispensations to the cleanliness of materials can be made almost instantly. In the pharmaceutical industry, a method of detection must be developed specifically for the compound being handled. Due to the nature of the pharmaceutical compounds being handled and their high potency, the methods must be designed to detect trace levels of material. There typically is a delay between the time samples are taken for analysis and when the results of these tests are obtained and communicated back to the personnel responsible for the decontamination. The delay associated with the testing makes it impractical to perform the analyses each time material or equipment is removed from the isolator. It is therefore recommended that this testing be done initially to ensure that the cleaning procedure works for the specific compound. The testing should then be performed periodically to ensure that cleaning procedures are being followed and performed correctly to ensure adequate cleaning and worker safety.

Additional Sample Precautions. Additional considerations in designing the isolator include accommodating the use of inert gas atmospheres (e.g., nitrogen or argon) for handling oxygen sensitive compounds. If inert gas atmospheres are utilized, appropriate precautions such as the installation and use of oxygen monitors in the room containing the isolator are needed to ensure worker safety. Special wavelength-specific lighting for photosensitive compounds should also be incorporated into the isolator and containment laboratory if needed.

17.4.5 Transferring Materials Into and Out of the Isolator

Moving materials such as samples, flasks and waste in and out of the isolator can be accomplished using ports or an isolator pass-through. The types and applications of ports and pass-throughs are discussed below.

Ports. Waste items (e.g., wipes, filters) can be removed from the isolator through ports such as bag-out ports or rapid transfer ports (RTP). The general principle of these ports is to allow the user to place waste products in the port. The port is then sealed and the bag or the RTP canister is then removed from the isolator. The bag or canister is then disposed of as hazardous waste. It is recommended that an isolator be equipped with at least one bag-out port and one RTP port. Bag-out ports, as shown in Fig. 17.4, allow for the removal of large equipment and filters as well as waste. RTP ports are typically more expensive than bag-out ports, and in addition to

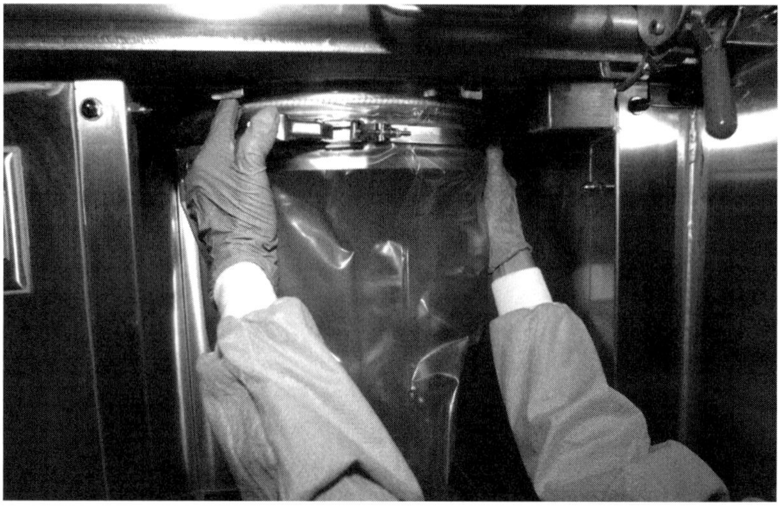

Figure 17.4 A typical bag-out port.

waste disposal they can be used to transport items from one isolator to another or to store hazardous samples or items.

Some of the advantages of RTP ports include the ease of use and the relative speed that materials can be moved into and out of the isolator using these ports. The RTP container itself can be made in a variety of different materials and, can serve as a secondary packaging container or as a long-term storage container for samples. The outside of the containers are easily labeled. When used for waste removal, adapters can be made for waste drums so that waste material can go directly from the isolator, into an RTP container and then directly into a waste drum without exposing the waste to the environment.

Drawbacks of the RTP ports are that they cannot be hooked into the isolator clean in place (CIP) system so, they must always be considered dirty until an adequate cleaning procedure is developed. There are also size limitations to the RTP ports and their corresponding containers. Once a certain size port is selected for the isolator, this is the only diameter container that can be used, unless the isolator port is modified. The port also requires an additional penetration of the isolator wall and serves as another potential point for air leaks. In addition, the RTP containers are not amenable to the transport of flasks into and out of the isolator; they require rotation and maneuvering of the RTP container to dock it into the isolator. Unless the port is mounted into the isolator floor, which will take up valuable space, the ability to transport liquids into and out of the isolator is limited to securely closed vials or bottles. The final limitation is the tendency of the seals on the mating surfaces of the RTP ports to become contaminated with potent material during transport operations. Procedures should be put in place to ensure that the mating surfaces of the RTP ports are thoroughly decontaminated as soon as the transport container is undocked from the isolator wall.

Pass-Throughs. Another mechanism of transporting materials into and out of an isolator is the use of a specially designed isolator pass-through. One type of pass-through, which is shown in Fig. 17.5, consists of an interlocking double door arrangement with a wash-down feature. First, the inside of the pass-through is automatically

(a)

(b)

(c)

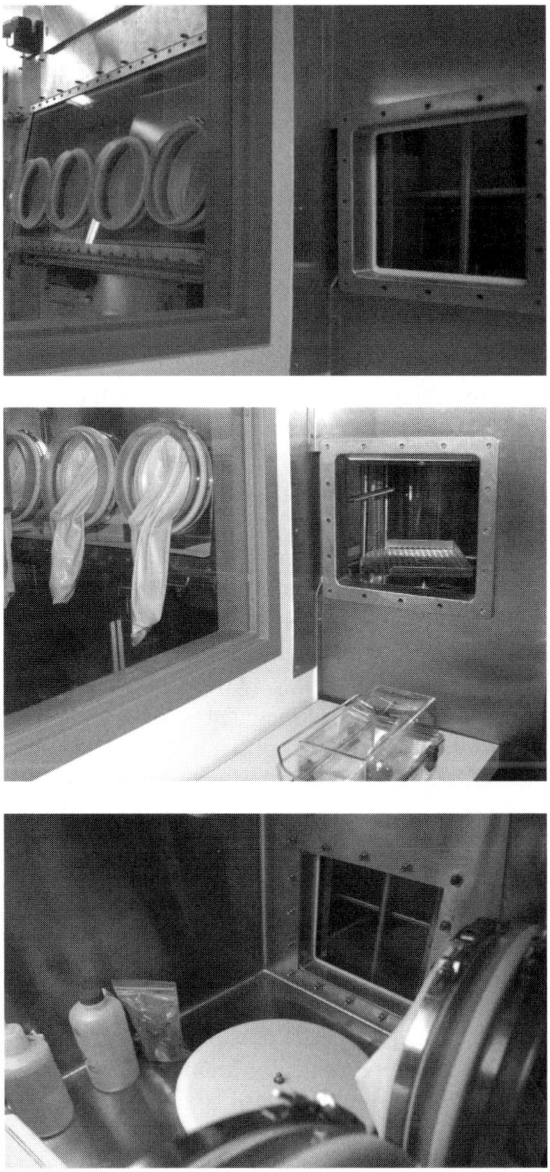

Figure 17.5 Typical isolator pass-through. (a) View of exterior door, closed. (b) View of exterior door, opened. (c) View of interior door, closed.

washed down with water or a wash solution to remove any particulate matter. The exterior door is then opened so that the operator can place an item into the pass-through compartment. The exterior door is then sealed and the interior door is opened. At this point, the operator can reach into the pass-through compartment, using the isolator gloves, and pick up the item and move it into the isolator. The doors are interlocked in such a manner that the interior and exterior doors cannot be opened, under normal use, at the same time. This prevents the contaminated air inside of the isolator from directly intermingling with the air inside the laboratory.

Whenever the interior door of the pass-through is opened, the pass-through has the potential to become contaminated from any residual material on the inside of the isolator. The wash-down, in this case, removes any residual potent material that is inside the pass-through or on any items to be removed from the pass-through. The wash-down is typically performed with water but other options such as various solvents and CIP solutions may be utilized, if these options are incorporated into the isolator design.

There are several advantages to the use of pass-throughs for the transport of materials into and out of the isolator. These benefits include the fact that the size of the pass-through can be built to meet one's needs. It is easier to transport flasks and other loosely sealed liquid containers in and out of the isolator with fewer concerns about spills. The wash-downs are typically easy to perform and are not technique dependent.

The disadvantages of the pass-throughs include the generation of potentially contaminated waste water from the wash-downs. Depending on the compounds handled in the isolators, the wash-down water may need to be treated before being discharged to a treatment facility. Since the pass-throughs require the use of a wash-down cycle to ensure worker safety, there is a potential for the materials being transported into and out of the isolator to become contaminated with the wash-down solution. The inside of the pass-through also tends to stay wet and is a potential site for microbial growth. The final disadvantage is that there tends to be ergonomic issues associated with the use of pass-throughs. It can be difficult to place materials into and remove them from the pass-through, leading to excessive bending and stretching on the part of the isolator user.

17.4.6 Operations Inside the Isolators

Operations performed inside of a glove box or isolator tend to be more difficult than those being performed in a standard laboratory setting. The main reason for this difficulty is that all operations are being performed through the glove ports. Two factors come into play when working in glove ports; the first is the loss of range of motion. The glove ports by their very construction limit the amount of motion that can be undertaken. Port size and shape play a key role in this and must be taken into account when designing the isolator. The second factor is loss of dexterity. The gloves used in the isolators are generally much thicker than would be used in a standard laboratory setting. They also tend to be bulkier and less form-fitting than standard gloves. If under-gloves are worn, they further compound the issue.

In general, operations performed in glove boxes and isolators tend to take much longer than the same operations in a standard laboratory setting. With experience, the time difference lessens, but is never eliminated.

Weighing. Weighing of dry materials in isolators tends to be problematic. Typically, in analytical testing, sample weights in the milligram range are used. Weighing such small quantities of materials can be difficult under the best of laboratory conditions. Performing this inside a glove box or isolator with swirling air currents and vibrations while wearing bulky gloves can seem a daunting task at best. Based on experience, the major issue with weighing operations inside an isolator is static. One solution is to control the relative humidity in the isolator. In general, higher relative humidity tends to reduce the amount of static in the environment. There are other ways to reduce the amount of static encountered during weighing operations. A Staticmaster® ion source containing Polonium 210 (NRD LLC, Grand Island, NY) can be placed in the weighing chambers of the semimicro balances. These devices can reduce the amount of static in the weighing enclosure of the balances, allowing them to come to a stable weight much quicker. Alternatively, electronic deionizers such as the Haug U-shaped electrode (Mettler-Toledo, Columbus, OH) can be used. This electrode works by dissipating the static charge on materials passed through the U-shaped electrode. These electrodes can be placed in front of the balance doors so that the sample is passed through the field prior to entering the weighing enclosure. This effectively dissipates any static charge that may be on the sample, container and gloves. Installing this ionizer in place inside of the isolator tends to reduce the amount of static in general, even when materials are not passed directly through the field.

In a typical laboratory environment, samples are often weighed onto glassine weighing paper and then transferred to flasks by pouring the material from the paper into a flask. Any residue on the weighing paper is then rinsed into the flask using a dissolving solvent to assure complete sample transfer. Using glassine paper for weighing operations inside the isolator is not a realistic option since the gloves used in the isolator are bulky and the operator typically lacks the dexterity to successfully handle the glassine paper and transfer material from the balance to the sample flask. Samples typically end up on the inside of the isolator rather than the inside of the flask.

There are several options for performing weighing operations. These include back-weighing (i.e., weigh container containing a sample before and after removal of material and use the difference to obtain the sample weight), using weigh boats, and developing dilution schemes to get samples to the proper concentrations. Based on experience, it was found to be easiest to utilize small aluminum weigh boats for weighing operations. These weigh boats are large enough to be manipulated using tweezers but small enough so that they are not excessively heavy for even the most sensitive microbalances. The analyst can accurately weigh the sample into the weigh boat that has been previously placed on the balance pan and tarred. After weighing the sample, the analyst can transfer the entire boat into a wide-mouth volumetric flask to be diluted to volume. In our experience, the volume of the weigh boats when left in the volumetric flasks is minimal and was found not to adversely effect the analytical testing.

Analysis of Samples. Any analytical testing that requires the handling of a high potency dry material should be looked at as a possible candidate to be moved into the isolator. Such testing can include Karl Fischer water testing, spectroscopic testing (e.g., sample preparation for IR, Raman and NMR), compendial testing such as residue on ignition and heavy metals, appearance testing, and HPLC and GC sample preparations. Some of the equipment used in this testing is too large to place inside an isolator. An alternative approach for these tests is to prepare the sample in the isolator and then take the prepared samples out of the isolator and to the test equipment in a safe manner. As soon as solid samples are put into solution, they are considered safe to transport out of the isolator, if placed into a sealed container. Further dilutions of materials in solution can then be done in a standard chemical fume hood using appropriate laboratory hygiene practices. In this way standard laboratory HPLC and GC systems can be used for the majority of the analytical testing without the need to place these instruments in an isolator or containment laboratory. Any waste materials generated during analytical testing including but not limited to vials, columns, syringes, GC inlet liners, and any solvent wastes should be disposed of in an appropriate manner.

17.4.7 Analytical Equipment Considerations

Isolators should have sufficient service port penetrations to allow as much equipment to be placed outside of the isolator as possible. Traditionally control boxes, chillers, keypads, and printers were placed as close to the analytical instrumentation being used as possible. The amount of equipment in direct contact with the samples should be minimized. If equipment needs to be placed in the isolators, the only way to remove that equipment later is to prove that the equipment has been cleaned to acceptable levels by swab testing. Based on experience, this cleaning is difficult to accomplish and in many cases the equipment needs to be considered contaminated and discarded if there is a need to remove it from the isolators.

When choosing instrumentation to place within the isolators, one should consider modularized instrumentation. By using modular instrumentation, parts of the instrument that do not have to be in direct contact with the sample can be located outside of the isolator. The benefits of this are twofold. The first benefit is that, by only placing the instrument modules that need to be in contact with the sample inside the isolator, one is effectively freeing up space in the interior of the isolator. This space can be utilized for additional analytical equipment or sample preparation. The second benefit is that, if the equipment malfunctions, you may only have to replace one module rather than the entire instrument.

Analytical equipment that is chosen for the isolators must be selected with care. In general, select instruments that are as compact as possible that still meet the analytical needs. For most analytical testing, sample sizes will be small, so micro- or semimicrobalances are routinely used. It is recommended to place balances on vibration dampening materials. Placing the balance on a vibration dampening mount not only helps to isolate the balance from vibrations that are being transmitted through the isolator, but also elevates them slightly and makes them easier to use. Based on experience, balances that are elevated to slightly below the glove port level are more comfortable to use than those which require the operator to reach further down. Consider having custom controls made for the balance which will allow the operator to tare, print and open the doors to the balance without removing her hands from the isolator gloves.

Install data capture devices such as PCs and balance key pads and printers outside of the isolator. Custom cabling may have to be made to accomplish this, but it minimizes the amount of equipment in the isolator and, if these devices malfunction or need repair, they are easily accessible and do not require decontamination. In general, due to the nature of analytical instrumentation, if equipment inside the isolator needs to be repaired, it must either be done inside of the isolator or the equipment must be scrapped and replaced. For large equipment, it might be worthwhile cutting the covers or service panels and reattaching them in such a manner that they can more easily be removed if service is needed prior to placing them in the isolator.

Below is a list of some analytical equipment that may need to be in the isolators and recommendations for how they can be used and/or protected.

1. *Balances:* If possible, work with the manufacturer to remove the control panel from the isolator and have a weight cell as an integral part of the isolator. If this is not possible it would be necessary to place a waterproof containment box over the balance to prevent water from damaging the balance during the wash-down and cleaning of the isolator.
2. *Magnetic stirrers:* A magnetic stirrer (e.g., IKAMAG®, IKA Works, Wilmington, NC) mounted underneath the base of the isolator can provide the stirring needed for solutions that are in the isolator, even through the half-inch stainless steel base. An overhead stirrer motor (e.g., EUROSTAR®, IKA Works, Wilmington, NC) can also be mounted on the outside of the isolator in the shroud area. With this arrangement, the flexible shaft(s) of the stirrer is the only part that resides inside the isolator and, these shafts can be moved within the isolator as needed.
3. *Chillers:* Chillers can be placed under the isolator in the shroud area. The connection to the isolator can be made through a quick-connect manifold. This arrangement also works well for utilities such as nitrogen and vacuum.
4. *Karl Fischer (KF) titrators:* KF titrators with special cabling can be placed into the isolator such that the cables run through a service port to an RS-232 or USB connection on the isolator. A laptop PC can then be plugged into the RS-232 or USB connection to collect data. The use of a laptop PC can be beneficial because it allows the PC to be stored out of the way when not in use.
5. *Differential scanning calorimetry (DSC):* A DSC instrument with a remote pressure cell can be utilized. This remote pressure cell will allow the bulk of

the instrument to be placed outside of the isolator, keeping it free from contamination. Chillers and utilities can be run to the instrument through service port penetrations.

6. *Physical properties test equipment:* Any physical properties testing that has the possibility of generating a dust or aerosol must be contained in the isolator. This type of equipment (e.g., tap density, friability, tablet hardness test equipment) should then be placed directly inside an isolator.

17.4.8 Fire Suppression System

Given the nature of the compounds being handled in the isolator and the fact that flammable solvents may be used to clean the isolator and the instruments within the isolator, consideration should be given to the installation of a fire suppression system within the isolator. While the building fire sprinklers will extinguish fires outside of the isolator, there should also be a fire suppression system for the interior of the isolator. It is recommended that UV/IR detectors be placed within the isolator itself. These detectors work by sensing both the heat (IR) and light (UV) generated when a fire is present in the isolator. Neither UV nor IR alone will trigger the fire suppression system.

For the suppressant, there are several choices. The two most common suppressants are dry chemical and carbon dioxide. Of the two choices, carbon dioxide is the suppressant of choice for use inside the isolator. If a discharge of suppressant does occur, either accidentally or in the event of an actual fire, carbon dioxide leaves no residue, and therefore cleanup is much easier. In additional, carbon dioxide is much less likely to damage sensitive analytical equipment when compared to dry chemical suppressants. It should be noted, however, that special considerations must be considered when deciding to use a carbon dioxide system. The isolator controls must be programmed such that, in a fire event, the air intake is dampered shut. The exhaust to the isolator should be programmed so that any mechanical exhaust blowers turn off and the exhaust valves are shut only part-way. This will allow excess pressure that builds up in the isolator to bleed off through the partially open exhaust valve. By dampering the exhaust valve in this manner, there will not be enough of a pressure buildup to inflate the gloves to the point where they might rupture, thereby increasing the likelihood of spreading contamination to the outside of the isolator.

17.4.9 Training

Training for potent compound handling should consist of training on the compound-specific handling guidelines as well as instructor-led training on the use of the isolators, glove boxes, and any needed PPE. A training regimen that has been found to work well consisted of having analysts first read handling guidelines and standard operating procedures related to the use of the potent compound handling facilities and isolators. This was then followed by a hands-on instructor-led training session, where the analysts learned how to operate the isolators, make glove changes (i.e., regular glove changes as well as emergency glove changes), troubleshoot isolator problems, and interpret isolator fault codes and how to respond to them. Users were also given training on the isolator fire suppression system and the use of the online closed circuit camera system that was used for remote monitoring operations inside the laboratory. In addition, compound-specific training was performed. This training included the handling practices needed for the specific potent compound an individual would be working with as well as a walk-through on what operations he/she would be doing in the containment laboratory. If training on any specialized equipment was needed, it was given at this time.

17.4.10 Ergonomic Issues

Ergonomics is a major concern with using isolators. There are limited choices in such things as isolator heights and isolator gloves, and the use of this equipment over an extended period of time can cause ergonomic difficulties. Some of these issues and strategies to address them are discussed below.

Isolator Height. In most cases, the isolators are at standard heights but, unfortunately, people do not come in standard sizes. Isolators become a challenge to use for the very short and the very tall. Although there are stand-alone isolators that have hydraulically controlled legs so the working height of the isolator can be adjusted, they are not practical in all instances. Adjustable height stands cannot be used if the intention is to fix and secure the isolators in place. Ways to address these issues include the use of an ergonomic sit–stand chair (Lyon Workspace Products, Aurora, IL) and/or a platform, such as an aerobics exercise step platform. The sit–stand chair helps the taller than average person use the isolator, but it is still somewhat uncomfortable for the shorter than average person to use. Standing on an aerobic exercise step adds approximately seven inches to the height of a person; this can be a benefit for a shorter than average person when using the glove ports and reaching into the isolator. The advantage of the aerobic step is that it is lightweight, easily moved, cleanable and inexpensive.

Some isolators are mounted on adjustable stands so that the height of the isolator can be adjusted to an individual's ideal working height. If vibration-sensitive operations are being performed, it is recommended that the isolator legs be pinned in place to prevent unwanted movement. There are several disadvantages to adjustable height isolators, including the possibility that the legs will not move equally, thereby leading to an isolator being out of level. This is very problematic when performing weighing operations. Other problems include the inability to utilize rigid piping for utilities. If the isolator moves up and down, supply and waste lines must be made from flexible material, which is more prone to breakage.

Isolator Gloves. Ergonomic issues are highlighted when using the isolator gloves. For ergonomic reasons, the isolators should be built so that the centerline of the glove ports is approximately 48 inches off the floor. This height is based on the ideal target working height (e.g., 2 inches below elbow height) and the average elbow height of 95% of workers (e.g., 46 inches).[2] Large size or oval ports make reaching around the inside of the isolator easier, while smaller circular ports can adversely affect one's range of motion. In general, hand-specific glove configurations should be utilized wherever possible, as these gloves tend to be more comfortable and easier to use. The smallest hand size glove that can be utilized is preferable as it eliminates excess material and increases dexterity. Due to the negative pressure in the isolator, operators can experience fatigue due the resistance to movement of the hands in the gloves. When outfitting a glove box or isolator for multiple users, care should be taken that gloves are not too small for the user with the largest hands or too big for users with the smallest hands.

Equipment Accessibility. Care should be taken to minimize the amount of bending or stretching that operators need to perform. Equipment should be placed directly in front of and centered between two glove ports if possible.

Ports and Pass-Throughs. Bag-out ports present an ergonomic issue. Due to the constraints of the location of bag out ports, it is difficult to get the full range of motion needed to make the changing of these bags easy. Analysts removing waste or changing bags may have to sit on the floor to perform these operations if the bag out ports are placed in the isolator floor. The use of a hydraulic table with an accommodating range of motion may or may not make this easier. There also tends to be ergonomic issues associated with the use of pass-throughs, as it can be difficult at times to place materials into and remove them from the pass-through from the interior of the isolator. These difficulties can lead to excessive bending and stretching on the part of the isolator user.

17.5 ADDITIONAL CONSIDERATIONS FOR HANDLING POTENT MATERIALS

A few additional considerations for handling potent materials are discussed below.

17.5.1 Shipping and Receiving Potent Samples

One area that is often overlooked in developing handling guidelines is the shipping and receiving of potent compounds. When shipping potent compounds, care must be taken to protect workers from accidental exposure to the compound. The outside of the primary package containing the sample (e.g., a screw-top amber glass bottle) should be thoroughly rinsed and decontaminated. Any labels that are placed on the primary packaging should be completely covered with clear tape to prevent the possibility that normal handling or cleaning of the bottle will cause the label to become unreadable. The primary package is then placed into a secondary package (e.g., plastic bag) which is then closed in such a manner as to reduce the risk of material escaping the secondary container in the event that the bottle containing the compound breaks. The outside of the secondary package should contain the same information as is on the label of the primary container. The sample should then be placed into a rigid packing tube, which contains a suitable cushioning material to prevent breakage of the primary container. The sample is now ready to be overpacked and shipped.

When receiving packages containing potent compounds, the package should be thoroughly inspected for any signs of damage that may have occurred during shipping. In all cases, a minimum of gloves, safety glasses and a laboratory coat should be worn when opening packages. Place the package in a laboratory hood or ventilated weighing enclosure when opening the outer package. If no damage is observed to the packing materials, the potent compound may be unpacked to the secondary packaging layer. If any visible damage is observed on any of the packaging or, if the secondary packaging needs to be removed, immediately move the package to a secure location and don appropriate PPE. Damaged packages should be placed into an isolator. If an isolator is not available, the package should be transferred into a laboratory dedicated to the handling of potent compounds and be placed into a ventilated enclosure. Once in a controlled environment and the proper PPE has been donned, the material may be completely removed from all packaging. If there is a chance that any packaging material has been contaminated with the potent compound, dispose of the packaging material in accordance with hazardous waste disposal practices.

17.5.2 Transportation of High-Potency Materials

Procedures for transporting high potency materials, including API, drug product, used glassware and waste, to and from the laboratory must be clearly established. For API and drug product samples, the sample container should be clearly labeled as to the contents, the hazards associated with the high-potency compound and a contact name of a person familiar with the handling requirements for the compound. The outside of the container should be wiped with a suitable solvent to remove any residue present on the container. If a decontamination procedure is in place to inactivate the compound, the outside of the container should then be decontaminated following this procedure. The primary sample container should then be placed into a clean secondary container and delivered directly to the final destination. Samples should not be left unattended when being dropped off; they should be delivered directly to the person requesting the sample, or their designee, to ensure the samples are secured and stored in an appropriate manner.

17.6 SUMMARY

Pharmaceutical materials, in general, are becoming more potent. Effects that are therapeutically desirable in a patient may present a health hazard to workers handling these materials on a routine basis. Care must be taken to address worker safety when handling active compounds. The use of PPE and administrative and engineering controls can be used to ensure worker safety when handling potent compounds in either a standard analytical laboratory or a containment laboratory. The different types of laboratories and approaches have advantages and disadvantages, which must be carefully considered when developing procedures and strategies for handling potent compounds.

ACKNOWLEDGMENTS

The authors would like to thank Joy Gaughan for the development of our potent compound handling training program and the rest of the PGRD Groton EH&S staff for their contributions to our efforts on handling high potency, low-dose compounds.

REFERENCES

1. Marsh D, Marshal P. 2007. Assembling the appropriate expertise for contained facility design and implementation, presented at Containment of Potent Compounds, sponsored by Executive Conference Corp., January 25–26, 2007, Philadelphia, PA.
2. American Glovebox Society. 1998. guideline for gloveboxes, 2nd ed. AGS-1998-G001.

PART IV

REGULATORY CONSIDERATIONS IN THE DEVELOPMENT OF LOW-DOSE DRUG PRODUCTS

CHAPTER 18

REGULATORY CONSIDERATIONS IN THE DEVELOPMENT OF LOW-DOSE SOLID ORAL DRUG PRODUCTS

*RAVI S. HARAPANHALLI, Ph.D
Branch V, Division of Pre-marketing Assessment and Manufacturing Science, Office of New Drug Quality Assessment, Office of Pharmaceutical Science, Center for Drug Evaluation and Research, Food and Drug Administration, Silver Spring, MD 20993

18.1 INTRODUCTION AND OVERVIEW

Regulatory considerations in the development of low-dose solid oral drug products are discussed in this chapter. While much of the chemistry, manufacturing, and controls information discussed here applies to conventional doses as well, it should be considered much more carefully while developing low-dose drug products. Low-dose vs conventional dose is not defined in any regulations. However, in 1973, the *British Pharmacopoeia* defined "microdose" preparations as dosage forms containing less than 2 mg or 2% w/w of active drug in a formulation, and introduced a requirement of individual tablet assay for "microdose preparations." For the purpose of this paper, a "low dose" means that the dose strength is less than 1 mg/dose and/or 1% w/w of active drug in a formulation. Regardless of the definition, it is important to understand that, as the relative percent of the active drug in a formulation decreases, many seemingly simple factors become critical and may affect the dose content uniformity and homogeneity of the active drug in a formulation. The following schematic describes content uniformity problems that are critical to the low-dose formulations (Fig. 18.1). As shown in Fig. 18.1, dosage units may be isopotent but display intraunit nonuniformity in the distribution of the active. This type of inhomogeneity may critically affect the rate of release of actives from large units such as lozenges. Similarly, dosage units may show inter-unit nonuniformity because

*Current address: Principal Consultant, PAREXEL Consulting, 4600 East-West Highway, Suite 350, Bethesda, MD 20814, ravi.harapanhalli@parexel.com

Formulation and Analytical Development for Low-Dose Oral Drug Products. Edited by Jack Zheng

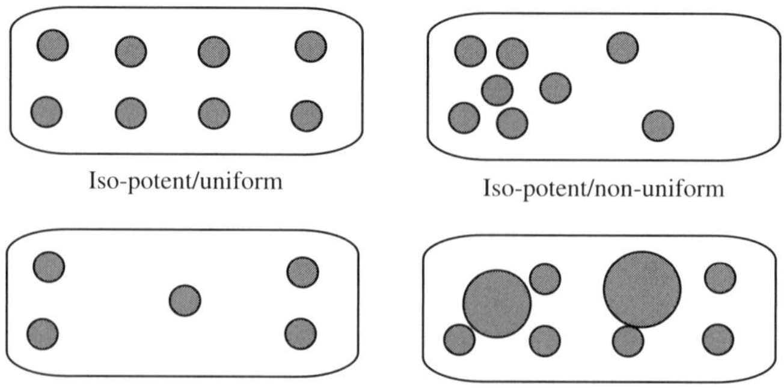

Figure 18.1 Schematic description of content uniformity of dosage unit.

of agglomeration of the active compound and/or other problems of formulation segregation.

Drugs formulated at low doses are often highly potent in nature, and they often display a narrow therapeutic range. A narrow therapeutic range is defined in 21CFR 320.33(c) as a situation where there is less than a two-fold difference in median lethal dose (LD_{50}) and median effective dose (ED_{50}) values or where there is less than a 2-fold difference in the minimum toxic concentrations and minimum effective concentrations in the blood. Additionally, drugs displaying narrow therapeutic range require careful titration and patient monitoring to ensure their safe and effective use. Some examples of narrow therapeutic range drugs include theophylline, carbamazepine, and leothyroxine. Drugs such as fentanyl display narrow therapeutic range within a given individual such that the lowest concentration at which clinical toxicity occurs may be the minimum or median concentration producing a therapeutic effect or vice versa. Therefore, for highly potent drugs, potency and content uniformity are often linked directly to safety and efficacy. Also, in some cases, if strengths are closely related; overlapping potencies of different strengths may also become an issue to reckon with. Therefore, special attention should be given to the formulation and analytical development, clinical trial material manufacture, and commercial manufacture of low-dose formulations. Variability in the manufacturing process needs to be minimized and stricter process controls are often required to be implemented. Potential for physical transformations of active drugs during manufacturing and its effects on product performance and bioavailability will have to be assessed. Two critical in-process controls, namely blend uniformity and dosage unit content uniformity testing by stratified sampling, must be established. Variability in content uniformity and assay may need to be tighter than the usual range of 90.0–110.0%, often accepted for conventional doses. Physical and chemical stability of the formulation with regard to polymorphic changes, hydration status, particle size, reactions with excipients and/or with the impurities in the excipients will have to be assessed carefully during stability assessments. Analytical methods with adequate sensitivities will have to be developed to assay microgram levels of actives and submicrogram levels of their impurities and degradation products. Interfering impurities from excipients may often pose challenges in the development of suitable analytical methods. Additional concerns such as cleaning validation and environmental containment and exposure limits need to be addressed from cGMP perspectives.

18.2 THREE-PRONGED APPROACH TO LOW-DOSE FORMULATIONS

A three-pronged approach consisting of quality-by-design (QbD), rigorous in-process testing, and end product testing with tighter assay ranges is recommended for the development and viable manufacture of low-dose formulations. A QbD approach that is woven using the principles described in the ICH Q8,[1] Q9,[2] and Q10[3] guidelines is highly desirable. Such an approach is particularly suited for the development of low-dose formulations because it ensures quality is built in by proper upstream controls and designs. Moreover, quality by end testing alone does not detect overpotent or underpotent batches up until the testing of the finished product has occurred. Therefore, efforts should be made to achieve robust product and process designs and to understand critical quality attributes and critical process parameters, including flow properties and segregation tendencies of powder and granulation blends so that appropriately engineered equipment designs may be utilized in ensuring content uniformity. Concurrent with QbD, quality should also be verified by adequate in-process and end product testing. ICH Q6A[4] recommends that in-process testing may be carried out in lieu of end product testing for certain quality attributes if such tests are shown to be at least as sensitive as the end product testing and if there is no reason to believe that quality attributes might change subsequent to such in-process testing. Consistent with this approach, the Agency released draft Guidance[5] in 2003. The Guidance is based on the recommendations of the PQRI working group on blend uniformity analysis. The Guidance states that the methods described are not intended to be the only methods for meeting Agency requirements to demonstrate the adequacy of powder mix and that traditional powder blend sampling and testing can also be used. The Guidance also states that the formulations with extremely low-dose and/or high potency may call for more rigorous sampling than is described in assessing the uniformity of powder blends or the uniformity of content of the finished dosage units. Therefore, for the low-dose formulations, additional sample testing intervals and events should be included to assure rigorous in-process testing. Also, it is recommended that both blend uniformity testing and dosage unit content uniformity testing by stratified sampling be carried out throughout process development and during routine commercial manufacture. Insofar as end product testing is concerned, tighter ranges such as 95.0–105.0% for assays and content uniformity testing are recommended, especially when overlapping potencies from closely related strengths are likely to result in overlapping safety concerns.

18.3 PHARMACEUTICAL DEVELOPMENT REPORT

A detailed pharmaceutical development report providing a justification for the chosen processing options, product and process development, critical quality attributes, critical process parameters, and scientific approach to process scale-up that is based on product and process understanding is expected in an NDA. Sufficient process understanding information to assure the Agency that the applicant will be able to manufacture the product reliably at the intended commercial scale is also expected in an NDA. The pharmaceutical development report should minimally consist of rationale for component selection, product development and its optimization, and process development and its optimization. The report should describe how risk management principles were applied during the development stages to identify failure modes relating to critical formulation variables and product quality attributes and how the process was developed to accommodate expected variability in the raw materials and processing parameters and controls. The following elements should be adequately described.

18.3.1 Salt Selection of Drug Substance

If the drug substance is being developed as a salt, appropriate discussion on the choice of the chosen salt form should be provided. It is expected that vigorous salt screening studies are performed to preferably identify a nonhygroscopic stable salt form. A summary table of salts screened based on a range of physico-chemical properties including hygroscopicity, stoichiometry, and physical stability may be provided. It is likely that a selected salt may have been suited for earlier prototypes such as oral powder for reconstitution, or capsules, but may not be suited for the final dosage form such as a tablet because of noncompatibility with the excipients and desired stability characteristics.

18.3.2 Solid-State Forms (Polymorphs, Hydrates, Solvates)

Adequate efforts to generate all possible solid-state forms of the drug substance should be documented in the pharmaceutical development report. Results of the detailed polymorph mining studies should be presented including various conditions of crystallization using solvents of wide polarity range. All crystalline and amorphous forms should be identified using complementary analytical techniques such as X-ray powder diffraction, FTIR, scanning Raman microscopy, DSC, and solid-state NMR. Detailed information on pH vs solubility profiles, stability, and manufacturability aspects of the polymorphs should be presented in justifying the selection of the polymorphic form for development. Generally, the most thermodynamically stable form is expected to be developed further. It is important to understand that polymorphic changes may lead to three areas of concern, namely, differential stability, differential biopharmaceutical properties leading to changes in bioavailability, and differential physical properties such as compaction and segregation affecting manufacturability. All these concerns should be addressed in the assessment and selection of polymorphic forms and their control. The drug substance should be monitored for polymorphic changes on stability using one or more complimentary analytical methods with adequate sensitivities. Polymorphic changes should also be monitored during the manufacturing process of the drug product and upon its storage using analytical method(s) with adequate detection and quantitation limits, and ICH Q6A (Decision Tree 4) may be referenced for assessing whether a specification to control polymorphic content in the drug substance and the drug product is necessary or not. Understandably, monitoring for polymorphic changes in a low-dose formulation is not straightforward. Libraries of reference scans of formulation components and drug substance polymorphic forms may have to be constructed and multivariate algorithms may have to be used to assess spectral data for morphic changes. Innovative approaches such as C-13 labeling to enhance sensitivity of C-13 solid-state NMR to study polymorphism[6] in low-dose solid formulations may also be used.

18.3.3 Hygroscopicity

The ability of the drug substance to gain, hold, and release moisture should be investigated by exposing the drug substance to humidity. Typically, such studies are carried out using automated vapor sorption instrument with relative humidity step increments. The results of dynamic water vapor adsorption studies should be presented to assess whether any special protection from humidity is needed during handling, shipping, or storage. For low dose formulations, it might be particularly important to assess if moisture causes any agglomeration.

18.3.4 Aqueous Solubility

A table showing solubility of the drug substance in various aqueous solutions at different pH values should be provided. It is important to assess whether the drug substance shows high or low solubility in the entire physiological range. The Agency Guidance on BCS-based waivers[7] may be referenced for details.

18.3.5 Permeability

The permeability of the drug substance should be established using in vitro Caco-2 cell model and mass balance studies in humans to assess percentage recovered in urine.[8] In the Caco-2 cell permeability assessment, drug substance at various concentrations should be used and various controls for high and low permeability, efflux inhibition, and for permeability and efflux inhibition should be utilized. The permeability should be presented as "P_{app} (nm/s)" for both the apical-to-basolateral and basolateral-to-apical directions. If pH difference between the apical and basolateral buffers is expected to result in artifacts in transwell assays, the experiments may need to be carried out at pH 6.5 and 7.4 to account for pH effects. The Caco-2 studies together with the mass balance studies should demonstrate whether the drug substance has high or low permeability.

18.3.6 Particle Size Distribution

A description of the desired particle size distribution[9,10] should be provided along with a justification. The particle size distribution should include $D\ (v,0.1)$,

D (v,0.9), and D[4,3] values with two-sided ranges and a span. If drug substance is obtained from a vendor who has filed a type II DMF, their certificate of analysis should be re-confirmed by the drug product manufacturer by retesting particle size distribution, appearance, and morphology on each batch of the drug substance. Analytical methods such as laser light scattering and sieve analysis may be used but they should be adequately validated. Theoretical models[11] may be used to estimate the effect of drug substance particle size on content uniformity. Typically, the computer models simulate the number, size, and mass of the drug particles in a batch and distribute them evenly across all unit doses. The input data usually include the lowest dosage strength, the drug substance density, and the geometric standard deviation. Based on achieving expected content uniformity, such computational models predict a geometric mean particle size D[4,3], D(v,0.1), and D(v,0.9) values. A discussion of how such theoretical models were used in the design of experiments (DoEs) in determining the desired particle size distribution to achieve a high content uniformity should be presented. Summary tables of particle size distribution ranges vs blend uniformity, in-process dosage unit tablet content uniformity, disintegration, dissolution, and where appropriate, bioavailability information should be provided in justifying chosen ranges for the particle size distribution. Particular attention should be given to D (v,0.1) and D (v,0.9) values and their ranges as fines tend to fluidize and segregate during processing as well as agglomerating, whereas the coarse particles tend to show hot spots due to poor blending.

18.3.7 Particle Shape and Morphology

A description of how the desired particle size and particle shape is achieved should be provided. It is desirable to achieve the required particle size distribution by controlling the conditions used to crystallize the drug substance. Crystallization conditions should be carefully chosen to minimize the formation of agglomerates. Design of experiments to investigate crystallization conditions may include nucleation, crystal growth, effect of agitator speeds, seeding amount, rates of addition of cosolvents, temperature controls, etc. to maintain desired supersaturation throughout the crystallization process. Photomicrographs of the crystals should be provided to assess the morphology of primary particles and extent of agglomeration during crystallization. Agglomerates should be adequately characterized in terms of their size and composition so that conditions to minimize their formation may be identified. Agglomerates may be simple clusters of primary particles that are friable, or they may be macrocrystalline forms that are not easily friable. For low-dose formulations, the drug substance should be devoid of any agglomerates to achieve proper blend and content uniformity results. Statistical DoE approach may be used to demonstrate functional relationship between crystallization parameters such as water content, agitator speed, antisolvent net content, addition rates and time, dilution, seeding, and reaction temperature to achieve controlled supersaturation vs size and shape of primary particles and agglomerates. Thus, based on such studies, proper conditions for crystallization may be chosen to obtain primary particles of desired size and shape while minimizing the formation of agglomerates. A summary of different crystallization conditions vs particle size distribution may be provided in support of the chosen process parameters for crystallization. If additional milling steps are incorporated in the drug substance manufacture, such steps should be only used to break the agglomerates and not to break the primary particles to achieve desired particle size distribution. For many drug substances, their plasticity may resist primary particle size reduction in low-energy mills such as wet mills or dry hammer milling. However, high energy milling such as jet milling may lead to significant primary particle size reduction and, in doing so, to loss of crystallinity and formation of amorphous regions within the primary crystal lattice, which may promote solid-state chemical reactions as well as to morphic changes and to secondary agglomeration. Therefore, for drug substances to be used in low-dose formulations, it is desirable to achieve primary particle size and shape via crystallization and to break agglomerates via low-energy milling. Also, various milling and formulation trials may have to be carried out to test jet milling, wet milling, hammer milling, etc., and formulations prepared by using drug substance that has been intentionally agglomerated or that has larger primary particle size and shape to assess the robustness of the formulation and the manufacturing process. Milled/micronized drug substances should be monitored on stability for potential agglomeration and morphic transformations.

18.3.8 Formulation Development

Development of a low-dose formulation requires careful considerations such as drug substance stability, drug–excipient compatibility, and desired rate and extent of drug release from the formulation matrix. Owing to a very low percentage content of drug in such formulations, the drugs may be much more amenable to physico-chemical interactions compared with those seen in conventional solid oral dosage forms. For example, even though excipients may be compatible with the drug substance, impurities and moisture content of the excipients may adversely affect the stability of drug substance in the formulation. Therefore, a detailed excipient-compatibility screening study should be carried out to demonstrate a stable and viable commercial formulation. Results from exploratory compatibility studies, which may include stressed storage conditions on dosage forms formulated with various pharmaceutical excipients, may be provided in justifying the choice of the formulation components. Such studies should assess both physical and chemical compatibilities of various components and their impurities.

Studies should be carried out to assess the effect of moisture on formulation, with respect to the hydration state of the active and the excipients and potential for agglomeration. Such studies typically include assessment of individual excipients as well as of the formulation. The hydration states of the components are assessed by crystallography studies. Visual examination of diffractograms and moisture sorption data indicate the presence of amorphous forms and the extent to which they may be present. Scanning electron microscopy (SEM) images show particle size and shape. Raman mapping shows whether individual crystals of excipients and actives can or cannot be distinguished. Isomorphous forms of excipients are preferred as they provide intimate mixing of components during mixing and handling. Moisture balance studies indicate the extent to which formulation components remain unchanged as a function of relative humidities and critical humidity at which they begin to absorb moisture. At high relative humidities such as 85% and above, often materials absorb significant quantities of water and may become deliquescent. X-ray analysis often indicates which component in the formulation is predominantly responsible for such deliquescence. When taken together, data from individual components and from the formulation should indicate whether any of the components can potentially absorb moisture under most ambient relative humidities (<75% RH). Similarly, stress studies using open dish experiments, where individual components are stored at high temperatures such as 50°C/75% RH for several weeks, should indicate whether weight gain is observed or not. Together, these studies should point out whether agglomeration due to moisture sorption is or is not expected to be a problem in the product formulation. Accordingly, suitable controls may be placed during manufacture and storage.

The physical compatibility assessment should also include hardness vs compression profiles, and incidents of capping, friability, disintegration, dissolution, etc for the tablet dosage forms. Design of experiments, if used, should be fully described and justified. It is also important to consider physico-chemical characterization, and acceptable processing properties in justifying the choice of a chosen salt form of the drug substance. All formulation changes should be bridged by proper CMC information and, as appropriate, by bioavailability/bioequivalence studies. Any biowaivers in support of formulation changes should be justified in light of BCS and other biopharmaceutical considerations.

Functionality-Related Characteristics (FRCs) of Excipients. Development of robust formulations entails proper selection of excipients and identification of their key properties[12] that relate to product performance. Therefore, special attention should be given to the selection of excipients and their grades for low-dose formulations. Excipients should be well characterized for various functionalities; they should be manufactured under well-defined controls, and they should have good batch uniformity and characterization. Premium-grade excipients designed for pharmaceutical use and supplied by manufacturers who have good change control and notification program should be used. Excipients FRCs are specific to a particular drug formulation and process, not to an excipient alone, and these should be determined experimentally, preferably via DoEs during formulation development. FRCs that directly impact the drug performance, including disintegration/dissolution and eventual in vivo dissolution, should be identified by a series of DoEs during formulation development. At times, performance FRCs identified by the drug product manufacturers may not be the properties typically controlled by the excipient maker's manufacturing process. Often, co-processed excipients with customized FRCs may need to be developed if off-the-shelf grades of excipients do not meet the desired FRCs. It is expected that FRCs are listed in a drug application and that specifications and certificates of analysis reflect them adequately. Demonstration of adequate formulation robustness with regard to FRCs is critical for the low-dose formulations since obtaining excipients which are consistent from lot-to-lot in desired functionality properties is not always possible. Therefore, during formulation development, excipient variation should be investigated to the extent possible, and robust formulations should be developed. Such studies may also point out critical FRCs and their acceptable ranges. In support of the chosen ranges for the FRCs of excipients, batches with extreme ranges should be utilized during the manufacture and the process should be shown to result in desired level of product content uniformity and homogeneity. Arbitrary selection of excipient batches and assessment of their fitness-for-use solely based on trial and error is discouraged.

As discussed above, testing to conform to pharmacopeia requirements may not be sufficient to assure excipient quality in the manufacture of low-dose formulations. Often, excipients make the bulk of the dosage form and if a dry blending and direct compression is utilized, the functional properties of excipients become even more critical compared to a granulation process. Typical functional properties to be tested for excipients include the following:

- powder X-ray diffraction patterns;
- differential scanning calorimetry;
- scanning electron microscopy;
- moisture sorption;
- porosity;
- density (bulk and tapped);
- surface area by nitrogen sorption techniques;
- particle size distribution and fines content;
- particle shape/morphology;
- near-infrared patterns;
- thermogravimetric analysis;
- water activity;
- water content by Karl Fisher, LOD;
- additional specific tests.

In essence, the test battery should include XRPD to characterize crystallinity of excipients, moisture analysis to confirm crystallinity and hydration state of excipients, bulk density to ensure reproducibility in the blending process, and particle size distribution to ensure consistent mixing and compaction of powder blends. Often three-point PSD limits are needed for excipients. Also, morphic forms of excipients should be clearly specified and controlled as changes may impact powder flow and compactibility of blends. XRPD, DSC, SEM, and FTIR spectroscopy techniques may often be applied to characterize and control polymorphic and hydrate composition critical to the function of the excipients. Additionally, moisture sorption studies, Raman mapping, surface area analysis, particle size analysis, and KF analysis may show whether excipients possess the desired polymorphic state and whether significant amounts of amorphous components are present. Together, these studies will ensure lot-to-lot consistency in the physical properties that assure flow, compaction, minimal segregation, and compunction ability of excipients used in low-dose formulations.

Physical Uniformity of Active with Excipients. Pharmaceutical development should document assessment of physical uniformity of the active with various excipients and excipient grades. Techniques such as FT Raman mapping[13–15] and SEM are often used to assess uniformity of distribution of the active and chemical assays such as blend uniformity analysis are used to corroborate the results of mapping studies. Surface features which are expected to affect the interaction between the active compound and the excipients may be assessed in these studies. These maps provide information on whether active compounds are uniformly dispersed in the excipient mix or not and the agglomeration levels. Favorable interactions such as active particles being attached to the surface and nestling in the crevices of excipients help bond the active with excipients in a powder blend and are less likely to lead to segregation. SEMs also reveal whether an ordered adhesive mix is formed with the excipient or not. Modifications such as pregelatinization and high moisture content of excipients usually impart better adhesive properties. The effects of moisture on forming stable and homogenous adhesive powder mixes is attributed to hydrogen bond formation due to the highly polar water molecules, where water may undergo chemisorption as well as physisorption.[16] The study results should reveal which excipient and what grade is suited to achieve better blend uniformity with minimal agglomeration of the active.

Common Problems of Material Flow. Content uniformity is affected by segregation, and segregation is affected by flow behavior of solids. Therefore, it is critical to understand common problems during material flow and transfer, namely, rat-holing, arching, and segregation.[17] Problems during material storage are the caking/agglomeration, time consolidation/dense packaging.

- *Rat-holing:* A rat-hole is a circular, cylinder-shaped hole that develops in a mass of bulk solids and, left undisturbed, can remain to form an integral part of the bin structure. A rat-hole usually forms above a bin outlet in that portion of a hopper that is not steep enough to maintain flow at the walls, such as conical hoppers. Generally, flow is limited to a central flow pattern. If the material is even slightly cohesive, material may stick to the walls and eventually become part of the bin structure. A collapsing rat-hole can severely compact material, which leads to arching.
- *Arching:* An arch is a stable obstruction to flow that forms over the point of narrowest cross-section of the bin (usually, the outlet). Bulk solids may arch by particle interlocking and cohesive arching. Particle interlocking occurs as particles lock together to form a mechanical bond. A cohesive arching occurs because of cohesion between the particles of a bulk solid. Because of cohesive strength, an arch (bridge, dome, etc.) may form which is strong enough to support the entire contents of the bin above. Therefore, the cohesive strength of bulk solids should be determined using, for example, a direct shear tester and the amount of stress required to collapse a cohesive arch should be assessed to prevent this type of arching. As the hopper span is increased, more stress is applied to the solid. Based on the flow function test results, one may determine the point at which

the stress applied (by the hopper span or opening) exceeds the cohesive strength of the material to prevent cohesive arching.

- *Caking or agglomeration during postprocessing storage:* Caking refers to the physio-chemical bonding between particles that occurs due to changes in humidity. Moisture in the air can react with or dissolve some solid materials. When the air humidity changes, the dissolved solids re-solidify and can cause particles to grow together.[18] Post-processing storage of materials prior to packing or out-loading is prone to caking or agglomeration. Four common ways of caking – mechanical caking, plastic flow caking, latent chemical reactions, and electrostatic charging – should be properly addressed during product and process development. Inter-particle moisture migration, latent maturing, and settling of particles during storage often results in caking. Therefore, appropriate procedures for handling and design of storage equipment to minimize caking should also be described for these products.
- *Time consolidation/dense packing:* For many materials, if allowed to sit in a hopper over a long period of time, the particles tend to rearrange themselves so that they become more tightly packed together. The consolidated materials flow less easily and tend to bridge or rat-hole.
- *Segregation:* This is another concern with the powders where different size and density particles tend to segregate due to vibrations and a percolation action of the smaller particles moving through the void space between the larger particles. Since, in a powder blend, particles are not identical, segregation is likely to occur to some extent during powder handling and manufacturing process. However, with proper procedures for handling solids, this can be minimized such that acceptable content uniformity results are obtained. Four modes of segregation are fluidization (air entrainment), dusting, sifting, and particle sliding. Fluidization can cause vertical segregation resulting in horizontal layers of fines and coarse material. Fine powders tend to retain air longer than the coarse powders because of their lower permeability. So, when a bin is being filled, the coarse particles are driven into the bed but the fine particles remain fluidized near the surface, creating a vertical or "top-to-bottom" segregation pattern. This type of segregation happens when powders are filled or discharged at high rates, or if gas counter-flow is present, such as during the initial fill of the feed system to the press. Also particles below 100 μm usually tend to develop air entrainment, leading to this type of segregation. Dusting results in airborne particles when powder is dropped and impacts onto a pile surface, causing release of finer particles into the air. Large pockets of air bubbling up through a stationary bed of material from below may also result in entrainment of fine particles. Suspended particles are carried by air currents to the least active portion of the receiving vessel's area, generally the lowest part of the pile surface furthest away from the impact point. Fine particles below 50 μm that do not readily adhere or strongly bind to larger particles usually tend to fluidize by this mechanism. It is expected that dusting segregation is accompanied by fluidization segregation. Sifting occurs when small particles trickle down through a body of larger particles. This is the most common means for particles to separate. In order

for sifting to occur, the particles must be free flowing, different sizes, fairly large (>100 mesh), and have some means of inter-particle motion (such as forming a pile). The particles segregate in a horizontal or "side-to-side" pattern. Particles sliding on a surface can segregate because fine particles tend to be more frictional than coarse ones. If a chute is used, the fine particles in motion settle to the bottom of the chute due to sifting. The increased friction of the finer particles causes drag and velocity differences between particles as they are sliding on the chute surface. When the particles discharge from the chute, the fine particles concentrate at the end, while the coarse ones have a trajectory which carries them further away. The segregation potentials of the powder and granulation blends are typically assessed using published ASTM methods.[19–22]

Factors Affecting Material Flow. Although material flow is a function of its cohesive properties, factors known to affect material flowability include moisture content, temperature, particle size, and time of storage at rest. Therefore, the flow properties of material should be measured to determine the effects of the environmental conditions discussed below.

- *Moisture content:* Increase in the moisture content of a solid leads to increased cohesive strength. Even slight increases in moisture content, for example, from 1 to 1.5%, may significantly increase the material flowability. Hygroscopic materials can experience significant moisture increases simply by being exposed to humid air.
- *Temperature:* Cohesiveness is also affected by the solid's temperature; typically, increase in temperature leads to increased cohesiveness. Flow properties testing at various temperatures may be carried out to optimize the right temperature for optimal flow.
- *Particle size and shape:* Finer particles tend to be more cohesive and hence more difficult to handle. Similarly, particle shape also affects flowability. Fibrous and angular particles are usually more cohesive than particles that are rounded.
- *Time of storage at rest:* As solid remains at rest in a bin or hopper, it can become more cohesive and flow less easily. At rest, the compaction loads due to head pressure can produce a strong cohesive bond. A chemical reaction, crystallization, or adhesive bonding can also cause this. Sometimes, after a cohesive arch is broken up by somehow initiating flow, the material can revert back to its original flow condition and not exhibit a similar cohesion if left at rest again. On the other hand, some materials may time and time again bridge and rat-hole even after flow is re-initiated.

Minimizing Segregation

- *Mass flow patterns (first-in-first-out):* Even though the material can segregate side-to-side, the coarse and fine particles will be reunited at the outlet because of mass flow.

- *Minimum head of material:* Keep a minimum head of material above the hopper section in a mass flow bin to reduce the velocity gradient that occurs as the material reaches the hopper section in a mass-flow bin.
- *Cohesiveness:* Make the material more cohesive by adding water, oil, or other functional excipients. One of the prerequisites for segregation is inter-particle motion. Increasing cohesiveness causes the particles to stick together and reduces this motion.
- *Tangential entry directions:* Creating a configuration of a tangential entry into bins when handling fine solids that segregate by air entrainment is highly recommended. Instead of filling the bin from the center of the top of the bin, one may introduce the material in at the top of the bin but on the side, tangential to the circumference of the bin. This may actually minimize a vertically segregating material by causing side-to-side segregation. The particles will be reunited when they are discharged at the outlet of mass-flow bin.

Minimizing Time Consolidation and Caking. If material is being loaded into the silos after having come from a process, it should be given sufficient time for thorough drying or for any residual reactions to take place in a controlled manner. Flash dryers may serve to drive off moisture from the surfaces of particles, but leave a core of moisture locked in the center. Once these particles have left the process, this core of moisture can be drawn to the drier outer layer. If there is a mass of particles, this moisture can migrate across particles and deposit a small amount of solid as it does so. Variations in ambient temperature (such as overnight cooling and subsequent warming during the day) can generate several reversals of this moisture migration, each of which deposits solids resulting in a stronger solid bridge forming between the particles—and ultimately a cake to form.

One approach to controlling the problem of caking due to moisture migration is to use a mass flow design of silo in which one or more plenums are installed in the cone area. The exact number of plenums required is dependant upon the determination of the safe upward air velocity that can be employed to condition the material without the risk of fluidization occurring. Fluidization data is typically derived from trials using a fluidizing test apparatus. The plenums may be in the form of an annular air inlet which is stepped back from the walls of the cone section to facilitate smooth material flow without obtrusion. A mass flow silo with conditioning plenum(s) can be operated equally well in either continuous or batch mode.

Physical Properties of Powder Blends and Granules. High-potency drugs are often formulated at low doses and, owing to the cost and convenience considerations, a direct compression process is often chosen as a processing option over wet and dry granulation processes. Empirically, one may rank these processes as "direct compression > dry granulation > wet granulation" in the decreasing order of blend and content uniformity problems. Regardless of the processing option, factors such as high-throughput productions, larger batch sizes, and smaller particle sizes of APIs may often result in poor blending, segregation, and poor flow of the blended material leading to unacceptable content uniformity. With high potent drugs formulated at low doses, such problems are often exacerbated into safety issues with underpotent dosage units compromising effectiveness and overpotent units leading to adverse events. Therefore, powder and granulation blends should be adequately assessed for their flowability, compressibility, tendency towards caking, arching, ratholing, etc. Similarly, consideration should be given to the equipment used for their handling and storage, such as blenders, hoppers, drums, chutes, silos, and feed frames. It is essential to understand the flow characteristics and storage requirements of the material being handled and to design the process equipment to take these factors into account.

Measurement of Bulk Solids Properties. Physical bulk properties of solids relevant to handling operations can be measured using several laboratory test methods. These include bulk density, tensile strength, and shear properties including cohesion, internal shear strength, wall friction on different equipment surfaces, permeability, and sifting and fluidization segregation testing. USP General chapter <1174> proposes the standardization of test methods that may be valuable during pharmaceutical development and lists the four commonly reported methods for testing powder flow-angle of response, compressibility index or Hausner ratio, flow rate through an orifice, and shear cell. Angle of response is the constant, three-dimensional angle relative to the horizontal base assumed by a cone-like pile of material formed by any of several different methods. The compressibility index is determined by measuring both the bulk volume and the tapped volume of a powder and has been proposed as an indirect measure of bulk density, size and shape, surface area, moisture content, and cohesiveness of materials because all of these can influence the observed compressibility index. The flow rate through an orifice is measured as the mass per time flowing from any of a number of types of containers. Shear cell methodology may be useful in obtaining a variety of parameters such as yield loci representing the shear/normal stress relationships, angle of internal friction, unconfined yield strength, and derived parameters such as the flow factor and other flowability indices. Therefore, summary studies and the results of determination of various flow properties should be presented in the NDA.

The formulation is expected to exhibit favorable mechanical properties.[19–21] Important compact properties to be studied include brittle fracture index, worst case bonding index, modified bonding index, and viscoelastic number. Additionally, dynamic indentation hardness, elastic modulus, tensile strength and powder flow performance indicators, namely uniform flow number, cohesivity, and flow variability should be assessed using appropriate test methods. Compressibility of the powder and granulation blends should be assessed by studying compression force vs hardness curves. A lower target compression force for a given target tablet hardness yields longer commercial tooling life (i.e., no tooling damage or breakage) as the required compression force may be below the metal fatigue limit of the tooling. Also, the increased granulation compressibility enables the manufacture of tablets with sufficient hardness to withstand tablet-to-tablet tumbling or attrition dynamics in commercial-scale film-coaters. Functional relationships between tablet average weight, hardness, friability, disintegration, dissolution vs compression forces (both precompression and main compression) and tablet press speeds should be provided to assess whether ranges in compression force and press speed have any significant impact on drug product performance. Similarly, ejection force vs compression force relationships should be studied to assess the impact of glidants such as colloidal silicon dioxide in reducing ejection forces. Tablet hardness may be considered a process parameter that influences the film-coated tablet appearance quality. Tablet hardness may directly impact logo legibility for large scale film-coating processing. Therefore, a tablet hardness study may be carried out to establish an acceptable range that produces film-coated tablets that meet the defect criteria for appearance test.

18.3.9 Manufacturing Process Development

A process description and equipment comparison information should be provided linking any process and/or equipment changes including any site changes that may have taken place during the investigational stages of the IND and the proposed commercial process and equipment. A description of how various process parameters functionally link to the material quality attributes of process intermediates such as dry blends, granulations, postgranulation blends, tablet cores, and tablet coating quality, should be provided. Process optimization efforts to maximize blend uniformity, minimize postblend segregation during storage and tableting/capsule filling operations, and to maximize content uniformity should be described in detail. It is desirable to use the actual drug substance in all developmental studies. Understandably, controlled substances such as opioids may not be easily available for investigative studies and if dyes are used as surrogates or placebo formulations are used during process optimization, such studies should be justified. In such cases, the optimized process parameters should be reconfirmed by the use of active formulations containing the active components. A discussion of whether alternative designs of manufacturing processes were investigated should be provided before presenting the chosen process. Although wet granulation may provide most desired content uniformity for the low-dose formulations, owing to stability and overage considerations, more often dry granulation and direct compression of powder blends is chosen as a processing option. For example, if a dry blending and direct compression process is utilized, options such as granulation, in which the active compound is incorporated in the granulation as a molecular dispersion spray to improve homogeneity, should be investigated and described. Overages of drug substances in the manufacture of the drug product should be justified and should be solely to compensate for losses during handling and unit operations and not to overcome any instability problems during manufacture or through product shelf-life. The need for overages should be assessed throughout the manufacture of conformance batches.

Drug Substance Milling/Micronization Process. Milling parameters such as equipment size and throughput, milling time, screw-feed designs, and residence time of drug in the mill, should be carefully considered during process development and scale-up. Disproportionate increases in the milling lot size and milling times relative to equipment size are often deleterious to the physical quality of drug substances, especially if this leads to increased residence time in void areas where material flow is limited. If smaller milling equipment is used for prolonged time, residual material from the void areas may harden and agglomerate into unfriable particles. Similarly, mill stoppages to empty receiver vessels may add to the residence time in the mill. High-energy milling process often resulting in heat generation may contribute to process-induced stress on the drug substance particles and to its physical transformation and agglomeration. Processing stress may lead to an activated surface on drug substance crystals, which may in turn create amorphous regions, surface energy changes, electrostatics, moisture sorption, and changes in flow/adhesion. Scale-up should therefore be commensurate with equipment size and capacity and overmilling should be avoided to eliminate formation of undesirable agglomerates. A robust milling process should be developed with optimized milling times and reduced residence times for any portion of the drug substance in the mill. Additionally, consideration should be given to eliminating need for stopping mills to empty receiver chutes. Collection chutes capable of containing an entire lot of drug substance help minimize operator exposure. Even though prevention of formation of agglomerates is desired, mitigating measure may include prescreening with an appropriately sized mesh to remove unfriable agglorémates in the drug substances before the mixing/blending step. Mesh size for prescreening should be calculated based on the density of the drug substance and acceptable fraction of the lowest strength dosage unit that may be accommodated as a single particle of drug substance. Typically, no more than 5–10% of the lowest strength of the dosage unit should be represented by a single particle of the drug substance.

Blending and Milling Operations. The type of equipment used, the ranges of blend times and blender fill volumes studied, and order of drug substance and excipient addition, geometric dilution procedures employed, etc. should be described and justification should be provided for selecting optimal conditions. Mixing times and speeds should be carefully evaluated for the preblends, main blends, and postlubrication blends. If process analytical technologies are used to continually monitor blend uniformity, the details of such processes should be provided in addition to the results from blend uniformity and in-process dosage unit content uniformity results. If DoEs are utilized, they should be described. They may include studies to evaluate blend uniformity as a function of blend time and fill volume. Any evidence of demixing or segregation of blends should be evaluated if blending process is continued past the time point when uniformity is achieved. Similarly, DoEs may be utilized in evaluating compression variables on the physical properties of the resulting matrix. Functional relationships, such as dependence or independence of tablet hardness, length, and friability on press speed, hardness and compression force relationships, friability and compression force relationships, and tablet dimensions vs compression force, should be assessed during pharmaceutical development.

Material transfer operations between process steps such as charging the final lubricated blend into the tablet press hopper have the potential to impact the blend content uniformity when drug and excipients are not evenly distributed within the powder mixture or granules as a function of particle size. Therefore, material transfers can lead to segregation of the blend, and may result in poor content uniformity of the tablets. The current best practice for detecting these issues is to monitor the tablet potency and content uniformity throughout the compression process, sampling most intensively at the beginning and end of the run, or other significant events during the compression process such as bin change-over. These samples are referred to as stratified tablet potency and core tablet uniformity.[5,22] The draft Guidance states that the methods described are not intended to be the only methods for meeting Agency requirements to demonstrate the adequacy of powder mix. It also states that the formulations with extremely low dose and/or high potency may call for more rigorous sampling than is described in assessing the uniformity of powder blends or the uniformity of content of finished dosage units. Therefore, stratified sampling from only 20 locations (registration/validation batches) and only from 10 locations (for the routine commercial batches) may not be adequate. Also, the premise that the historical data (three validation lots) is a predictor of the performance of the future may be a risky proposition for low-dose formulations. Hence, in-process content uniformity testing alone may not replace blend uniformity testing for routine commercial manufacture. Also, for low-dose formulations, there is often a link between blend uniformity testing, in-process content uniformity testing, and dissolution testing results. Agglomeration of the drug substance in the formulation is reflected by the failure of one or more of these tests. Therefore, for low-dose formulations, all three tests are recommended as continuous in-process controls. Also, in view of the potential risk with the low-dose formulations, postapproval switching from existing testing to PQRI/FDA-recommended procedures or vice versa may not be filed as annual-reportable changes and may require FDA assessment to ensure robustness of testing. Special consideration should therefore be given to the stratified sampling locations, sample size, location mean potency, individual tablet potency, and uniformity (relative standard deviation). Blend uniformity criteria for low-dose formulations may include the following acceptance criteria when using tumbling blenders.

Stage 1: $n = 10$; RSD $\leq 5.0\%$, all individuals $\pm$ 10.0% of mean (absolute)

Stage 2: $n = 30$; RSD $\leq 6.0\%$, all individuals $\pm$ 10.0% of mean (absolute)

Stringent criteria may be used if justified. Also, for ribbon blenders, at least 15 stratified locations and triplicate sampling from each location are recommended with similar acceptance criteria. If any blend uniformity out of trend results is observed, appropriate investigation should be conducted to identify the root cause and to implement corrective and preventative actions. Some of the investigational techniques include variance component analysis, described by Prescott and Garcia.[23] Factors such as blend sampling techniques, blend sample handling, processing, and analytical testing of blend samples may likely contribute to blend uniformity out of trend results. The analysis should clearly demonstrate sampling errors vs true blend homogeneity problems and how such problems have been corrected. True sampling errors should be clearly documented and should be free of blending errors. Often, it is argued that blend samples may be more variable and less representative of the finished product than a stratified sample of the corresponding in-process dosage units. This kind of thinking leads to proposals to drop testing for blend uniformity testing past validation stages and/or to minimize the sample size for blend uniformity testing and to increase the sample size for dosage unit content uniformity testing. However, for low-dose formulations, it is important to test both blend uniformity and in-process dosage unit content uniformity by adequate stratified sampling and the batches should pass both the tests to demonstrate control over segregation and inhomogeneity. Sources of sampling error may be related to a "clean thief" effect or to a "sampling depth." "Clean thief" effect is seen if blend samples collected with the first few thief stabs may be significantly lower in drug content than samples collected with subsequent thief stabs. This may be considered a sampling bias if the drug content of samples changes when the order of blend sampling is reversed. In other words, if a "clean thief" effect exists, drug content of the blend samples become a function of the order in which a sample is collected rather than the location in the blender from which it is collected. In such cases, one should determine the number of thief stabs to be taken to condition the thief to a point in which a blend sample is representative of the powder. If a "sampling depth" problem exists, samples collected from the bottom of symmetrical mixing vessel may be significantly and consistently higher in drug content than samples collected from the top of the mixing vessel. This may be considered a sampling bias rather than poor blend homogeneity if, when mixing, the vessel is inverted prior to sampling and the depth affect is still observed. In other words, samples collected from deeper depths within the bed may be higher in drug content regardless of whether they are derived from the bottom or top of the mixing vessel. Manufacturers should evaluate techniques to minimize the artifacts associated with these two sources of sampling error and bias.

In-process dosage unit content uniformity testing by stratified sampling is critical to the testing of content uniformity of low-dose formulations. Recommended sampling and acceptance criteria include 30 stratified sampling intervals covering start-up, run, and end of the run. Also, additional events such as stoppages longer than 5 min, hopper changes, adjustments made to fill depth, and compression force or tablet height parameters, should also be sampled. Each event and location should be sampled at least in triplicate. More sampling is recommended at press startup and at intervals close to the press shut-down because blend segregation is more likely to happen during the beginning and end of a compression run. The following acceptance criteria are recommended.

Stage 1: $n \geq 30$, location mean of 90.0–110.0%, RSD $\leq$ 4.0%, all within 85.0–115.0% of target

Stage 2: $n \geq 90$, location mean of 90.0–110.0%, RSD $\leq$ 5.0%, all within 85.0–115.0% of target

Depending on batch size, one to seven individual matrix samples may be assayed per location and the location mean and overall mean should be calculated. Additionally, a composite sample of 30 dosage units may be tested from the bulk units after the completion of the manufacturing process. Different sampling size and acceptance criteria may be recommended if justified based on safety considerations and overlapping potencies. If segregation of blend occurs during compression/capsule filling operations, appropriate measures should be established to minimize such segregations. Segregation is more likely to occur at the end of compression run because of inadequate feed systems used in the tablet press. Table 18.1 illustrates some potential failure modes related to blend and tablet core homogeneity problems seen with low-dose formulations and how to investigate them.

TABLE 18.1 Potential Failure Modes Related to Blend and Tablet Core Homogeneity Problems for Low-Dose Formulations

Root Cause for High Potency	Failure Mode	Outcome	Investigation
Nonuniform final blend prior to compression or filling	Following final blending, drug substance dines settle on the top layer of the blend	Top layer of the blend is superpotent	Prior to tablet compression, samples taken from top layer of blend in IBC for analysis
Segregation of blend during tablet press operation	During compression, drug substance fines segregate and remain in the IBC	Residual powder in the IBC is superpotent	Sample of residual blend in the IBC is analyzed as a composite sample for blend potency
	Routine starting and stopping of the tablet press could introduce blend segregation	Tablet potency variability observed immediately before and/or after tablet pres shutoff	During tablet compression, shut down the tablet press and take samples immediately before tablet press shut down and immediately after tablet press restart
Segregation of blend by tablet press feed system at the end of batch	During compression, drug substance fines segregate and remain preferentially in the tablet press hopper at the end of the batch	Remaining blend in tablet press hopper is superpotent	Take stratified samples during compression of residual blend remaining in the tablet press hopper
	At the end of the compression process, the hydrostatic pressure on the blend in the tablet press hopper is diminished	Reduced hydrostatic pressure coupled with the design of the feed system could result in segregation of the residual blend	Remaining blend at the end of compression is removed from tablet press die channels and assayed as a composite sample

As mentioned above, often, the high potency dosage units result at the end of a compression/fill run where hydrostatic pressure is reduced and the feed system is unable to handle such a variation. To ensure high potency tablets do not enter the batch, it may be advisable to define the end of the compression process when a sufficient quantity of residual blend remains on the hopper. Also, stratified dosage unit samples should be taken at frequent intervals approaching the completion of the compression process to verify that the final tablets compressed in the batch are not superpotent. It is recommended that compression force changes be monitored continually during tableting process and percentage of RSD values be assessed. Variations in the compression force exceeding certain established limit may be an indication of blend segregation.

It should be noted that a certain level of regulatory overlap and redundancy between the center vs field is expected in the review and inspection of low-dose formulations to assure adequate product quality. Therefore, blend uniformity and in-process dosage unit content uniformity testing may be seen as in process controls under 21CFR314.50(d)(1)(ii)(a) and 314.94(a)(9)(i). Similarly, according to cGMPs, under 21CFR211.110(a)(3), drug product blend uniformity testing should be carried out to demonstrate adequacy of mixing of formulation components. Accordingly, drug product sampling plans for these tests may be reviewed by both center and field offices.

18.3.10 Dissolution and Bioequivalence Studies

A detailed discussion of how a dissolution method was developed and validated should be provided. Data demonstrating the method robustness and discriminating power and bio-relevance of the chosen test method should be provided. In setting specifications for dissolution, collective data at different time points may be used in a distribution-free bootstrap calculation (Monte Carlo simulations) or other models to determine probability of failing an acceptable batch at any given Q value. The bootstrap approach may be acceptable for making inferences when distributions are not well defined. If such approaches are used, sufficient information on the exact method used to assess replication of bootstrap calculations should be provided. Justification should also be provided for applying bootstrap distributions to estimating extreme values of the distribution of dissolution data. If a two-point dissolution specification is being set, a discussion on independence or dependence of failure at the two time points should be provided, including an explanation of why this leads to additive probabilities of failure. The general expectation is that Q should be set such that a significant number of batches (e.g., 20–30%) go to stage 2 testing on a routine basis.

If disintegration is proposed in lieu of dissolution, summary data should be provided showing that disintegration is at least as discriminating as is dissolution in identifying batch failures. Such studies may include making various side batches and aberrant batches showing different dissolution and disintegration profiles. A summary of an overall bioequivalence strategy for the drug product throughout various stages of development[7,8] should be provided linking the prototypes with pivotal and the to-be-marketed formulations. *In vitro* and *in vivo* correlations or rank orders, if developed, should be summarized.

18.3.11 End Testing for Drug Substances and Drug Products

The following are typical quality attributes for drug substances used in low-dose formulations.

- appearance—absence of unfriable oversized agglomerates;
- morphology—polymorph control by FTIR, DSC, PXRD, etc.;
- particle size distribution (two-sided, D_{10}, D_{50}, D_{90}) by sieving and laser light scattering.

Acceptance criteria for end testing of low-dose drug products are expected to be tighter than usually expected of the conventional dosage strengths. The "one size fits all" USP standard for content uniformity, " $\pm 15\%$ ranges with $n = 10$" may not be adequate. Permitted variation in drug content must be considered against the following:

- the range of clinically used dosage increments for the drug;
- if dosage is routinely adjusted in $+25\%$ increments, a $\pm 15\%$ permissible variation in tablet content is a concern with NTR products.

The usual range of 80.0–125.0% (i.e., -20% to $+25\%$) for bioequivalence does not match with $\pm 15\%$ permissible variation in tablet content. Hence tighter assay ranges of 95–105% and tighter variability are often needed instead of the usual 90–110% range.

18.4 FACILITY CONTROLS FOR HIGHLY POTENT DRUGS

There is no FDA definition and/or policy on highly potent drugs. Current GMPs do not require separation or dedication of equipment and facilities. However, 21 CFR 211.42(c) states that there shall be separate or defined areas or such other control systems as are necessary to prevent contamination. Also, 21 CFR 211.67(b) states that written procedures must be established and followed for cleaning and maintenance of equipment. Therefore, appropriate environmental controls including containment and worker exposure issues need to be addressed for high potency drugs including cytotoxic agents. Dedicated facilities may be appropriate for material of an infectious nature, or of high pharmacological activity or toxicity. If validation inactivation and/or cleaning procedures are established and maintained, the need for a dedicated facility may be offset. It is the responsibility of the manufacturer to minimize health risks due to cross-contamination and to document them appropriately. Also, it is the responsibility of the manufacturer to define and justify safe exposure thresholds for such drugs based on toxicological assessments of exposure – response relationships.

18.5 CONCLUSION

As discussed in this article, the low-dose formulations are usually highly potent drugs, and they often display narrow therapeutic range. Consequently, potency and content uniformity are directly linked to safety and efficacy. Overlapping potencies for different strengths may often be related to product safety. Several challenges of formulating low-dose formulations have been discussed, including the importance of implementing a robust pharmaceutical development program based on a three-pronged approach of quality by design, rigorous in-process testing with stratified sampling, and end testing with tighter acceptance criteria for assays and their variations. The need to develop a robust drug substance milling process was also discussed. Scale-up issues such as equipment, milling time, batch size, and feeding rate to minimize overmilling were highlighted, since overmilling may lead to the conversion of the polymorphic forms and to agglomerates. It was emphasized that proportionate process scale-up that is commensurate with the equipment size and capacity is critical to the physical quality of the drug substance used in low-dose formulations. Prescreening with an appropriate mesh to remove unfriable agglomerates, if formed during milling, was also discussed as an interim measure to control agglomerates in drug substances and excipients. Consequently, important tests to control the drug substance include appearance to ascertain absence of unfriable oversized agglomerates, morphology tests by FTIR, DSC, PXRD, etc., and two-sided three-point particle size control by sieving and laser light scattering. Controls on the functionality-related characteristics of the excipients were emphasized. The pharmacopeia testing alone may be inadequate, and additional testing such as particle size, bulk and tapped densities, and morphic forms may be critical for excipients as these properties impact the manufacturability of low-dose formulations. the importance of documenting mechanical and physical properties of formulations was also discussed. The significance of testing for powder flow (PSD, shape, size, static charge and charge duration, density, hopper geometry), flowability—angle of response measurements, moisture (hygroscopicity, hydration state), compaction properties, Hiestand tableting indices (bonding, brittle fracture and strain indices), etc., was also discussed in the light of designing proper equipment to ensure desired material flow and to prevent segregation. The need to clearly document and justify the chosen manufacturing process was mentioned, since content uniformity issues may be critical in going from wet granulation to a direct compaction process. Therefore, direct compression blends would have to be carefully tested for segregation potential of the blend, that is, fluidization and sifting segregation testing and testing for cohesive properties by Jenike shear testing or equivalent methods. Hopper designs (mass flow, cone flow, gravity feed, centrifugal feed, etc.) and increased testing at the end of compression runs and tablet press shutdown at appropriate times were also discussed as being critical to assuring product quality. The FDA may be glad to involve proactively at earlier stages of drug development and may provide scientific feedback as part of the critical path initiative to facilitate faster industrialization of developmental drugs. A clear opportunity exists for process analytical technologies for highly potent drugs formulated at low strengths.

REFERENCES

1. International Conference on Harmonization (ICH) Q 8—Pharmaceutical Development.
2. Internal Conference on Harmonization (ICH) Q 9—Quality Risk Management.
3. International Conference on Harmonization (ICH) Q 10—Pharmaceutical Quality System.
4. International Conference on Harmonization (ICH) Q6A—Specifications: Test Procedures and Acceptance Criteria for New Drug Substances and New Drug Products: Chemical Substances (Including Decision Trees).
5. Draft Guidance for Industry: Powder blends and finished dosage units—stratified in-process dosage unit sampling and assessment. U.S. Department of Health and Human Services, Food and Drug Administration, Center for Drug Evaluation and Research (CDER), October 2003.
6. Booy KJ, Wiegerinck P, Vander J, Kaspersen F, Lambregts D, Vromans H, Kellenbach E. 2005. The use of ^{13}C labeling to enhance the sensitivity of ^{13}C solid-state CPMAS NMR to study polymorphism in low dose solid formulations. J. Pharm. Sci. 94(2): 458–463.
7. Waiver of In Vivo Bioavailability and Bioequivalence Studies for Immediate-Release Solid Oral Dosage Forms Based on a Biopharmaceutics Classification System, August 2000.
8. Bioavailability and Bioequivalence Studies for Orally Administered Drug Products, General Considerations, March 2003.
9. Allen T. 1992. Particle size measurement, 4th ed. London: Chapman & Hall.
10. Rowle A. Basic principles of particle size analysis. Malvern Technical Paper, MRK034.
11. Zheng Y, Johnson KC. 1997. Effects of drug particle size on content uniformity of low-dose solid dosage forms. Int. J. Pharm. 154: 179–183.
12. Schoneker D. 2007. Excipient Functionality; an IPEC Americas Perspective. American Association of Pharmaceutical Scientists Annual Meeting and Exposition, San Diego, CA, November 11–15, 2007.
13. Sasic S. 2007. Raman mapping of low-content API pharmaceutical formulations—1. Mapping of alprazolam in alprazolam/xanax tablets. Pharm. Res. 24, 58–65.
14. Housman DS, Cambron RT, Sakr A. 2005. Application of Raman spectroscopy for on-line monitoring of low dose blend uniformity. Int. J. Pharm. 298: 80.
15. Kauser N, Cornelius V, Snowden MJ, Mitchell J, Mwesignwa E, Do N, Farell T. 2006. Assessment of low-dose content uniformity of indomethacin in excipient blends using FT-Raman mapping spectroscopy. AAPS Annual Meeting and Exposition, San Antonio, TX, November 2, 2006.
16. Ahmed H, Shah N. 2000. Formulation of low dose medicines—theory and practice. Am. Pharm. Rev. 3(3): 9–14.
17. Marinelli J. Solids Handling Technologies—Practical Solutions to your Solids Handling Problems. Available at: www.solidshandlingtech.com. 2001–2008.

18. Griffith EJ. 1991. Cake formation in particulate systems. New York: VCH.
19. Standard Practice for Measuring Sifting Segregation Tendencies for Bulk Solids (D 6940-03).
20. ASTM. 2003. Annual book of ASTM standards, Vol. 04.08.
21. Standard Practice for Measuring Fluidization Segregation Tendencies of Powders (D 6941-03).
22. Boehm G, Clark J, Dietrick J, Foust L, Garcia T, Gavini M, Gelber L, Geoffroy J, Hoblizell J, Jimenez P, Mergen G, Muzzio F, Planchard J, Prescott J, Timmermans J, Takiar N. 2003. The use of stratified sampling of blend and dosage units to demonstrate adequacy of mix for powder blends. PDA J. Pharm. Sci. Technol. 57(2): 64–74.
23. Prescott JK, Garcia TP. 2001. A solid dosage and blend content uniformity trouble shooting diagram. Pharm. Technol. 25(3): 68–88.

INDEX

Formulation and Analytical Development for Low-Dose Oral Drug Products. Edited by Jack Zheng